W9-BJP-069

# Is your training working?

Do you *really* have some progress in muscle and might to show for your efforts over the last few months? If not, your training is not working and it is time to make major changes—time to put into practice the advice given in this book.

This book's sole purpose is to teach *you* how to achieve *your* drug-free potential for muscle and might. It is not concerned with perpetuating myths and falsehoods, or promoting anything that will not help *you* to achieve *your* potential.

Out of necessity this book does not promote conventional training methods. The reason for this is very simple—most conventional training methods simply do not work well for most people.

Open your mind, set aside the ingrained traditions that have been limiting your progress, be prepared for radical if not revolutionary training concepts, apply what you learn, and then you will achieve what you crave—*terrific gains in muscle and might*.

## But where are the photographs?

There is no shortage of photographs in the training world. But there *is* a shortage of training instruction that is 100% relevant to the training masses. Nearly 500 pages of text are needed in this book to provide the necessary in-depth instruction. Many photographs would have made the book even larger, and considerably increased the costs of production, printing and mailing, and thus the cost to you. Photographs are vitally important, however, for teaching exercise technique, and nearly 250 of them are included in a companion text—i.e., THE INSIDER'S TELL-ALL HANDBOOK ON WEIGHT-TRAINING TECHNIQUE—which focuses on correct exercise form.

# Here's what others are saying about BEYOND BRAWN...

"I want to say without hesitation that BEYOND BRAWN is the greatest book ever written on how to train with weights. And it is the greatest book ever written on how TO LAST while training with weights. It is the greatest—period!"
  – Dick Conner, veteran strength coach and 25-year-plus proprietor of The Pit, a famous no-frills gym in Indiana

"Everyone who yearns to maximize their genetic potential for muscle and might owes it to themselves to read, grasp and apply the training information contained in BEYOND BRAWN. This book is the bible of rational strength training...Page after page is jam-packed with practical real-world training information that you just cannot find anywhere else...This book has my highest endorsement—it is without a doubt the very best book on strength training I have ever read."
  – Kevin R. Fontaine, Ph.D.
  Assistant Professor of Medicine
  Johns Hopkins University School of Medicine

"BEYOND BRAWN is an encyclopedia of information, detail upon detail, of all of the subtopics related to weight training...It is information upon information about how to train properly and effectively...I obviously liked it a lot and recommend it highly."
  – Dr. Ken E. Leistner
  Co-founder of Iron Island Gym, New York

"BEYOND BRAWN is packed with what I consider real information on how to build your body. This book provides all the information you will ever need to develop slabs of muscle safely and effectively. It's like having your own personal coach and mentor guiding you to bodybuilding success. BEYOND BRAWN is the definitive Encyclopedia on Bodybuilding—a superb book that is truly very special."
  – Bill Piche
  Triple-bodyweight deadlifter in drug-free ADFPA competition

"BEYOND BRAWN is the most comprehensive, helpful and honest book on natural strength training today. With great care and in extraordinary detail, this book covers every training-related topic you can imagine, and without any hype or commercial messages. It will surely help everyone who reads it and I will strongly recommend it to all of my clients."
  – Bob Whelan, M.S., M.S., C.S.C.S.
  President, Whelan Strength Training

"BEYOND BRAWN shows you in intricate detail the most productive and safe ways to train. This is the book we all wish we had years ago. It is an absolute MUST READ."
  – Richard A. Winett, Ph.D.
  Publisher, MASTER TRAINER

**THE INSIDER'S ENCYCLOPEDIA ON HOW TO BUILD MUSCLE & MIGHT**

**CS PUBLISHING LTD**
NICOSIA, CYPRUS

# Beyond BRAWN

**Stuart McRobert**

Copyright © 1998 by Stuart McRobert
All rights reserved. No part of this book may be used, reproduced or transmitted in any manner whatsoever—electronic or mechanical, including photocopying, recording or by any system of storing and retrieving information—without permission from the publisher, except for brief quotations embodied in reviews.

CS Publishing Ltd., P.O. Box 20390, CY-2151 Nicosia, Cyprus
tel + 357-233-3069  fax + 357-233-2018  e-mail: cspubltd@spidernet.com.cy
web site: www.hardgainer.com

US office: CS Publishing Ltd., P.O. Box 1002, Connell, WA 99326
tel 509-234-0362  fax 509-234-0601  web site: www.hardgainer.com

Cover illustration by Stephen Wedan copyright © 1998
Cover design by Nicholas Zavallis

First printed in 1998
Reprinted in 1998, 1999 and 2000, with minor changes and corrections
Revised edition printed in 2001, and reprinted in 2003, and 2004 (with minor
    changes and corrections)
Printed by J. G. Cassoulides & Son Ltd., Nicosia, Cyprus

## Publisher's Cataloging-in-Publication
### (Prepared by Quality Books, Inc.)
McRobert, Stuart.
        Beyond brawn : the insider's encyclopedia on how to build muscle
    and might / Stuart McRobert. --1st ed.
        p. cm.
        Includes bibliographical references and index.
        ISBN: 9963-616-07-0 (hardcover)
        ISBN: 9963-616-06-2 (softcover)


        1. Weight training.   2. Bodybuilding.   I. Title.

GV546.M33 1998                          796.41
                                        QBI98-853

# Contents

## Warning—Safety

Every effort was made in this book to stress the importance of proper technique and safety when using bodybuilding and strength-training programs. Regardless of your age, check with your physician to ensure that it is appropriate for you to follow such programs. Proceed with caution *and at your own risk*. The author, CS Publishing Ltd. or distributors of this book cannot be responsible for any injury that may result from following the instruction given in this manual.

## Warning—Disclaimer

The purpose of this book is to provide you with information on bodybuilding, strength training and related topics. It is sold with the understanding that neither the publisher nor author are engaged in providing legal, medical or other professional services.

Every effort has been made to make this book as thorough and accurate as possible. Despite this, all information on the subject matter has not been included, and there may be mistakes in both content and typography. CS Publishing Ltd. and the author shall have neither liability nor responsibility to any entity or person with respect to any injury, loss or damage caused, or alleged to be caused, directly or indirectly, by the material given in this book.

*If you do not wish to be bound by the above, you may return your copy to the publisher for a full refund.*

Where it has been cumbersome to use both genders of a pronoun, only the male one has been used. With the exception of exercise poundages, muscular girths and dietary quantities that are specifically targeted at males, this book is aimed at both sexes. Both men *and* women can benefit enormously from the instruction here.

## Acknowledgments

Without the publicity arising from being published in newsstand bodybuilding magazines, the interchange with the authors and readers of HARDGAINER, and feedback from readers of my articles, this book could not exist.

Specific gratitude, in alphabetical order, is owed to John Balik, Steve Downs, Steve Holman, Bob Kennedy, Chris Lund, Peter McGough, Dave McInerney, Bill Phillips, Peary Rader and Joe Weider for publishing my articles.

I want to thank Jan Dellinger, Brooks Kubik, John Leschinski and Efstathios Papadopoulos, DC, for providing feedback and a sounding board during the production of this book. A special debt of gratitude is owed to Dave Maurice for his consistent rigorism, thoroughness and patience when critiquing draft copies of individual chapters.

Debts of appreciation are also owed to Carolyn Weaver for the index, Stephen Wedan for the cover illustration, Nicholas Zavallis for the cover design, and J. G. Cassoulides & Son for its dependability and expert printing.

## Trademarks

All terms mentioned in this book that are known to be trademarks have been marked as such. But CS Publishing Ltd. cannot attest to the accuracy of this information. There may be unintentional omissions in acknowledging trademarks. The publication and use of this book does not affect the validity of any trademark or service mark.

> As far as instruction goes, there is very little that is truly new in the weight-training world. Here is how I expressed this point in BRAWN: "Charles A. Smith, over the time I knew him before his death in January 1991, used to remind me that what we have today we owe to the past. How right he was. As Chas used to put it, 'It's upon the pioneers' shoulders that we have to stand in order to be as tall as they. We're merely the heirs of those who have gone before us.'"

# Introduction

Thank you for buying BEYOND BRAWN. This book was written with one objective in mind—to teach you how to build a superbly muscled, strong, lean and healthy physique. BEYOND BRAWN can change your life!

If you are a genetically typical bodybuilder or strength trainee you will have gotten little or no satisfaction from your training. Despite having faithfully followed conventional training instruction you will have become frustrated and disillusioned. Conventional training methods—those which are vigorously promoted in almost all gyms today—only work *very well* if you are one of the very few who are naturally highly gifted for muscle building, or if you are propped up with dangerous bodybuilding drugs. But if you train as this book advocates, you can make drug-free gains that may astound you, *regardless of how average or otherwise your genetic inheritance is.*

This is a very serious book dedicated to people who are *impassioned* with their training. In the best interests of your education this book presents information in a very detailed and direct manner, and it confronts many traditional opinions.

The education needed to write this book came from many sources. My own training experiences and a life that has been consumed by weight training make up only a part of the education. As an obsessed youngster I digested much of the nonsense and confusion that abounds in the bodybuilding world. But because I did not have an excellent genetic inheritance, and would not use drugs, this led to years of unrelenting frustration. Finally I came across training methods that *do* work for most people. This book details those methods.

The publishing of HARDGAINER since its inception in 1989 has given me a unique insight into training for genetically typical people. The education was bolstered by a great deal of writing for newsstand bodybuilding magazines, and extensive research. With practical training for drug-free people being my *full-time* employment, it has focused my mind on bodybuilding and strength training like nothing else ever could. Much of the acquired knowledge has been distilled for inclusion in this book. In it you are getting a wealth of information you can really use.

This book builds on the foundation constructed by BRAWN. The latter focused on appropriate role models, the inadequacies of conventional training, genetic realities, and the rationale behind drug-free training for typical people. BEYOND BRAWN goes into far greater depth on exercise program design, and covers much that was never even mentioned in BRAWN. BEYOND BRAWN also takes some of the most important topics that were only touched upon in BRAWN, and covers them in great depth. While BRAWN and BEYOND BRAWN are ideal companions, along with THE INSIDER'S TELL-ALL HANDBOOK ON WEIGHT-TRAINING TECHNIQUE, each can stand alone.

BEYOND BRAWN is an encyclopedia on *how to build* muscle and might, for adults of both genders and all ages, and trainees of all levels of experience other than the competitive elite. It is *not* an encyclopedia on the whole of weight training. The omitted aspects are readily available elsewhere and include physiology, pondering on the mechanism of muscle growth, detailed descriptions of micronutrients, nutritional breakdown of food, updates on the ever-changing food supplement scene, and history of the Iron Game. As interesting as these concerns are, they are either irrelevant as far as your individual pursuit of muscle and might is concerned, or only *marginally* relevant.

BEYOND BRAWN focuses on information that is not easily found elsewhere. It is devoted purely to that which will help *you* to further *your* progress to the realization of *your* potential.

A thorough student of both BRAWN and BEYOND BRAWN will find differences of opinion or emphasis between the two works. BEYOND BRAWN was completed nearly seven years after BRAWN was first published, and during those years I added a great deal to my understanding of training. And I am still learning.

To your training success,

Stuart McRobert

# How this book will help you

This book can save you years of wasted training toil. It will propel you into the practical know-how needed to turn even a novice into a tremendously informed bodybuilder or strength trainee. You can learn all this from just a few weeks of serious study. Then apply it and you will develop a degree of muscle and might that will make a mockery of what you would have achieved had you stayed with conventional training methods.

By the time trainees get to grips with what works for drug-free, genetically typical and genetically disadvantaged people, they have usually wasted many years, and often have acquired permanent legacies of injuries from unsuspectingly following harmful training instruction. The vast majority of trainees, however, give up long before ever understanding what training reality is all about.

While the journey towards any goal will teach you much about the activity in question and you as an individual, you will not travel far if you experience a heavy burden of failure.

You no longer have to waste years of your life, and risk giving up in the process, before acquiring an in-depth understanding of weight training. But if you have lost a chunk of your life by following terrible instruction, this book will teach you how to make the most of your training future.

## Not the final word

This book is *not* the final word, but it is more than enough to provide the how-to instruction (*excluding* exercise form, which is covered in a companion text) for nearly everyone who lifts weights. While the book specifically targets hard gainers and extremely hard gainers, its instruction can pack muscle and might onto easy gainers in even greater quantities, and in less time.

This book does *not* cover the honing, refining and "polishing" needed by competitive bodybuilders, because those concerns are relevant to only *very few* trainees. This book is about priorities, down-to-earth realities, and what matters most to nearly everyone who wants to improve physique, strength and fitness. BEYOND BRAWN is targeted at the huge majority of trainees, not at the highly gifted minority.

## Drug-free ethos

The rampant use of muscle-building drugs is the worst calamity that has ever hit the training world. Drugs have produced dishonesty of untold proportions. The first casualty of drug use is the truth.

Some bodybuilders and strength athletes who only got to the top because they had drug assistance are still claiming that they never took chemicals. Usually they are dishonest because they are ashamed of their drug use, and do not want to tarnish their clean public images. And some even promote the charade that they were hard gainers.

While the harm to health that the chemicals have wreaked is a huge problem, as are the criminal implications of illegal drug use, these are *nothing* relative to the immeasurable harm done to the *drug-free* training masses.

Rampant but generally secretive drug use since the early sixties, when steroid use really took off, led to drug-assisted training methods being promoted as suitable even for the drug-free training masses. This produced the almost universal belief that these training methods are the ones for everyone to follow.

But these conventional training methods do not work for drug-free genetically typical trainees. Because these training methods are so unproductive, most people are quickly propelled into the well of frustration and disappointment.

To make conventional routines work *very well*, harmful anabolic chemicals usually need to be used. Dissatisfied bodybuilders looking for quick fixes to their training frustrations and disappointments have produced huge markets for drug pushers. But the drug route is not the only solution for training woes!

If people would train on routines like those promoted in this book they would get results that would astound them. They would not experience the frustration and disappointment that are usually standard when using conventional training routines. Then they would not feel pressured to take dangerous drugs in order to make their training work.

Abbreviated training routines need to be combined with the candid understanding that out-of-this-world strength and muscular development are only possible for genetic phenomena. Then ultimate expectations will be modified accordingly, and no comparison made with the development of the competitive elite.

Keep your integrity, sanity and health. Absorb with every atom of your being the paramount fact that your health is your most important possession. And your integrity is not far behind in importance. *Train drug free, always!*

## Where you stand in the spectrum of potential

Dividing a *random* sample of drug-free weight trainees into degrees of "hardgainingness" cannot be done accurately because of the difficulty of specifying, identifying and then quantifying with consistency the characteristics of "gainingness." But for the purpose of getting at least an approximation, here are some suggested figures.

At the "hardest" end of the gaining spectrum are the near-zero gainers who, for reasons of health or extreme structural problems, find it almost impossible to gain (but *not impossible* if they train properly). They number fewer than 5% of any random sample from the training masses.

At the "easiest" end of the spectrum are the super easy gainers who have phenomenal genetics and fantastically-responsive bodies. The phenomenally blessed—the genetic freaks, and I am not using "freaks" in a pejorative sense—number much fewer than 1% of the *whole* training population.

The genetic freaks have a blend of bodytype, muscle insertion points, neuromuscular efficiency, muscle belly length, muscle fiber type and number, tendency for leanness, and recovery abilities that give them a *tremendously* responsive body. For competitive bodybuilding there are pivotally important aesthetic factors that are also genetically determined. See BRAWN for a detailed discussion on how genetic freaks are assembled.

Behind the extremely responsive easy gainers are the "regular" easy gainers who are able to gain to some degree on most programs, though they do not have the talent to become fantastic *unless* pumped to their jowls with chemicals. There is a considerable number of these easy gainers, perhaps as many as 10% or so of a random sample of weight trainees. It is this group that provides gyms with most of their successes. But these successful trainees use programs which are training suicide for genuine hard gainers. Many trainers and coaches belong to the category of "regular" easy gainers. But these easy gainers often have a body part and an exercise or two they struggle in, relatively speaking. While easy gainers typically adhere to conventional training routines, and often gain well from them, they gain *far* more when they adopt programs like those described in this book.

Near-zero, easy and extremely easy gainers total about 15% of a random sample of trainees, leaving 85% or so who are "regular" hard gainers that get nowhere using popular routines. (These approximate percentages are strictly for a drug-free population. Drug use would distort the percentages.) Hard gainers have *a lot* of potential for growth, but to realize it they must train *appropriately.* The harder a gainer you are, the less room for error you have in your total exercise, rest and nutrition program, and the more educated you need to be. This book will educate you.

Though "hard gainer" is a well used term in the bodybuilding world in particular, and also used in this book, it is actually a misnomer. Because hard gainers are the majority it would be more accurate to call them "normal" gainers. As it is, the term "hard gainer" implies a condition that is abnormal.

Whatever genetic potpourri you have been dealt is all you are going to get. Whatever shortcomings you may have, you have to live with. Rather than spend time complaining about your genetic fate, pour your energy into achieving your genetic potential. An average or even a less-than-average potential for bodybuilding, *if achieved*, is stunning to an untrained person, and respected by almost any trained individual.

Focus on achieving *your* potential, *not* on comparing yourself with ideals. Apply yourself intelligently and you may discover that what you thought was a modest potential is actually a lot more.

If you are consumed with the achievements of others, enviously look at the natural talents of a gifted but tiny minority, and bemoan your own genetic fate, you will never deliver the consistent and savvy dedication needed to do what will satisfy you most of all—*the achievement of your own full potential for muscle and might.*

## Application of training reality

BEYOND BRAWN will take you right "inside" weight training, to study the practical reality of applying knowledge. It is not a theoretical treatise or pack of pseudo-scientific claptrap. It provides the real-life, adaptable, flexible and step-by-step instruction needed by *typical* people who have demanding jobs and family lives.

This book provides extensive details of the nitty-gritty practical application of training. Without a thorough understanding of the practical application of training, even a good program will fail for most followers. Only *you* can truly know how to train yourself, but you can only do this if you know enough about training. This book will teach you in extensive detail how to design your own training programs, so that you can become the best trainer you will ever get—your own.

Though all the material that can be useful for typical trainees is not included in this book, if you cannot get big and strong from following the advice given in this text, there is no drug-free alternative that can get you big and strong. This applies no matter how expensive or hyped up the alternative may be, no matter who endorses it, and no matter how "scientific" the results of some jiggery-pokery with numbers, "research" and data may appear.

## How to get your money's worth from this book

You cannot get an education in a subject without investing in very serious study. Weight training is no exception. To dip into this book, and selectively pull statements and segments out of context, will neither do the book justice nor your weight-training education. There is so much vital information crammed into this work *and it is all interrelated*. The book needs to be studied from cover to cover. Because it contains so much information, a considerable investment of time is required if you are to benefit fully from the book.

To experience the full force of this book you need to read it more than once, and then, in both the near and distant future, review parts of it. There is so much to learn and master. As you read this book do not hesitate to turn back to re-read parts. The more thoroughly you grasp the material as you go along, the easier you will understand the rest of the book, and the quicker that all the pieces will fall into place.

Use this text like a workbook, i.e., highlight parts, and make notes in the margins. But only do this if the book is yours. If you have a borrowed copy, contact the publisher and get your own book to mark up and make notes on.

## The depth, breadth and eclecticism you need

This is not a quickly written book of simple prescriptions and proscriptions, or a single plan that is supposed to work universally. Cut-and-dried, neat-and-tidy programs are misleading. There are important components common to all programs that work for typical trainees, but people respond differently to the same program even assuming that each person interprets the program in the same way. Generic "one size fits all" programs are utterly unfit for mass use.

This book presents different interpretations of abbreviated training routines that focus on core exercises. This versatile eclecticism produces a great depth and breadth of instruction. Draw upon this to educate yourself about how best to exploit weight training. While there is always the trial-and-error component of weight training, this book teaches you enough to spare your having to go through the degree of trial-and-error that most trainees have to before learning what works for them.

This book intentionally provides radical training strategies, and even some methods and tips that are downright blasphemous relative to gym norms. This is done for *one reason only*—to provide all hard-gaining trainees, even *extreme* hard gainers, with the instructional tools they need in order to make good progress. Building impressive physiques and strength levels should not be the right of just the gifted minority.

Learn from the very costly experiences of those who have been through the mill of desperate frustration with conventional training advice. This book is not based on only one man's journey, but is a distillation of the experiences and acquired wisdom of generations of people.

### READ – GRASP – APPLY – PERSIST – *ACHIEVE!*

The revised edition of this book includes a new chapter—in Section 3—and many revisions throughout the book.

## Note on the Trap Bar and shrug bar

Where the Trap Bar® is referred to in this book, you may also read "shrug bar." The shrug bar came on the market after BEYOND BRAWN was first published. The two bars are produced by different manufacturers. Both are excellent training tools. The shrug bar provides more knee room because it has a hexagonal shape as against the rhombus shape of the Trap Bar. Please see page 481 for how to find more information on the shrug bar. You may, however, find the *standard* shrug (or Trap) bar too restricting for safe bent-legged deadlifting, and require a custom-made bar with gripping sites placed wider apart.

There are few photographs in this book because nothing is included on exercise technique. Exercise form is covered in unique and extensive detail (including 244 photographs) in a companion book—THE INSIDER'S TELL-ALL HANDBOOK ON WEIGHT-TRAINING TECHNIQUE.

You will benefit from BEYOND BRAWN in direct proportion to how seriously you study the book, how thoroughly you grasp the contents, how well you make the understanding one with you, and how resolutely you apply what you learn.

Before thinking something important has been missed out of this book, please wait until you have read every page. There is an extensive amount of information here, and it is all interrelated.

Excluding the introductory material, each paragraph of this book is itemized. For example, 4.23 means that that particular paragraph is number 23 of Chapter 4. Itemizing each paragraph makes it almost effortless to find whatever you are looking up in the index.

## Statement of intent

I have absolutely no interest in drug-assisted training. But I am not naive. I know a great deal about the appalling mess of drugs in the world of weight training. Because I am only interested in drug-free training, and primarily concerned with satisfying the needs of the hard-gaining masses, some of the methods and values promoted in this book are heretical relative to much of what is customary in gyms today. There is no other approach to take if training methods that are practical and helpful for drug-free typical people are to be promoted.

Never forget that the phenomenal success enjoyed by so few bodybuilders is primarily due to their great genetic advantage compounded by drug assistance. Anyone who tries to tell you otherwise is either ignorant, or confused between fact and fiction. And all drug-assisted (*and* drug-free) genetic phenomena do not have a clue how to train drug-free genetically typical people. Always keep that in mind when you hunt for help with your own training. The imitating of inappropriate role models has been largely if not totally responsible for the poor bodybuilding progress had by most *serious* gym members throughout the world.

## The pivotal truth

Achieving your potential for muscle and might demands extraordinary discipline and dedication. There is no place for half measures, corner cutting, laziness or lukewarm enthusiasm. If you do not train well, rest well, sleep well and eat well, you will get nowhere or make only minimal progress. And you need the full package on an unrelenting basis if you are to make the fastest progress possible. There is no room for compromise!

You alone are responsible for your dedication and discipline. The buck stops with you. How much do you want a terrific physique? Are you prepared to do everything necessary other than use drugs? Are you prepared to give your absolute best shot? If you are, you are reading the right book.

A Chinese proverb says that a journey of a thousand miles begins with one step. By choosing to study this book you have taken the first step—a huge step—towards the strong, well-developed, fit and lean physique you crave.

Apply what this book teaches and you will be off and running for a lifetime of very productive training. You will experience the exhilaration from anticipating great physical change, the thrill of accumulating strength gains, and the euphoria from achieving physical transformation.

# Section 1

## Establishing a secure foundation

Break away from training methods that do not work. Open your mind and find out from this book how to get in charge of your training. If you are new to training you will learn how to sustain your initial great enthusiasm and expectations. If you have been frustrated by poor results for a long time, you can return to those early and heady days when you were gung-ho about training and could not wait to get into the gym for a workout. But first you need to learn how to channel that vigor into productive training.

You have got to make the necessary changes now. You cannot keep chucking away chunks of your life on unproductive training routines. Life is in short supply and the years quickly slip by.

# 1. Setting the Scene for Building Muscle & Might

1.1 Unless you have a terrific genetic inheritance for muscle building, the conventional approach that prescribes a *traditional* split routine, more weight-training days than non-weight-training days, lots of isolation exercises, multiple exercises per body part, and a great many sets per workout, delivers little or no gains. Full-body routines of too many exercises performed too frequently are also unproductive for most trainees. Hundreds of thousands of people are living testimony to this stark reality.

1.2 Bodybuilding, and strength training in general, are wonderfully rewarding activities *so long as you get satisfactory results*. Regardless of genetics, gender or age, each of us has tremendous power to improve physique, fitness and health; but very few people fully exploit this power because so few people train in a way that is truly appropriate to them.

1.3 The way most people train it is no wonder there is such a huge failure rate and rapid turnover of members in most gyms. If only people would adopt the radical and abbreviated format right from the start, rather than first having to waste perhaps many years of their lives on conventional and inappropriate training instruction. Then the success rate for weight training would spiral hugely, and the turnover rate in gyms would plummet.

1.4 Stop following instruction that you know is not working. You do not need to be an expert to know if something is not helping you. *More of what did not help you over the last few months is not going to help you over the next few months.* Stop imitating the training of people who have genetic talent you do not. And stop thinking that anything other than the basic combination of training, food and adequate rest is going to make much if any difference to the results you get from your efforts in the gym.

1.5        Get in charge of your training! If you do not start now to do something that works, when are you going to start building the physique you want? Bodybuilding and strength training are not hit or miss activities. You have tremendous control over your physique development, *if only you would start to employ it.*

1.6        There are no quick fixes in drug-free training. It is a long and demanding journey to achieve your genetic potential, unless you are one of the *very few* who are genetically gifted and have little trouble getting big and strong. You will never be able to compete with the awesome elite physiques, but you *can* build a physique that will be stunning to untrained people. To do this you need to start training productively, and you have got to start *now*. Put the instruction of this book into action!

## Responsibility and commitment

1.7        Irrevocable willingness, commitment, determination—call it what you want—is a huge part of making training deliver the goods. You must stay the course and resist peer pressure and the herd instinct that push you towards conformity. And you need to have a mind that is open to investigating the radical.

1.8        While the circumstances of life make some decisions more likely than others, and at times almost force your hand, the reality is that each person is responsible for his or her own exercise program's results. *You* decide which exercises you use, how you perform them, and how often you train. *You* decide when you quit a set, when you go to sleep, how well you eat, and whether or not you cut corners in general. Though life's circumstances influence those decisions, and test your resolve and stickability, you alone are responsible for your progress in the gym. The buck stops with you.

1.9        Accept responsibility for having created the current state of your physique and fitness. Then assume the responsibility for changing what you do not like.

1.10       Let your dissatisfaction with your current physique propel you into furiously motivated, determined and dedicated action to improve it.

1.11    But first you need to have an open mind and the willingness to do what needs to be done (drug-free, of course). You must never be put off by apparent setbacks and difficulties. It will not be smooth sailing, but if you want it badly enough you will get there. You will overcome obstacles, and setbacks will become challenges. Persist, and eventually you will get there.

1.12    We are concentrating on an area where genetic restraints have great influence. Keep your goals very challenging but realistic, achieve them, and then set more specific and challenging goals.

1.13    You must be willing to do all that is necessary—in your training, diet, and rest schedule, and ignore the negative vibes of others. If any of this willingness disappears, so will your progress.

## Thought control

1.14    Do not allow negative thoughts and negative people to drag you down. Negative thoughts and negative people will harm all your endeavors. If you imagine failure, dwell on it, and prepare for it, then you will fail.

1.15    This book gives you a step-by-step plan for bodybuilding and strength training success, but you will ruin it if your mind dwells on the wrong things. While a poor program and a good attitude are not going to help you, unless your good attitude keeps you persisting until you find a good program, a good program together with a poor attitude is no good.

1.16    Be alert to your thoughts. Stand back from your mind and watch what goes on in there. Notice how much negativity there is. Put the negative thoughts aside as soon as they appear. The ability to concentrate on the positive will come without trying, so long as you focus on getting rid of the negative.

1.17    With a good plan, and no time for negativity, you are set for the confidence and persistence that lead to success. But the journey there will be neither trouble free nor easy.

## The "hard gainer" tag

1.18    A hard gainer is the genetically average or disadvantaged drug-free person, usually male, that typifies gym members. Hard gainers are usually naturally thin, though there are fat hard gainers. Hard gainers respond poorly, or not at all, to conventional training methods.

1.19    Those who play down the importance of genetics are almost always those who were dealt a better-than-average or even an excellent hand of genetics. Few people care to think that they got something *relatively* easily. They prefer to give the impression that they really had to suffer for every pound they gained. As a result, few people in the weight-training world will admit that they got a head start from their inheritance. Anyone blessed with terrific inheritance and a very responsive body can never, *ever* get in the shoes of a true hard gainer. Sometimes the easy gainers' arrogance, conceit and gross misunderstanding of the plight of the true hard gainer is nauseating. But, ironically, it is often the easy gainers who preach training instruction to the gullible and impressionable hard-gaining masses. It is no wonder that the masses get nowhere—the blind are leading the blind.

1.20    Of course, as easy gainers close in on their drug-free potential for muscle and might they can find gains hard to make. But until they got to that point they found gains easy to make, *almost regardless of what type of program they used.* They trained, and they grew. But the "hard gaining" they "suffer" from as they get near their maximum potential is totally different from the hard gaining that true hard gainers have to deal with. Real hard gainers find gains hard to make right from day one, *unless they train as this book teaches.*

1.21    Can a "hard gainer" tag create a mindset of negativity? Does it set up an "I cannot do much" attitude that may set a self-fulfilling prophecy in motion? If you bemoan your genetic inheritance, stack yourself up against the competitive elite, and adopt role models light years away from your own reality, then of course you are not going to have the right mindset for becoming the best you can. But if we go into this further we will see how liberating and positive the "hard gainer" tag really is.

1.22    Once you recognize you are a hard gainer you set the stage for adopting realistic role models, sensible and practical training methods, and a sane drug-free long-term strategy. Then, while keeping training in its place, you will put into practice time-proven programs and start getting good results.

1.23    While realism is the hard gainer's watchword, you do not know how far you can go until you try—by investing in sensible instruction and dogged determination for many years.

Even average genetics can go a *long* way. Train as this book advises, pay your dues for a period of years, and then you will go as far as your genetics will allow—and perhaps much farther than you may currently think is realistic.

1.24    During the pre-steroids era, when the-then conventional training advice was much more useful for typical people than today's standard gym guidance is, sky-high goals were not promoted to the masses. Then, taking off in the sixties and accelerating thereafter, the widespread but usually secretive use of steroids greatly elevated training expectations. This led to increasingly unrealistic goals being promoted to the masses. (Bodybuilding drugs were around since before the sixties, but their influence did not really take off until during the sixties.)

1.25    Nowadays, consider yourself anything other than a hard gainer, and you are almost certainly *not* going to train according to your ability to respond to exercise. You will be swallowed up by popular routines and advice. You will be consumed by despair as you invest so much for so little return. You will be easy prey for being ripped off by charlatans, especially those who accuse hard gainers of being whiners and underachievers. These charlatans are the same individuals whose models of people who "overcame" genetic shortcomings are usually pumped to the jowls with steroids, but who never mention the contribution that drugs made.

1.26    Unless you see through all the fraud you will become another training failure and possibly take the drug route because conventional training methods do not work for typical hard gainers. Today's well-intentioned or, in some cases, the

> **Some influential writers and coaches will never "get it." They will never admit they have superior genetics, thinking that because they are not elite competitive bodybuilders they must be genetically typical. And many of these influential people do not have typical family lives, but have almost optimal training conditions, and often even have a background in drugs. It is no wonder that their training advice has little or no connection with practical reality for typical drug-free people. So the training masses continue to be led astray!**

unscrupulous "forget about genetics" and "you can do it too" mentality fuels training failure, supports the ripping off of the masses, and encourages drug abuse. As soon as anyone plays down genetics and drugs, you should hear alarm bells ringing.

1.27    Understanding that you are a hard gainer *frees* you from distorted aspirations, absurd training routines, and a life of obsessive ruin. It makes you cautious, skeptical and discriminating, thus sparing you from being misled by those who promise far more than they can ever deliver.

## Hard gainer creation

1.28    Conventional training advice creates permanent hard gainers, and shackles them in stagnation and frustration. Because the conventional advice works for so few people, it makes most people believe that getting bigger and stronger is much more difficult than it is, impossible even.

1.29    The instruction in BEYOND BRAWN is primarily aimed at people who cannot grow on conventional advice, but the irony is that by following the advice in this book you can realize terrific gains and, *relatively speaking*, make yourself into an easy gainer.

## The modern travesty

1.30    As the numbers of sham gyms and instructors increase, so does the drivel that is promoted as training instruction. Gyms concerned with maximizing profit—wrapped up in sales of their various accessories, food supplements and fashion clothing—have made a mockery of the gym business. It has got to the point where the last place to look for good coaching is in a modern well-equipped gym.

1.31    Many gyms should issue the following notice to their members. Keep this notice in mind should you ever hope to get good instruction from an appearance-first gym.

> This gym is all appearance and no substance. It is only because we have a lot of fancy-looking equipment that we impress everyone who knows little or nothing about training. Because we have spent a lot of money on marginal, useless and sometimes dangerous equipment we must encourage our members to use it. We never encourage the old-fashioned basic exercises. In fact, to save you from being tempted to use the latter, you will never find a power

rack or lifting platform here, and the squat racks we have are flimsy and unused. Who on earth wants to squat? Too much like hard work. Our instructors are as useless as we are, though some of them have very good physiques due to excellent genetics and use of steroids.

To deter you from using the time-proven most productive (but most uncomfortable) exercises, we have joined ranks with other gyms to perpetuate the hokum that basic barbell exercises are dangerous and, at best, only useful for beginners who are not fortunate enough to train in a modern well-equipped gym like ours. This is convenient for us, though, because we barely know the first thing of instructing safe and productive technique in the biggest and best barbell exercises. We promote the idea that you need a wide variety of isolation and machine exercises in every workout.

We make exercise fun. You can watch yourself in the many mirrors we have, listen to the music we entertain you with, talk while you train, and ogle the skimpily clad bodies of the genetically blessed, sensual female instructors we employ to keep you (men) interested in renewing your membership. Training here is fun, and fun means lots of members, though few of them stay long term. We depend on a constant influx of new members to make a profit.

Welcome to this gym. We promise we will not push you hard, and we hope you will enjoy your time here. That is, you will enjoy it until you realize that the methods we promote will not help make you big and strong unless you have fantastic genetics or are pumped up with steroids. Or like our regulars you will decide to forget about getting big and strong, and come here only for social contacts and visual kicks.

## Grit and character

1.32  No matter how you look at it, if you want to get much bigger and stronger you have got to pay your dues. This means knuckling down to hard work in the gym, and, when out of the gym, being conscientious and disciplined enough to ensure good daily nutrition and adequate rest and sleep. The buck stops with you. You either deliver, or you do not.

1.33  While your training and related activities should not obsess you to the detriment of your health, family and career, you have to be addicted to the iron, sights and sounds of the gym, the challenge of "one more rep," and the accumulation of small bits of iron on the bar. You need to almost worship the soreness you suffer on the days after a hard workout. And you need the required patience in order not to rush and ruin your progress. You must find training to be heaven on earth and, when in the gym, live to train.

1.34    You *will* have serious setbacks. You *will* get injured. You *will* overtrain for long periods. You *will* get misled. You *will* have sustained periods of desperate frustration. Family, education, personal and career concerns *will* get in the way. Through all of this you must maintain your zest for training.

1.35    Never will you even contemplate packing it in. Even if temporarily you cannot train, your desire will never be extinguished. You will find something positive in all apparent misfortunes—and there nearly always is something positive if you look hard enough. During "down" times you will prepare yourself for getting back into training with greater zeal, commitment and organization than ever before.

1.36    Grasp with the inner core of your being the highest training truth for hard gainers—progressive poundages in good form using abbreviated routines dominated by the big basic exercises. Then gear everything you do to ensure that you live this simple truth. And keep delivering the application *for year after year after year.*

1.37    You cannot buy or hire the desire and discipline that drives you to do all this. Others can encourage you, motivate you, and perhaps even bully you along for a short while. But if you cannot *stand alone* and deliver the goods by yourself, you are *never* going to realize your potential for muscle and might. The desire has got to be so intense that your body and soul are steeped in it for the long haul.

1.38    It is you who has to struggle in the gym. It is you who has to drive yourself to do more, and more again, and yet more again and again. It is you who has to deliver the sustained good diet

> **You must find training to be heaven on earth and, when in the gym, live to train.**

and five or, even better, six meals each day. It is you who has to ensure you rest and sleep enough. To do all of this you need exemplary grit and character.

1.39    Deliver this grit and character and become the best that you can. Do not compare yourself with others. It is bettering yourself that matters, not stacking yourself up against others. Focus on bettering yourself—again, and again, and again.

## The thrill of training

1.40    The power to change one's own physique is one of the biggest appeals of weight training, if not *the* biggest. Lifting weights is a solo activity over which you alone have the power of control. Once you know what to do, you need rely on no one.

1.41    No matter where you are now—big or small, strong or weak, young or not so young—you need only compete with yourself. It is you, against you. Progress is measurable, and concrete. It can be as little as just one more rep than last week in a given exercise, with the same poundage. Or it could be the same rep count but with an extra pound on the bar. Or it could be one of several other indicators of progress.

1.42    All of these small doses of progress are little thrills you will never tire of. They make weight training a fabulous activity. But you cannot experience this unless you implement a rational and productive interpretation of weight training.

1.43    Physique improvement and strength training are not just about getting bigger and stronger muscles, though, of course, they are hugely satisfying in themselves. Training is also about enjoying exercise, and making yourself fitter, more flexible and healthier, and about strengthening your mind, self-esteem and confidence.

1.44    Though physically hard to do, training satisfies a basic human need for physical effort. No matter where you are now, you can take delight in realizing some new goal in the physical sphere.

1.45    But none of this can happen unless you rate exercise high in your priorities. Resolve, *now*, to give your exercise program and dietary discipline the priority they deserve. Get on course for realizing the physical qualities you admire. Put a spark in your life through productive training.

1.46     Not only will you look and feel great, and maintain your
         physical youth while others around you are getting old, but
         you will love the journey there and the knocking off of all the
         little targets; and revel in the pleasure that exercise brings.

1.47     Each of us can create a utopia of training sanity. By doing this
         we can keep our own houses in order, and develop ourselves
         so that we are outstanding in the minds of untrained people.
         We can then present ourselves as examples of how training
         works for "average" people.

1.48     Resistance training is one of man's finest discoveries. Do not
         miss your chance to benefit from it.

## In praise of bodybuilding

1.49     Bodybuilding gets some bad press because many people
         consider bodybuilding as the exclusive territory of excessively
         narcissistic, drug-using, all-appearance-and-no-function,
         frivolous freaks. For sure, some bodybuilders do give weight
         training dreadful publicity because of their gym antics, drug
         use and dealing, and appalling ignorance of the type of
         training that is needed by drug-free typical people. But this has
         *nothing* to do with what I consider bodybuilding to be.

1.50     Because most commercial gym training instruction is usually
         called "bodybuilding," and because it is usually so paltry, it
         gives bodybuilding a bad name.

1.51     I have great respect for any drug-free person who can lift huge
         weights. But because I have a strong bias towards appearance
         and aesthetics, I see appearance first and lifting performance
         second. If appearance is heavily compromised I have little
         interest in the strength achievements.

1.52     To my mind, bodybuilding is about molding your physique so
         that you are satisfied with its appearance *and* performance. It is
         nothing to do with drugs, excessive narcissism, obsessive
         concern with bodyfat percentages, conventional bodybuilding
         routines, or training frivolity.

1.53     Bodybuilding *as I interpret it* is very healthy, but a pure-strength
         focus can become unhealthy. The bodybuilding that I promote
         encourages muscular and strength balance throughout the body,
         mostly achieved through focusing on compound exercises.

1.54    The bodybuilding I promote never puts health second to appearance or performance. Aerobic conditioning, and maintaining a bodyfat level below 15% (for a male), are usually neglected by pure-strength devotees. Some big modern-day strength supermen seriously neglected their health and appearances, and are dead as a result.

1.55    Rational bodybuilding keeps appearance at the forefront. This is good. When appearance matters, overeating is out, and bodyfat is never allowed to exceed 15% (for a man). When health is the number one concern, aerobic work is not neglected, and nutrition is not just about protein, protein and more protein. An excessive focus on animal products is unhealthy.

1.56    Rational bodybuilding is about selecting exercises that are best *for you*. While this should always mean a focus on the big basic exercises, it does not mean a rigid adherence to a fixed prescription of exercises. Even the great exercises are not equally suited to all trainees. Never lock yourself into using an exercise if it does not suit you. The number one priority for any exercise is that it does you no harm. For example, squat darn hard if you know how to squat, and if you are at least reasonably well suited to the exercise. But if you truly have knee and/or back problems, or if you have a terrible structure for squatting, then to battle on with the squat is foolish. (Note that nearly all the "you *must* squat" advocates are themselves blessed with very good mechanics for the squat.)

1.57    Some people are simply not designed to become *very* strong, though of course most people can become *much* stronger. But many of these people have a very aesthetic body structure. So rather than try to make themselves into something they are not designed to be—powerhouses—they should focus on something they are suited to, i.e., bodybuilding, with the emphasis on appearance. Do not focus on what you will never be able to do well. Instead, focus on what you can do better.

1.58    But if you are a natural powerhouse, and that is where your interests lie, then go for it, full-bore. But make sure that you keep an eye on your appearance, and do not neglect your health in the pursuit of getting ever stronger.

1.59    Given the choice between reducing bodyfat substantially, or increasing strength substantially, most people would prefer the former. Fat loss will do more to improve their appearance. But the best choice would be to become substantially leaner *and* substantially stronger. This would hugely improve appearance. It *is* possible to stay strong while becoming lean, so long as you do it properly. The conventional overtraining route to a leaner physique can strip off more muscle than fat.

1.60    Most men who start training when over age 30 are unlikely to have a gung-ho zeal for *huge* size and strength. They are more likely, at least to begin with, to want to add 20–30 pounds of muscle, and get their bodyfat under 15%. To get there they will have to invest in very serious basics-first training dominated by progressive poundages.

1.61    Whether categorized as a bodybuilder, strength buff, or any other type of weight trainee, the bottom line of productive weight training is *the same*—a focus on basic exercises, abbreviated routines, hard work, and progressive poundages.

1.62    Properly done, bodybuilding is one of the most rewarding activities around. Changing your appearance for the better, in a substantial way, is bliss. And bodybuilding can do this better than any other activity.

1.63    Use a rep count for a given exercise that best suits *you*, get as strong as you can in exercises that suit *you* and which *you* can perform safely, keep your bodyfat levels to below 15% (or below 10% if you want an appearance that is stunning— assuming that you have some muscle), eat healthfully, perform aerobic work two or three times per week, stretch every other day, and then you have got the full bodybuilding package.

## Dedication vs. obsession

1.64    Not only is tempered enthusiasm for training a healthier approach than an obsessive enthusiasm, it actually ends up over the long term in being *more productive*. I do not want you to avoid obsessive enthusiasm just because it creates a seriously imbalanced life. I want you to avoid obsessive interest because *only then will you actually have the chance to achieve your natural physique and strength potential*.

1.65    I know a lot about an obsessive interest in bodybuilding. I had one for several years. Had I not had the character and discipline to resist the temptation to take bodybuilding drugs, I may have destroyed myself. I never ruined my health by drug abuse, but I certainly damaged my body as a result of doing many things wrong in my training.

1.66     As a teenager I cut myself off from everything I thought would have a negative effect on my bodybuilding. I became a recluse. I enclosed myself in a bodybuilding shell. I lost interest in my academic studies. I swallowed all the training and dietary nonsense that abounded at that time (in the mid seventies). I was very gullible and knew of no one who could keep me on the training straight and narrow. I was at the mercy of whatever literature I found, but could not distinguish between good and poor instruction. If it was in print, I believed it.

1.67     I had no time for anyone who talked or wrote about realistic goals, overtraining, or the dangers of certain exercises and specific exercise techniques, or the need to be prudent with intensity enhancers. I labeled those people as "wimps" and "underachievers." Who wanted to be conservative? Who was interested in being "realistic"? *I wanted to be huge!*

1.68     Being very young at the time I could apparently get away with harmful exercises, techniques, and abuse of intensity enhancers, *at least over the short term.* So I continued with those harmful practices. Those dangerous practices included gross overtraining, squatting with my heels raised on a board, performing hack machine squats, squatting with the bar too high on my shoulders, bench pressing with a very wide grip, bench pressing to my upper chest, performing deep flyes and lying and standing triceps extensions, performing stiff-legged deadlifts with an exaggerated full range of motion, and including specific "cheating" movements. Some of those techniques came to haunt me a few years later, when knee and back problems permanently limited my training.

> **It is not just the elite of the bodybuilding world who have very responsive bodies and the ability to tolerate a volume and frequency of training that most people cannot. Very successful performers in any athletic activity usually have this gift. Their training methods, too, should not be copied by drug-free typical trainees.**

1.69      Had I listened to those "wimps" who urged a conservative approach to training, and had I listened more to my own body, then I would not have caused the long-term damage that I did. Today I promote a conservative approach to training in general, and to exercise selection and technique in particular. Experience has taught me that the conservative approach is not only the safest way, *it is actually the most productive and satisfying, over the long term.*

1.70      The conservative approach is not just limited to exercise selection and technique. It also concerns exercise program design. Most people train too much. Not only is this counterproductive for short-term results, it produces the overtraining that wears the body down and causes long-term structural problems.

1.71      All this assumes that you actually keep training over the long term. An obsession leads to burnout because it produces poor results for most people. It causes so much frustration that most people give up training after a year or few, or they turn to drugs.

1.72      When you are obsessed you tend to discard reason and intelligence, and become all passion and emotion. This leads to gullibility and following poor training programs, skewed diets, bad exercises, and destructive ways of performing exercises that should be safe and super productive. This is precisely what happened to me. I trained too much (and thus wasted a big chunk of my life), followed skewed diets, used harmful exercises, and when I did use the best exercises I often used perverted and destructive variations.

1.73      Had this obsessive interest produced a great physique, then maybe I could argue that the price was worth paying. I suffered so much in the quest for a great physique, but did not get what I thought would make all the dedication worthwhile. When it finally dawned on me that after years of rabid dedication I did not have the physique that I had targeted, I was devastated. To invest so much into one target, and then fail to get to that target, produces extreme frustration and disappointment.

## The best way

1.74      So much for doing things in the wrong way. What you want to know is how to do things the right way. That is what this book is all about. The right way does not mean being obsessed. It means being highly dedicated but while remaining critical and discriminating, and while keeping a balanced approach that does not neglect the more serious aspects of your life.

1.75    Learn the lessons taught in this book and then you can get on with making the most of the magnificent benefits of weight training, but without doing yourself any short-term or long-term damage. You can then train for a lifetime without having to spend time working around injuries and joint problems. Then you can continue to train on the most important exercises—you will *not* have to drop the best exercises.

1.76    In this way you will be securely on the best program to achieve your full physique and/or strength potential, *and* you will not have compromised on the rest of your life. Then training will have enriched your life rather than robbed you of a big chunk of it and perhaps left you with permanent scars.

## The biggest champions

The biggest champions of the training world are *not* the drug-enhanced genetically blessed competitive elite. The biggest champions are the unsung heroes who applied years of dogged determination in order to build themselves up against the odds, without ever using drugs, without seeking or finding publicity, and without divorcing themselves from the rigors and responsibilities of everyday working and family life. Genetically gifted and drug-enhanced super achievers who have near-perfect training conditions and lifestyles cannot hold a candle to the real heroes of the training world.

# Training Jargon

1.77    Weight training has its own characteristic lingo. Here is a brief
        tour through the most fundamental terms and words you need
        to understand before continuing—a glossary in use. As
        necessary as it is to understand the lingo of the training world,
        watch out for the pseudo-scientific and nonsensical jargon that
        bamboozles the unaware into a chaos of confusion. No matter
        how much you know about the razzmatazz of the training
        world, if you do not consistently deliver what is needed for *you*
        to make progress, you will never make decent gains.

## Reps

1.78    The basic unit of weight training is the rep, or repetition. If you
        hang from an overhead bar and pull yourself up, and then
        lower yourself to the starting position, you would have done a
        single rep of the pullup or chin. A series of reps comprises a
        set. A set can consist of one rep (a single), very low reps (2–4),
        medium reps (5–12), high reps (13–25), or very high reps (25+).
        These divisions are subjective. Different people may have
        different definitions of low, medium, high and very high reps.

1.79    Reps can be done slowly, quickly or somewhere in between.
        But one person's "slow" can be another's "fast." More than
        one rep cadence works, at least for some people, but fast and
        explosive training carries a very high risk of injury. This book
        focuses on a *controlled* cadence and exercises where speed is
        *not* a necessity. This means lowering the weight under control
        and then pushing or pulling the bar smoothly *and* with good
        biomechanics. There should be no throwing, bouncing,
        yanking or jerking.

1.80    Reps can be done with a pause of a second or a few seconds
        before each, or they can be done continuously, or they can be
        done with exaggerated pauses of as much as 30–60 seconds
        between reps, i.e., rest-pause work. The exaggerated pauses
        permit heavier weights to be used.

## Sticking point

1.81    Most exercises have a point, often about halfway up, where the
        resistance seems to get magnified. This is the point where the
        resistance seems to stutter, or even get stuck if you are at your
        hilt of effort, hence the term "sticking point." If you make it
        through the sticking point, the rest of the rep should be easy
        (but the sticking point could actually be at the end of the rep).

## Concentric and eccentric phases

1.82    A rep has two phases, i.e., the positive or concentric (pushing or pulling) part when the muscle shortens, and the negative or eccentric (lowering) part when the muscle lengthens. Sitting down to a chair is the negative or eccentric phase of a squat, while standing up is the positive or concentric phase.

## Sets

1.83    An exercise is usually done for multiple sets before moving onto the next exercise. Sets come in two basic types: warmup sets and work sets. Warmup sets are done with weights lighter than those to be used for work sets. Warmup sets prepare you for work sets.

## Flexion and extension of joints

1.84    Bringing together the bones associated with a joint is flexion, e.g., sitting is knee flexion because it brings the bones of the upper and lower leg closer together. Joint extension brings the bones into alignment, e.g., straightening the legs.

## Range of motion

1.85    Reps can be done with a full or partial range of motion. Usually the full range is performed—all the way up, and all the way down. But a few exercises are usually done with a partial range of motion. For example, very few people squat to where their rear thighs fold over their calves. So most squatters only do a partial movement. To squat to a position of full knee flexion, with a weight that is heavy for the lifter concerned, can be injurious, especially to the lower back.

1.86    Short-range movements of just a few inches are intentionally used in some programs. These are called partial reps, or partials. A partial rep could start at the beginning, middle or end point of an exercise, or specifically from or to the sticking point. If the partial is over just the final few inches of a rep, it is often called a "lockout."

## Body parts

1.87    Exercises target specific body parts, or muscle groups. In a simplified format here are the main body parts:

   a. abdominals (abs) and obliques of the front midsection

   b. biceps and brachialis (front of the upper arm)

c. buttocks or glutes (glutei muscles)

d. calves (gastrocnemius and soleus)

e. chest (pectorals, or pecs)

f. erectors (columns of muscle on either side of the spine)

g. forearms

h. lats (latissimus dorsi, muscles on the back under the arms)

i. neck

j. shoulders (deltoids, or delts)

k. thighs (quads or quadriceps on the front, hams or hamstrings on the rear, and the thigh adductor muscles)

l. triceps (rear upper arm)

m. upper back (small muscles around the shoulder blades, and the large trapezius covering much of the upper back)

*Anatomy charts are provided at the end of this chapter.*

## Exercises and equipment

1.88    Exercises can be done with free weights (primarily long-bar barbells and short-bar dumbbells), or machines. The former are the traditional and most versatile way of training. Machines reduce the need for instruction and the chance of acute injury. It is harder to lose control with a machine than free weights.

1.89    Free weights properly used *are* safe, but they require more expertise and skill than does a machine. While some machines are valuable if used properly, most are a hindrance to progress for the serious trainee. Some are even dangerous because they lock the user into a movement pattern that may not fit individual parameters such as height and limb lengths.

1.90    Though the risk of acute injury is usually reduced in machine exercises, there is often an increased chance of chronic injuries and irritations. And for home trainees, machines are usually prohibitively expensive.

1.91    An important distinction needs to be made between machines that lock you into a fixed groove, and those that involve cables which allow some freedom of movement. A lat machine, for example, allows plenty of individual freedom of motion and positioning, but a pullover machine offers much less.

1.92    As far as barbells go, there are "exercise" bars that are the same diameter (usually a tad over an inch) over the whole length and can be as short as about 4 feet, or as long as about 7 feet. There are Olympic and power bars that have revolving sleeves of about 2-inch diameter at their ends. These bars are about 87 inches long, depending on the manufacturer. All these bars are straight. Then there is the cambered squat bar (bent like a yoke), the Trap Bar® [and shrug bar, see page 16], and thick bars.

## Compound and isolation exercises

1.93    Exercises come in two basic types: compound (i.e., multiple-joint movements), or isolation (i.e., single-joint ones).

1.94    The squat is a multiple-joint exercise because it involves movement at more than one joint, and hence involves a lot of musculature—primarily the quads, glutes and erectors.

1.95    The leg extension—straightening your leg while seated—is a single-joint exercise because it involves movement at only one joint (the knee). The leg extension primarily targets the quads.

1.96    To train the whole body using only isolation work means you need a lot of different exercises. But most of the body can be trained using a mere handful of compound movements.

## Core exercises

1.97    Compound movements are usually tagged "basic exercises," though some people include a few single-joint exercises under that description. The term "basic exercise" does not have a standard definition. This inconsistency leads to confusion.

1.98    The most important exercises are the *core* movements, i.e., squat, bent-legged deadlift (usually referred to as "the deadlift"), sumo deadlift (arms held *between* the legs), stiff-legged deadlift, leg press, bench press (flat, incline and decline), parallel bar dip, shrug variations, pulldown, row variations, pullup (pronated grip) and chin/chinup (supinated grip), pullover using a machine, and overhead press.

1.99      These core exercises are the primary ones you must focus on
          (only a select few in each routine) in order to develop bigger
          and stronger muscles. Each abbreviated training routine
          usually has between two and five core movements in it.

## Secondary exercises

1.100     The most important of these are calf raises, crunch situp, side
          bend, shoulder external rotator work, back extensions, and
          specific neck and grip work (including finger *extensions*). Curls
          can be included if you do not get enough biceps development
          from rows, pullups or pulldowns. A mix of core and secondary
          exercises covers all the body.

## Builders and refiners

1.101     The core exercises are the ones that will build the substance of
          your physique. The secondary (or "accessory") exercises plug
          the gaps left by the core movements. But there are many
          isolation exercises, e.g., leg extensions, pec deck work, lateral
          raises, concentration curls, cable cross overs, and triceps
          kickbacks that are rampant in gyms worldwide. These are the
          detail exercises. The top physiques use them, and need them,
          because they are working on details.

1.102     Hardly any gym members, even very experienced ones, have
          built enough muscle mass to be concerned with detail isolation
          exercises. Some of these, however, may be appropriate for
          rehabilitation purposes following injury or accident. This type
          of use is for a rehabilitation professional to prescribe.

1.103     Generally speaking, the detail exercises distract you from
          what you should focus on if you want to get big and strong.
          Not only that, but they rob your recuperative system (your
          recovery "machinery") of some of its reserves, thus
          restraining if not curtailing your progress in the big building
          exercises. Also, because some of the detail exercises are so
          hostile to joints and muscles, they can cause injuries that lead
          to training regression.

## Safety first

1.104     Your specific choice of exercises is not only restricted by the
          limited number of really productive building exercises. It is
          greatly influenced by which specific exercises, or variations of,
          you can perform safely, consistently and long term, with
          progressive poundages.

1.105    The biggest exercises *are* uncomfortable to do. If they were easy to work hard on they would do little or nothing for you. But do not use an exercise that is harmful for you.

1.106    Most people can do most if not all the best exercises, so long as good form is used; but "most people" does not mean everyone.

## "Heavy" and "light" weights

1.107    These words are used confusingly. Some people use "light" to mean a poundage that permits a lot of reps to be performed, even if done to failure. Others use "light" to mean any poundage that is substantially less than what could be used for the rep count under consideration, e.g., if a trainee is capable of bench pressing 250 pounds for ten reps, and performs ten reps with 200 pounds, the 200 pounds would be considered "light." Some refer to the "light" weights a weaker person uses even if that person is training with maximum intensity.

1.108    In this book, "light" weight generally means that the set's rep target can be met easily, with little or no strain. A "heavy" weight is one that demands much effort to complete the set's rep target, regardless of how many reps that is.

## Routines

1.109    Training routines are comprised of groups of exercises. They can be either full-body, divided, or split routines. A full-body routine trains the entire body each workout. A divided program takes a full-body schedule of exercises and divides it into two or three smaller routines to be spread over seven days, or perhaps a longer period. A conventional split routine divides the body into two or three parts, and each part is usually trained twice every 6–8 days or so.

1.110    The "week" is not necessarily the calendar one. The "biological" week is more important. Someone with good recuperation may have a six-day biological week, while someone with slow recuperation may have a ten-day biological week. Some people need more time between workouts than others. The idea of the biological week is a way to understand this.

1.111    A training program can be comprised of a single training routine (for a one-routine program) or multiple routines (for divided programs). Many people use "routine" and "program" synonymously.

## Cycles

1.112    Training routines are usually slotted into cycles. A training cycle varies the training intensity, typically over a period of about 10–12 weeks. Cycles can be shorter, or longer.

1.113    A cycle has a comfortable initial few weeks where you focus on exercise technique and ironing out any flaws. Also during this stage you get used to any exercise changes you may have incorporated into the program. The comfortable start gives your mind and body a break from the intensity of full-bore training. You get mentally and physically restored, and that provides the springboard for moving well into new poundage territory later on. A gaining momentum is created.

1.114    Over the cycle's initial few weeks you should fairly quickly increase your exercise poundages. Then you hit the intensive stage, which you should drag out for as long as possible with small and gradual poundage increments. The more poundage gains you clock up, the more muscle gains you will make.

1.115    On the surface, beginners do not have the need for cycling that experienced trainees usually do. This is largely because beginners have yet to develop the ability to train very hard, and are using only very light weights relative to their ultimate potential strength. Despite this, beginners should never push themselves hard until they have learned good form, and slowly built up their weights while maintaining good form.

## Degree of effort

1.116    "Training to failure" means taking a set to the point where you cannot move the bar any further against gravity. (Some people call this "training to *momentary* failure." You need to realize that there is no universal agreed definitions of "failure" in its different contexts. This causes confusion.) At that point of failure you either lower the resistance to a safe resting place, or a training partner helps you to complete the rep. In practice, most people could extend their "to failure" sets by several reps if they were well supervised and motivated.

1.117    Intensity can be taken further with the assistance of a training partner who provides just enough help to enable you to do reps you otherwise could not do by yourself. These are called forced reps. There are other intensifiers, including static holds, pre-exhaustion, negatives, back-to-back sets, and drop sets.

## Grip options

1.118    In some exercises you have a choice of grips to use. A supinated grip has both palms facing you during the course of the exercise. A pronated grip has both palms facing away from you. A mixed or reverse grip (for deadlifts and shrugs, primarily) has one hand facing away and the other facing towards you, for greater gripping strength. A parallel grip positions your hands parallel to each other.

1.119    Other grips include the regular one where the thumb is securely *around* the bar and *on top* of the index finger, as against the "thumbless" one where the thumb rests on the bar alongside the index finger. Then there is the hook grip, a specialized grip that places the thumb *between* the bar and your fingers.

## Spotting

1.120    Spotting is help from one or more assistants while you perform a set. The primary function of spotting is to prevent injury. Spotting can come from a training partner or anyone who is in the gym at the time and who is willing and able to spot for you. A spotter stands by ready to provide help if needed.

## Categories of weight training

1.121    Weight training is a broad activity in which there are several specializations. Most trainees are usually interested in more than one specialization, and there is overlap among the different classifications. Here are five categories, in no particular order.

    a. *Bodybuilding:* Development of the musculature in a proportionate manner, with appearance and aesthetics being more important than performance.

    b. *Strength training:* Development of strength and function taking priority over aesthetics, often with a sport in mind.

    c. *Olympic weightlifting:* Two lifts, i.e., the snatch, and the clean and jerk, as performed at the Olympic Games, with performance being all important.

    d. *Powerlifting:* The three powerlifts, i.e., the squat, bench press and deadlift, with performance being all important.

    e. *All-round lifting:* Over one hundred official lifts, with performance being all important. BB

*Some of the musculature shown on the right side of each anatomy chart is different from that on the left. This occurs where the outer layer of muscle has been omitted in order to show some of the deeper musculature.*

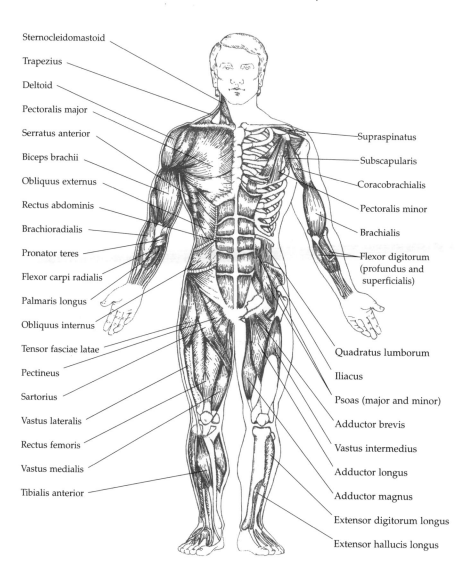

Sternocleidomastoid

Trapezius

Deltoid

Pectoralis major

Serratus anterior

Biceps brachii

Obliquus externus

Rectus abdominis

Brachioradialis

Pronator teres

Flexor carpi radialis

Palmaris longus

Obliquus internus

Tensor fasciae latae

Pectineus

Sartorius

Vastus lateralis

Rectus femoris

Vastus medialis

Tibialis anterior

Supraspinatus

Subscapularis

Coracobrachialis

Pectoralis minor

Brachialis

Flexor digitorum (profundus and superficialis)

Quadratus lumborum

Iliacus

Psoas (major and minor)

Adductor brevis

Vastus intermedius

Adductor longus

Adductor magnus

Extensor digitorum longus

Extensor hallucis longus

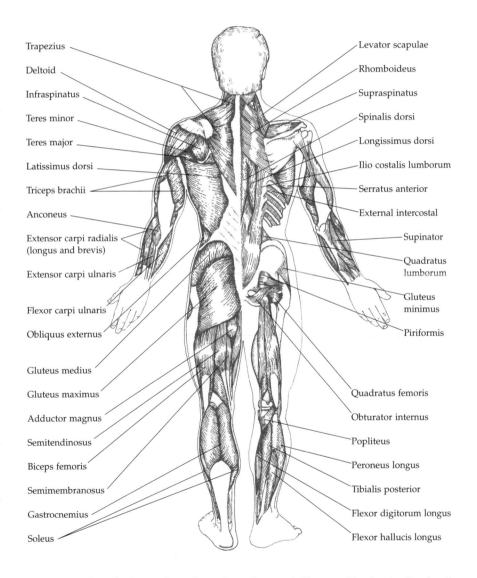

Trapezius

Deltoid

Infraspinatus

Teres minor

Teres major

Latissimus dorsi

Triceps brachii

Anconeus

Extensor carpi radialis
(longus and brevis)

Extensor carpi ulnaris

Flexor carpi ulnaris

Obliquus externus

Gluteus medius

Gluteus maximus

Adductor magnus

Semitendinosus

Biceps femoris

Semimembranosus

Gastrocnemius

Soleus

Levator scapulae

Rhomboideus

Supraspinatus

Spinalis dorsi

Longissimus dorsi

Ilio costalis lumborum

Serratus anterior

External intercostal

Supinator

Quadratus
lumborum

Gluteus
minimus

Piriformis

Quadratus femoris

Obturator internus

Popliteus

Peroneus longus

Tibialis posterior

Flexor digitorum longus

Flexor hallucis longus

*Drawings by Eleni Lambrou based on those of Chartex Products, England.*

One of the biggest and most disastrous errors in the training world today is the belief that basics-first abbreviated programs are only for beginners.

As Charles A. Smith told me shortly before his death, "You never know how important good health is until you no longer have it." Think about this. Dwell on it. Make it one with you while you still have your health, not when it is too late. Avoid all harmful habits, activities and environments. Look after yourself!

The first reading of this book will teach you a huge amount. A second reading will produce another big leap in your understanding of how to train effectively. This will occur because the second reading will build on the first. It will deepen your grasp of each topic, and knit everything together to provide all the know-how you need to achieve your potential for muscle and might.

# 2. General Philosophy for Outstanding Development

2.1     This book hammers away at the most important matters you need to stubbornly hold onto for as long as you want to make the most of your weight training. Here is the point-by-point general philosophy you need to train and live by if you want to develop outstanding muscle and might. (This philosophy is largely, but not entirely, described in the book BRAWN.)

2.2     There are countless novices and intermediates who are swimming around in a sea of marginal issues while neglecting the cardinal ones. There are young people who have been training for over ten years and yet still cannot squat much over their bodyweight for 20 reps. Yet they are agonizing over anything and everything related to training *except* for progressive poundages in the big exercises.

2.3     Bodybuilding and strength training are almost laughably simple; but simple does not mean easy. All that really matters is focus, and progressive poundages in good form. Pick a handful of the biggest and best exercises *for you* and then devote *years* to getting stronger, and then stronger still in them. You can use variations of the basic movements for variety, but you do not have to. There is even danger in using variety because you can lose focus and get caught up in an excessive assortment of exercises.

2.4     Do not search for the "definitive word" on basic gaining training. Once you have found something that works well, and so long as it keeps working, why spend time trying to find something else? Like so many other people, I wasted many years trying to study all the maybes of training instead of just applying one single certainty. What matters more to you, knowing all of the possible alternatives but being way below your potential development, or, knowing much less but being far bigger and stronger?

2.5    Especially in the beginning and intermediate stages of
       training, a dislike of change, and being old-fashioned and
       stubborn, are desirable characteristics. Only once you are
       already big and strong should you explore "new" opinions, *if*
       you have got the time to risk wasting. But even then, once you
       are advanced, if you venture too far into the myriad opinions
       about training you risk losing sight of what matters for most
       typical people. But at least by then you should be able to
       separate the wheat from the chaff.

2.6    Personal achievement is where it is at for those who lift weights,
       but most trainees get so little out of their own training largely
       because they are preoccupied with the achievements of others.

2.7    The bodybuilding and strength-world elite almost all had
       incredibly responsive bodies while they were building
       themselves up. They applied a very simple formula: train and
       grow. Almost no matter how they trained, they grew. It was
       never a case of whether or not they would grow; it was just a
       case of at what rate. That easy-gaining minority have
       absolutely no personal understanding of how the "train and
       grow" formula can be applied but not produce. But this lack of
       productivity is the outcome when conventional training
       routines are used by hard gainers. Not only that, but many
       hard gainers applied the "train and grow" formula with *far*

---

Ever-increasing weight on the bar in good form is not
the only type of progression. For pure strength training,
poundage increase is far and away the most important
form of progression. For building muscular size,
however, there is more to consider than just poundage
progression—as will be made clear much later on in
this book—but still, poundage progression is very
important. After all, how many well-developed men
struggle to squat with just bodyweight on the bar?

Though the biggest muscles are not the strongest, and
the strongest are not the biggest, for the great majority
of people there is a very strong relationship between
strength and muscular size, *providing* that strength is
not built using specific strength-focus techniques like
very low reps, partial reps and low-rep rest-pause work.

---

*more* determination and dedication than the super-responsive easy gainers ever did, but *still* the hard gainers got nothing from it. Clearly there are other factors at play.

2.8 Being genetically typical means you have a body that is light years removed from the elite's. Imitating the training of the elite will have you following routines that will not get you even half way to achieving your genetic potential.

2.9 Training an easy gainer is a cinch, relatively speaking. Training hard gainers is where the real challenge is. Of course easy gainers have their difficulties, but these are trivial concerned with those of bona fide hard gainers. Genuine hard gainers have a real battle to develop "mere" 15-inch arms. Rampant easy gainers will get 17 inches with little trouble— they train and they grow. Only thereafter *may* they have trouble gaining. But some phenomena will clear 18-inch arms before their growth rate seriously slows down. Legitimate hard gainers have a battle to get to 250 pounds in the bench press. Easy gainers will only really start to have serious trouble well after they have cleared 300 pounds, and in extraordinary cases not until after 400 pounds has been topped. A 300-pound bench press by a genuine hard gainer is a far greater achievement than a 400-pound one by an easy gainer. But the easy gainer can never understand this because he can *never* understand the plight of the hard gainer. And knowing how to successfully train easy gainers does not provide the experience and know-how for being able to *successfully* instruct hard gainers. Please pause and allow the last sentence to sink in real deep.

2.10 Genetics matter a heck of a lot—*big time!* Just anyone cannot become a top champion.

2.11 Muscle and might are truly great, until taken to extremes. When bodybuilding and lifting become drug-fueled obsessions, they become destructive. Some of the world's most successful bodybuilders and powerlifters are testimonies to lives ruined by obsession. Their former (or current) awesome physiques and strength levels are nothing relative to the unpublicized chaos of their private lives, major problems with drink and drugs (steroids and often "recreational" drugs too), serious health problems, no career prospects, and lack of happy family lives. And those are the "successful" ones. For each "success" there are hundreds if not thousands who ruined their lives but without the fleeting compensation of fame arising from winning a big title. There may even be criminal activities to fund drug habits; and the drug habits themselves may be illegal, depending on the country concerned.

2.12    The high-set, lots-of-exercises, high-frequency, almost-live-your-life-in-the-gym advice that claims to be training instruction for the masses comes from at least three sources. First, from the *very few* bodybuilders who are so gifted that they can gain very well from this instruction even without the assistance of drugs. Second, from the far bigger number of trainees who have learned that almost any training program will work if they get into serious drug abuse; but these people rarely mention the importance of drugs. Third, from armchair trainers who have absolutely no idea of what constitutes effective training for the typical hard gainer.

2.13    In an activity where the vast majority of its participants are genetically typical, we have the amazing situation of instruction that is appropriate for the masses being very hard to find. Generally speaking, the training world focuses on the achievements and training of the competitive minority. Even when instruction appropriate for the masses is publicized, it is usually downright misunderstood by those who are buried in conventional dogma.

2.14    The number of people who have tried weight training is astonishing. Out of almost any random selection of adults you will find a big number who have been members of a gym at some time. Hardly any of them, if any, will still be training, and probably none of them will have obtained even a small fraction of the results they were led to believe they would.

2.15    Of course the lack of adequate application and persistence accounts for part of the failure the masses experience with weight training. But it is the lack of consistent, practical and effective information for typical people that is mostly to blame.

2.16    Training instruction does not just have to be effective; it has to be *practical*. Most adults have demanding jobs and family lives. Time and cash to devote to training are in short supply. Instruction must not make excessive demands upon time and money if it is to be practical for the masses.

2.17    I am only one of the many who had the perseverance—or
        insanity, depending on how you look at it—to find out what
        *does* work through years of personal experience and
        observation. To have come through all this, to have "seen the
        light," to know the huge cost involved, and then see others
        following the same path of misery, is heart-rending.

2.18    Few people have the perseverance to stay the course (drug-
        free) before "seeing the light." Nearly all of them will give up
        training, or resort to "staying in shape." There is nothing
        wrong with training to "stay in shape," if that is what you
        want. But if big and strong muscles are what matter to you,
        then to resign yourself to "staying in shape" is a disaster.

2.19    Getting muscularly bigger and stronger is not complex. While
        finding the fine-tuned interpretations that work best for you
        can take time, and involve some trial and error, the essence of
        how to get bigger and stronger is simple enough. But if you
        are not willing to work hard at most of your workouts, you
        will never be able to develop big and very strong muscles.
        Fortitude, determination, persistence and dedication are
        needed in abundance.

2.20    If you are not developing bigger and stronger muscles, it is the
        basic combination of your training, rest, sleep and food
        consumption that is at fault.

2.21    Women who want to get bigger and stronger should train in
        the same way that men should.

2.22    It is not the training equipment that matters. It is what you do
        with it that counts.

2.23    It is not the training facility that counts, but what you do with
        the gear that is in it. Most people will never get their own
        home gym, and will only use commercial facilities. Someone
        who has a home gym that is full of good basic gear will get
        nowhere with it if he does not use it properly. Someone can

> I knew so much about that which I did not need, but
> knew so little about that which I needed. Therein lies
> the plight of most bodybuilding junkies.

train at a commercial gym loaded with frivolous and even dangerous equipment, but so long as he only uses the decent gear—and almost every gym has some decent gear—and uses that decent gear properly, he can make great gains. If your attitude is right, if you do not get distracted by any of the training madness that may be going on around you, and if you are knowledgeable enough to be independent of pseudo instructors, you can make great gains in *any* gym.

2.24     See abbreviated training as the first resort, not the last resort. Do not waste years of your life trying anything and everything else before finally trying abbreviated training.

2.25     Be sure to keep your exercise form tight. Training to get big and strong does not mean using loose form and getting injured. Make excellent exercise technique the creed that you train by, with no compromises!

2.26     Never train through injuries. If an injury does not clear up quickly by itself, see a training-orientated injury specialist. Investigate the probable trigger of the injury (incorrect training), correct it, and do not let it happen again. And when you get an injury, investigate non-intrusive and non-drug therapies.

2.27     If you lift Mickey Mouse poundages, all you are going to get is a Mickey Mouse body.

2.28     Those who hoist the biggest poundages do not necessarily have the biggest muscles. It is not just sheer poundage that matters. Individual leverages, type of training used, lifting support gear (in powerlifting), muscle composition factors, neurological efficiency, and lifting technique, among other elements, account for differences in muscular development among individuals of similar strength levels. But for every individual—keeping all other factors constant—if bigger weights are built up to, then bigger muscles will be developed.

2.29     Focus on the big basic lifts and their variations. Do this for most of your training time. Do not try to build yourself up using tools of detail. Leg extensions do not build big thighs, and pec-deck work does not build big chests.

2.30     You cannot get very powerful in the big and key basic exercises without getting impressive throughout your body.

2.31    For appearance-first bodybuilders, only when you are already big and strong (but without having gotten fat) should you even consider concerning yourself with attaining outstanding definition, and the finishing touches of perfect balance and symmetry. Build the substance before you concern yourself with the detail. Perfectly proportioned and well cut up "bags of bones" do not look impressive. If you concern yourself too soon with detail work, as is nearly always the case with bodybuilders, you will never be able to apply the effort, focus and recuperative ability needed to get big in the first place. What is by far the biggest deficiency in a typical sampling of gym trainees? Plain muscle and strength. Despite this most trainees arrange their training so that the last things they will ever develop are lots of muscle and strength.

2.32    If you want to add two inches to your arms, bank on having to add thirty or more pounds of muscle to your whole body. You cannot do that by focusing your attention on your arms. Get your body growing as a unit, concentrating largely on leg and back work. About two thirds of your body's total muscle mass is in your legs, buttocks and back. The shoulders, chest, abdominals and arms only make up about a third of your muscle mass, so do not go giving those areas in total any more than one third of your total weight-training attention.

2.33    Impressive for us is not the awesomeness of the easy-gaining top liners. Hard gainers of average height who build to (or very near) a muscular 16-inch arm and 45-inch chest, with other girths in proportion, are worthy of more applause than are the super-easy-gaining elite. This sort of muscular development, along with good definition, is enough to set you apart from over 95% of the members of almost any gym anywhere in the world. And it is more than enough to stop untrained people in their tracks if you reveal your physique at a pool or beach. This is a magnificent achievement, and most typical hard gainers who really want it can get there or thereabouts. You can do this, too, if you are not limited by age or health; but you must have the *extraordinary* will, persistence and know-how needed. Depending on your genetic inheritance, and degree of application to your training, you may be able to develop an even more impressive physique than that outlined here.

2.34    While keeping your ultimate goals believable (but challengingly so), do not get carried away and expect too little of yourself.

Demand a realistic lot of yourself, and you will get a lot. Even the hardest of hard gainers can perform near miracles if they train correctly for long enough. Break your long-term goals into small ones and bite off one bit at a time.

2.35    There is no single universally effective training routine that caters for all individual needs and purposes. Neither is there one that will consistently deliver results for you cycle after cycle, and for year after year. You need to use different interpretations according to your needs, age, level of development, and out-of-the-gym lifestyle factors. You have to adjust routines to fit you and your uniqueness, but do it *within the confines of rational training*.

2.36    Few people train hard. There is a lot of grimacing and noise making in gyms, but only a little of it is coming from true hard work. The rest is acted. An irony here is that those few who can deliver full-bore work may produce it in too great a volume, and with too great a frequency. They get as much out of their training as do volume-first trainees, unless they have the genetics needed to grow from almost any type of training, or they are into steroids to compensate for genetic shortcomings.

2.37    To be able to go to the gym and train hard is a joy and a privilege, even though the hard work necessitates driving yourself through considerable discomfort. Savor this privilege and blessing, and revel in it.

2.38    Never train if you do not feel systemically rested from your previous workout. While some local soreness may remain, you should be systemically rested and mentally raring to go for every workout. If in doubt, train less often—always.

2.39    Muscle does not atrophy if not trained within ninety-six hours. The ninety-six hours falsehood has caused untold harm because it has produced so much excessive training frequency, and overtraining. Some exercises trained in some ways, at

> **See abbreviated training as the first resort, not the last resort. Do not waste years of your life trying anything and everything else before finally coming around to using abbreviated training.**

least for hard gainers, need more than ninety-six hours of rest for systemic recovery, and then some *more* time for the body to grow a bit of extra muscle (i.e., overcompensate).

2.40    All body parts do not need the same recovery time. For example, you need much more time to recover from a hard squat or deadlift session than from hard calf or abdominal work.

2.41    Training a single exercise or body part three times a week is too much other than for beginners who are acclimatizing themselves to working out, or for rehabilitating after an injury. Twice a week per exercise, or three times every two weeks, is a better *maximum* standard. Once-a-week training for the biggest exercises is a good rule of thumb. Fine-tune your training frequency according to your individual recovery ability.

2.42    Do not train flat-out all the time. Cycle your intensity to some degree. How you interpret cycling depends on your age, recuperation abilities, motivation, tolerance to exercise, out-of-the-gym lifestyle factors, quality of diet, poundage increment scheme, supervision (if any), and style and volume of training, among other factors. A very few people can train full-bore most of the time. Others can only do it in short, infrequent spurts. Most people are somewhere in between. The bottom line is poundage progression. So long as you keep getting stronger in good form, then what you are doing is working.

2.43    The value of increased training intensity is not the actual effort per se. What counts is the progressive resistance that the high-intensity training can produce. Just pushing yourself to your absolute limit in the gym will not in itself make you bigger and stronger. The very hard work will only yield gains if you fully satisfy your recovery needs, and avoid injury and overtraining. When your poundages stagnate or regress, you are doing something wrong, even if you are training full-bore.

2.44    Intensity heightening techniques such as forced reps, drop sets, and negatives are likely to do more harm than good. Ordinary straight sets pushed all the way to muscular failure, or near to it, are the way to go for nearly all your training.

2.45    To achieve the progressive poundages that produce gains in strength and muscular development, your body must recover *fully* from your training. As boring, unexciting and mundane as rest and sleep are, they should be right at the top of your priorities if you are to progress as quickly as possible. Everyone knows that sleep and rest are important, but almost everyone shortchanges themselves in this department. Unless you wake every morning feeling *fully* rested, and *without* having to be awoken, you are not getting enough sleep. And even if you are making gains in the gym, more rest and sleep could substantially increase your gains.

2.46    Only compare current attainment to the same stage of your previous cycle that used the *same* style of training. You cannot, for example, compare bench presses done rest-pause style from pins in the rack in one cycle, with those done touch-and-go in the next cycle.

2.47    Add small poundage increments when you are training full-bore. Do not go short-circuiting a cycle by adding a minimum of 5 pounds to the bar at a shot. Get some pairs of little discs.

2.48    Dependable training for typical people with regular lives is about doing things slowly, safely, steadily and surely. It is not about trying to do in two months something that needs half a year. It is about patience and knowing that getting there slowly is the quick way, in the long run, because the chance of injury and mental or physical burnout is much less. Quick gains bring a higher chance of injury and burnout. And if you cannot maintain the enthusiasm to train over the long term, how can you keep the gains you have made over the short term? Patience is one of the priority qualities needed for training success.

2.49    What matters is what works. If you can only gain on a routine that is absurd in its brevity and simplicity by conventional standards, fine. If you can gain well using a routine that most hard gainers would not gain an ounce on, that is fine too. When gains dry up, investigate radical alternatives with the general belief that less is best (without taking it to the extreme and giving up working out), and that harder training is better than easier training.

2.50    Train hard, but avoid overtraining. Then when you leave the gym you will be tired and well worked, but not exhausted. There will be no more struggling just to recover from the systemic fatigue from training, and never actually getting around to doing any growing. You will recover from the workout quicker, and stimulate more growth for your less-stressed recuperative abilities to respond to. You will put in more productive workouts over the long term, and thus clock up more progress.

2.51   Low-rep work can be very productive, at least for some people, so long as it is carefully worked into, form is kept tight, and absolute-limit poundages are used only very rarely.

2.52   High reps, especially in leg and back work, have been proven to pack on loads of muscle.

2.53   Do not neglect your calves, abdominals, grip, or the external rotators of your shoulders. This accessory work matters. So long as it is done in moderation, it is not systemically demanding and should not interfere with your progress on the big mass-building exercises other than perhaps during the very final stretch of a training cycle. At this stage the accessory work can, if necessary, be temporarily dropped in order to keep progress happening in the big exercises. Some neck work is mandatory if you are involved in contact sport, and still a good idea if you are not. And back extensions will help keep your lower back in good order.

2.54   There is a multitude of different interpretations of abbreviated and basics-first training—enough variation to satisfy you for the duration of your training life. Staleness with any single approach should not happen. But do not flit from one interpretation to another. Stick to one for long enough to be able to judge the worth of the interpretation as you have understood it, and put into practice. Then analyze the results, learn from what you did, and do it better next time around.

2.55   Nutrition matters, but forget the notion that it is 80% or even 50% of training success. Sitting down and eating and drinking is the easy bit. Knuckling down in the gym to very intensive work on the big exercises is the hard bit. That is the over-50% bit. Rest takes up a percentage and then nutrition comes out of the portion that is left. There are hundreds of thousands of gym members who slept well, had jobs that were not particularly stressful physically, and had more than adequate diets. They did not realize their physique and strength potentials because they did not train hard enough and progressively enough on the exercises that matter.

2.56    Nutrition is about food, not supplements. Food supplements are not panaceas for training woes. Only once you have a good working formula of training, food and rest should you consider topping up with supplements. Tons of muscle have been built without using food supplements.

2.57    Many hard gainers—especially the very young—do not consume enough calories and nutrients to pack on muscle. Regardless of your age, consume as much nutritious and healthful food as you can without getting fat.

2.58    While what you read in this book is geared for genetically typical and drug-free bodybuilders, powerlifters and general strength trainees, it will work even better if you have better-than-average genetics. People blessed with better-than-average genetics for building muscle and strength should not lose that advantage by seeing how much training they can tolerate and yet still make moderate gains. They should train like a regular hard gainer should, and then revel in the greatly increased gains their natural gifts will bring them.

2.59    Spare yourself the misery that countless people have gone through as a result of following conventional training methods. Spare yourself this while applying the methods that work for the masses—those described in this book.

2.60    If you have trouble getting bigger and stronger using abbreviated routines of basic exercises, you will make a difficult task into an impossible one if you change to longer and more frequent routines infested by lots of little exercises. Focus on getting a better understanding of how to make the basic formula work for you. Do not change philosophies.

2.61    Mistakes, lost time and bad judgements are part of the business of getting bigger and stronger muscles. Learn from them, and do not keep repeating them. But persist at all times. As Calvin Coolidge noted, "Nothing in the world can take the place of persistence." If you persist in applying poor training advice you will still get nowhere but into a mess of frustration. But if you have the persistence that ensures you never give up, you should also have the intelligence to root out the training methods that work. Once you have a good grasp of training, all you need is persistence and time. Then the realization of your potential for muscle and might is almost guaranteed.

2.62   No matter how much good advice you are given, only you can implement it. You are on your own when you are in the gym. All the best information, equipment and food in the world will yield nothing unless they are combined with an abundance of diligence, planning and determination.

2.63   Do your own thing, in your very important, drug-free, non-obsessive but yet so-satisfying way, knowing that whatever you do, you do by yourself and for yourself. Be into weight training for a lifetime. Demonstrate what weight training should be about—physique, strength *and* health, together with personal enjoyment and comradeship with fellow trainees.

2.64   Be a credit to the Iron Game. Train, but do not make a fuss and commotion. Leave the bragging and showing off to those who do not know any better. Practice modesty. And never forget that there is a lot more to life than training and muscles.

2.65   If you have invested a lot of time and effort on conventional training, you may feel attached to it despite it having delivered so much frustration. To start over with a radically different approach is an admission that you previously had it wrong. Have the courage to acknowledge the errors of the past, and the fortitude to start anew. Break away from the crowd who stick with the norm, even though they are going nowhere on it. What you want most of all is personal progress, not the contentment from being one of the crowd. There is no more time to waste. Clean the slate, and do not harp on about mistakes made in the past. Then start anew, and with passion.

2.66   To keep yourself on the track of abbreviated and basics-first training, stroll into almost any gym. A glimpse of the skinny youths imitating the training done by the elite should be enough to remind you of the mess that conventional training is in. The youths follow hyped-up routines and isolation exercises. They spend lots of money on food supplements but

> **Mistakes, lost time and bad judgements are part of the business of getting bigger and stronger muscles. Learn from them, and do not keep repeating them. But persist at all times. As Calvin Coolidge noted, "Nothing in the world can take the place of persistence."**

too little on quality food. They use all the paraphernalia that bodybuilders are supposed to—gloves, belt, fashion clothing and expensive training shoes. And they consume special workout drinks. But they will still have their sub-15-inch arms if you visit them in six months time, or even six years time supposing they have not long since given up.

2.67    Serious hard gainers are not lazy. We would like to be able to train a lot, because training is enjoyable. But much more enjoyable is experiencing good results. We use abbreviated and basics-first training because it delivers the best results, not because it is a cop out from long and frequent workouts.

2.68    There is not much *if anything* that is really new in the training world. What is "new" is usually just a twist on an old idea. With a dose of creative lingo and modern-day advertising hoopla, even something that has been around for decades can appear new. If you could go back to the early twentieth century you would be surprised at how much of bodybuilding and lifting as we know it today was being routinely done in those days. And the roots of plenty of today's training equipment and ideas go back much further. But because ideas and equipment are often presented today as being "new" and "modern," and because so few people know anything about the history of the training world, the pioneers are forgotten. Even the people who today claim the "new" training ideas and equipment designs are usually totally ignorant of the fact that men long-since dead came up with the original ideas and designs ages ago.

2.69    As Charles A. Smith told me shortly before his death in January 1991, "You never know how important good health is until you no longer have it." Think about this. Dwell on it. Make it one with you while you still have your health, not when it is too late. Avoid all harmful habits, activities and environments. Look after yourself! (Charles Smith was one of the major figures at Joe Weider's magazines in the fifties.)

## Failure of "one size fits all"

2.70    The training world is forever churning out "new" approaches that are claimed to be "the" way to train. Never mind that what is claimed as "new" is only a rehash of something that has been around for decades. What is dangerous is the claimed universality and definitiveness of whatever is being touted.

2.71 Many programs are not to be taken seriously because they were devised only for a quick commercial killing, and a few are outrageously expensive. Some programs do have specific aspects that may have practical value. But these aspects can only be selected by people who are highly knowledgeable about weight training.

2.72 A single program, even if it works well for some people, will not work well for everyone; and some heavily hyped programs are dangerous for all but a very small minority of trainees, and thus should never be promoted for mass use.

2.73 Avoid seeking the "perfect" training routine. Once on that slippery slope you will join the mass of trainees who are buried in all the peripheral, downright irrelevant or even destructive aspects of training. Instead, knuckle down, *long-term*, to paying the necessary dues on basic, straight-forward, sound and abbreviated training programs as described in this book. These programs cover trainees of *all* levels of experience who want bigger and stronger muscles. *One of the biggest and most disastrous errors in the training world today is the belief that programs like those in this book are only for beginners.* BB

---

There is a huge amount of vital information crammed into this book, and it is all interrelated. To dip in and out of it will neither do the book justice, nor your training education. The book needs to be studied from cover to cover, and more than once, if you are to benefit fully from it.

*My life should have been geared around poundage gain on each exercise. Initially it would have revolved around adding 10% to each exercise. Later on, I would have focused on gaining the next 5%, and then the next, and the next, etc. Nothing (except using good exercise form) should have entered my training mind other than achieving the next target percentage gain on my exercise poundages. This may be crude, primitive and basic, but this is what was needed.*

*Something does not have to be "the last word" for it to be of benefit to the masses. Apply something that works well, i.e., the priorities given in this chapter, and you may never even want to bother looking for "the last word."*

# 3.  All-Time #1
## Practical Priorities

3.1     Here is a summary of the practical priorities I wish I had
        riveted myself to during my early years of training. Had these
        priorities been implemented I would not have wasted years of
        my life following unproductive training methods. Of course I
        am not you. But any drug-free trainee of typical genetic
        potential will have much in common with me. Learning from
        the major lessons I picked up over the years will help *you* to get
        in control of *your* training.

3.2     I wish I could have had a wise and uncompromising mentor to
        have watched over me. Someone to have given me hell if I
        dared even to think of anything other than the abbreviated and
        basics-first approach. I should have been forced to have
        committed the essence of this training to memory. Such
        mentors are very rare. Use this book as the best alternative.

### Focus and progression

3.3     If I had chosen the squat, deadlift (both the bent-legged and
        stiff-legged variations, though not both in the same cycle),
        bench press, seated press, and the pulldown (or a row with my
        torso supported), and dedicated myself for five years to
        progressive poundages on those five core movements as the
        linchpin of my training, I would have gotten near to realizing
        my full size and strength potential *before* I was but 20 years
        old. I would have been better off if I had never heard of any
        other exercises. (A different fivesome of core exercises may be
        more appropriate for you.)

3.4     Of these big movements the deadlift is by far the least popular
        in gyms today. Though over recent years the deadlift has been
        getting some respect and publicity, it is still not getting
        anywhere near enough. The deadlift, properly performed, and

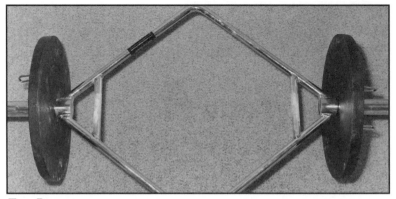

*Trap Bar*

especially when done with a Trap Bar, is a wonderfully productive exercise. For people who do not squat well, the Trap Bar bent-legged deadlift is likely to be a more productive exercise. If you do not have a Trap Bar, then the sumo-style bent-legged deadlift may be safer, easier to perform, and more productive than the conventional-style deadlift. But the sumo deadlift is not the equal of the Trap Bar deadlift.

3.5     My mentor would have taught me that body*building* is not about individually hitting all the bits and pieces of the physique to ensure complete and balanced development. Only by applying myself to getting stronger and stronger still in the big exercises would I have gotten big all over. Even the little areas would have come along. Once I was big and strong *then* I could have focused on fixing the relatively minor imbalances.

3.6     My training life should have revolved around adding a little more iron to each exercise every week or two. "A little" would have meant 1 or 2 pounds, except very early in a cycle when I could have added a larger increment each week. Bigger but less frequent poundage jumps could have been applied if I was working with a rep range where, for example, I built up the reps from say 12 to 20 in the squat. Then, I would have increased the poundage by 10 pounds, dropped back down to 12 reps, and worked up to 20 again over several weeks. Both progression methods work well.

3.7     Focus and progression, *focus and progression*, FOCUS AND PROGRESSION—these are the watchwords I should have lived by. All that irrelevance I swallowed about isolation exercises for the thighs, back, chest and shoulders, pre-exhaustion, pumping, volume training, conventional split routines, beyond-failure training, etc. All of it was useless for me, and almost certainly for the masses of typical trainees too. It cost me years of my youth.

3.8     I was a walking encyclopedia of information about Larry Scott, Arnold Schwarzenegger, Franco Columbu, Casey Viator, Frank Zane, Mike Mentzer, et al (the top bodybuilders during my teens and early twenties). *I knew so much about that which I did not need, but knew so little about that which I needed. And therein lies the plight of most bodybuilding junkies.*

3.9     If I had been cut off from the training media I would have been ignorant of what was going on in the bodybuilding and lifting worlds, and of all the discoveries that were supposedly being made in weight training and nutrition. But I would have been blissfully satisfied in steadily, safely and surely getting stronger and stronger, and bigger and bigger.

3.10    My life should have been geared around poundage gain on each exercise, but while maintaining excellent exercise form. Initially it would have revolved around adding 10% to each exercise. Later on I would have focused on gaining the next 5%, and then the next, and the next, etc. This is crude, primitive and basic; but this *is* what was needed.

## Rate of progress

3.11    When I first started weight training, age 15, I used about 50 pounds in the squat and bench press. (In my ignorance I never deadlifted regularly until many years later.) Moving to close to 100 pounds in the squat and bench press was straight-forward and linear, but then it started getting difficult.

3.12    With 100 pounds reached in the squat and bench press—and more in the deadlift, which I ought to have included—I should have focused on adding the next 10% (i.e., 10 pounds). Once I got to 110 pounds, I should have lived for the next 10% gain. When there I should have focused on the next 10% gain, and so on. Once I got to 200 pounds for reps in the squat I should have switched from targeting the next 10% gain, to the next 5%.

3.13    Going from 100 x 6 in the bench press, 100 x 20 in the squat and 135 x 20 in the deadlift (with the other members of the mighty fivesome progressing in proportion) to 150 x 6, 150 x 20 and 200 x 20 respectively (moving there in 10% shots) would have made a big difference to my physique. Spending the next 6–12 months moving to 200 x 6, 200 x 20 and 250 x 20 would have made another big difference.

3.14    Investing obsessive focus over the next 6–12 months, and using the 5% mentality to build up to 240 x 6, 245 x 20 and 300 x 20, would have built quite a fine physique. After investing another 6–12 months to work slowly up to 265 x 6, 275 x 20 and 340 x 20, I would have been going places for a hard gainer. Then, *still* centering on the same mentality and the same key exercises, had I concerned myself with nothing other than getting to 285 x 6, 300 x 20 and 365 x 20, I would have experienced another important step forward. I would have become bigger and stronger than nearly all drug-free trainees in any gym of the world, and all before my twentieth birthday. And if I had wanted to get bigger still, I would have kept the poundage-gain mentality going and going and going.

## Beyond the big five exercises

3.15    In this ideal world I would not have concentrated solely on the mighty fivesome. Another few areas would have gotten some specific attention. Midsection work, i.e., side bends and crunch situps, would have been done almost every week, once a week for each movement. Specific work for my shoulder external rotators, using a dumbbell, would have been done once a week when I was experienced enough to be bench pressing my bodyweight for 6 reps. Calf work would have been done once or twice each week. Some thick-bar grip work would have been included, together with some other specialized hand and finger exercise. Direct neck work could have been included once a week, along with a set or two of back extensions on non-deadlifting days. Curls would have been done if supinated lat-machine pulldowns were not in the current routine.

3.16    In my teens and twenties I had no interest in the leg press, falsely believing it to be an exercise only for people who were looking for an excuse not to squat. My imaginary mentor would have known better. I should always have given the squat the highest priority, but I should have realized the assistance value of the leg press. That I never pursued the leg press seriously until after I was forced to by knee injuries, is one of the regrets of my training life. But not having fully exploited the squat is a much bigger regret. The knee injuries I suffered were caused by poor squatting form, including using a board under my heels. At the time I was doing this form of squatting I was unaware of the eventual consequences. My imaginary mentor would never have allowed me to squat with a board or plates under my heels.

3.17    Though my body structure is better suited to deadlifting than squatting, with the expert coaching of my mentor I would have managed to squat well, and certainly much better than what I managed as I struggled along in ignorance during my actual youth. By being able to exploit the magnificent potential of the squat I would have taken a giant stride towards excellence in muscle and might.

3.18    At least in some cycles I should have given serious attention to the parallel bar dip. As it was I had a bench press fixation. The dip, done in good form, is a terrific exercise that is much underused. It is at least as productive as the bench press.

3.19    The great majority of my training focus should have gone on the primary fivesome, and the balance should have covered the secondary exercises (the accessories). Secondary work would only have been done after the scheduled exercises from the major fivesome had been trained. When intensity was so high on the primary fivesome that I would have little energy left for anything else, I would have cut back elsewhere.

3.20    I should have stayed with the same exercises for year after year, and persisted with the same productive formula. My wise dictator would have shielded me from anyone who might have offered negative comments on my training. I would have been unaware that any other exercises or training methods existed.

3.21    I would have done a moderate amount of stretching a few times a week. I would not have got hung up on it, but neither

> **I should have stayed with the same exercises for year after year, and persisted with the same productive formula. My wise dictator would have shielded me from anyone who might have offered negative comments on my training.**

would I have neglected it. I would have ignored aerobic work until I was into my thirties, preferring to keep almost total focus on what meant the most to me—weight training.

## Sets and reps

3.22     With progression being the key I would not have gotten myself hung up on sets and reps. I would have stuck with the rep number I preferred at the time for each exercise, changing it from cycle to cycle if I felt like it. Generally speaking, 5–8 reps would have been used for most exercises; but squats and accessory movements would usually have used higher reps.

3.23     With adding poundage in good form being the sovereign priority, the number of sets used would have been secondary. So long as I added a little iron to the bar each week or two, all would be well. Most of the time I would have done one, two or *at most* three work sets per exercise, reducing the number of sets at the end of a cycle when intensity was at its highest. Periodically, and usually for no more than just two of the exercises included in any given cycle, I would have been directed to use a six sets of six reps format with a fixed poundage for all sets, and a rigid one minute rest between sets. This cumulative-fatigue training would provide a variation in growth stimulation, and help keep me from growing stale.

3.24     My workouts would not have been rushed—about four minutes would have been taken between work sets of core exercises, and 2–3 minutes between work sets of accessory exercises. Rests between warmup sets would have been shorter, but the full rest period would have been taken prior to the first work set of an exercise. For occasional short spells—to give my musculature a variation in stimulation, and a mental change of pace—I would have taken shorter rest periods between work sets of some exercises, with corresponding poundage reductions.

3.25     My mentor would not have had me use a time-controlled very slow rep speed. But I would have been informed that very-

> **Everything would have been geared for making my body able to withstand another small dose of iron on the bar for each exercise every week or two, even if it was just a few ounces.**

slow-cadence training, properly applied, can be an effective way to train and especially valuable in some specific exercises, e.g., neck and shoulder rotator work. Lifting my maximum poundages *in smooth controlled form* would have been the focus. My rep speed would have been about three seconds up and about another three seconds down, but perhaps five seconds or so on the concentric of the very final rep or two of each set.

3.26    My reps would have been done with a brief pause between them, and never rushed. In many cycles the bench press, squat and overhead press would have been done "from the bottom," using a power rack, thus producing a pause at the bottom of each rep *and* at the top.

3.27    The deadlift, too, would often have been done "from the bottom." But for this particular exercise a partial movement from knee cap height upward would have been preferred.

## Long gaining cycles

3.28    I would have cycled my training intensity to some degree, but because of the *slow* but consistent poundage increment scheme I would have been using, I would not have burned out like most people do (even on cycled routines), and thus I would have worked at full-bore intensity nearly all the time. I would not have needed to have had much in the way of layoffs and "breaking-in" periods because I would have been handling the progression scheme properly, and not changing my exercises around much. My dictatorial mentor would have kept me from getting greedy about adding too much poundage at a time.

3.29    I would have added poundage slowly and in line with the rate at which I could build strength. This would have made my gaining cycles long, and reduced the amount by which I would have needed to cut back to start a new cycle.

3.30    I would have been trained very hard, and at times extremely hard. But I would never have been pushed so far that I would have become fearful of training; and I would never have been driven to vomiting during a workout. Poundage progression in good form would have been the criterion for training success, not intensity per se. My mentor would have repeatedly stressed that effort is merely the tool to stimulate strength gain and muscular growth, and not an end in itself. So long as my strength was increasing, then I was training hard enough.

3.31    My mottos would have been "less is more" and "less is best."
        Whenever in doubt I would have chosen less rather than
        more— fewer sets, exercises and workouts, but lots of effort.

3.32    I would have trained only twice a week. The deadlift and squat
        would have been trained just once per week each. The three
        other major exercises would usually have been trained twice a
        week or three times every two weeks. But I would not have
        hesitated to train each exercise only once a week in order to
        provide increased recovery time when needed. At such a time I
        would have done two of the mighty fivesome at one workout,
        and the other three on the second workout each week.

3.33    *Everything would have been geared for making my body able to
        withstand another small dose of iron on the bar for each exercise
        every week or two, even if it was just a few ounces.*

## Form and avoidance of injury

3.34    My dictatorial mentor would have been a stickler for good
        exercise form, even on the final rep of each set which, as my
        ever-reliable spotter, he would have assisted me on, if necessary,
        in order to ensure perfect form. Woe betide me if I relaxed my
        form. The weekly or biweekly poundage increment would have
        been small enough, however, so that I would never have
        perceived an increase in load, and never have had to loosen my
        form to compensate for an excessively sized increment.

3.35    Under the uncompromising eye of my mentor I would never
        have lost training time due to injury or overtraining. I would
        simply never have been permitted to overtrain. I would have
        regularly experienced the good type of muscular soreness from
        great workouts, and only very rarely would I have suffered
        from mild muscular strains. Due to perfectly supervised
        workouts I would have been prevented from doing the things
        that cause injuries. I would always have thoroughly warmed
        up for each exercise. I would not have been permitted to use
        poor exercise form or inherently harmful exercises. I would
        always have been obliged to work into new exercises gradually.
        I would never have been dropped into any full-bore work
        without a preparatory period. I would never have been
        allowed to let ego and bravado get the better of me. I would
        always have been fully prepared before performing singles or
        very low-rep work with limit poundages, and even then I
        would have used them only occasionally and very prudently.

## Nutrition

3.36    My mentor would have ensured that I never compromised my
        gains in muscle and might by cutting corners with my diet. I
        would have eaten a diet composed of nutritious food rich in
        protein—the most food I could eat without getting fat. I would
        not have had a phobia of fat in my diet, and would have eaten
        generously of foods containing the essential fatty acids. I would
        only have eaten natural foods while avoiding junk, hard fats,
        fried food, and overheated oils. Protein powder and vitamin
        and mineral tablets would have been the only supplements I
        would have consumed. Never would I have been permitted to
        get caught up in fad diets and extremes. My mentor would
        repeatedly drum into me the belief that anything that sounds
        too good to be true is usually exactly that.

## The rewards

3.37    I would have been experiencing the most motivating feedback
        possible from my unrelenting efforts on the mighty fivesome—
        bigger muscles from month to month. I would never have
        forgotten that results are what count most of all.

3.38    Never would I have been allowed to waste time fiddling with
        my training according to fads. By denying me this freedom my
        mentor would have kept my attention where it needed to be,
        enabling me to make almost continuous gains. "And what's
        training all about?" he would ask me each week, but never
        actually let me answer. "Progressive poundages in good form,
        m'lad—getting bigger and stronger muscles."

3.39    Of course everything cannot be plain sailing, not even in the
        utopian training world just described. I would still have had
        out-of-the-gym constraints to cope with. But because these
        constraints would have been on the back of a sound training
        program, I would still have made steady progress towards the
        realization of my strength and size potential. But if I had had

> The points in this chapter may seem dictatorial. But if
> all of this chapter was written in stone, and laid down
> as law in all gyms the world over, the instruction
> would work for so many people for so much of the
> time that it would probably be the most important
> contribution to Iron Game history.

these constraints on top of the sort of training program that most people use, I would have made little or no progress towards the strength and physique I craved.

## Putting it all together

3.40    The clear vision on hindsight presented in this chapter specifically applies to when I was in my late teens and early twenties. This was a time of my life when I had few responsibilities, and the chance to be well rested all of the time. I also had gung-ho motivation and good recuperation. Thus I could push my body full-bore for longer periods than I could later in life, and I could productively train each exercise more often. Applying the same perspective to a body twenty years older would be the same in principle, but there would be some modifications. These may include a reduced volume of work, shorter workouts, reduced training frequency for the big exercises, and greater attention to keeping overlapping exercises on the same day each week rather than spreading them over the week.

3.41    Regardless of what you have or have not done in the past, today is the start of the rest of your life. Now you have the chance to train correctly and start to make the progress you could only dream about while being lost in inferior training approaches.

3.42    The points in this chapter may seem dictatorial. This chapter is not, however, the definitive word on weight training. It does not have to be. But if all of this chapter was written in stone, and laid down as law in all gyms the world over, the instruction would work for so many people for so much of the time that it would probably be the most important contribution ever to Iron Game history.

3.43    Something does not have to be "the last word" for it to be of benefit to the masses. Apply something that works well, i.e., the priorities given in this chapter, and you may never even want to bother looking for "the last word."

3.44    Never, EVER let your attention waver from progressive poundages in good form. Never, that is, until you no longer want to build stronger and bigger muscles.

3.45    There are many interpretations of the abbreviated and basics-first training philosophy that this book is all about. No matter

which interpretation you use, the bottom line is the same—
progressive poundages in good form.

3.46    Apply this "progressive poundages in good form" dictum to
        your own training, *now*, and make the most of the next few
        years of your training life. You cannot correct the errors of the
        past, but you can get your act together for the future.

3.47    BEYOND BRAWN will teach you everything you need to know to
        put the "progressive poundages in good form" dictum into
        practice. Knowing the dictum is one thing, but organizing your
        life in order to *apply* the dictum is something else. This is where
        you need the in-depth understanding this book provides. [BB]

---

## Consistent vs. sporadic 100% dedication

You may not be able to deliver *consistent* 100%
dedication to your training, nutrition, rest and sleep
schedules. While 100% dedication on a consistent basis
is the ideal, good progress can still be made without it.
But you must *at least* provide consistent 100%
dedication *in spurts*.

Maintenance training, though demanding, is much
less demanding than that needed for building new
strength and development. You can relax *to a degree* in
your total approach *without* losing size or strength.
During maintenance work you should make no effort
to increase reps or poundages. But after a period of
maintenance work you must crank yourself up for 6–8
weeks of consistent 100% dedication. Get absolutely
everything in perfect order for just that short period.
Achieve a spurt of progress and then follow it with
another maintenance period. This is a very practical
approach for many people to adopt.

If you have only very short and infrequent growth
spurts you will make minimal progress. But if you
alternate a six-week period of 100% dedication with an
equal period of maintenance work, and do this
consistently over the course of a year, you could
achieve fine progress.

Draw motivation from elite-level accomplishments, but get your feet firmly back to earth when it comes to designing your own training program. If you do not do this you will be bang on course for treading the same road to training ruin that millions have already travelled.

There is a lot of promotion in this book of the deadlift, squat and bench press. This is simply because they are three of the most productive exercises any bodybuilder, or strength or fitness trainee can perform, SO LONG AS THEY ARE DONE WITH GOOD FORM. But they are not the only exercises worthy of special status as core movements.

# 4. Expectations—How Much Muscle & Might You Can Expect to Make Real

4.1      How good and strong a physique you can build, and how long it will take, depend on many factors including age, gender, genetics, training methods used, motivation, diet, and your rest and recovery schedule. Only you can find how far you can go by *actually going as far as you can go*.

4.2      To achieve your potential you need to invest *years* of effort, investigate different interpretations of sensible training, find what works best for you, and fine-tune it according to changes in your lifestyle and level of development.

## Real-world targets

4.3      Gauge your long-term goals on the basis of what *is* realistic for most typical people who train with weights, *provided* they give their pound of flesh and deliver the dedication, determination, effort and persistence that are needed.

4.4      Long-term goals, however realistic they may be, can seem so impossibly far off that they lead to discouragement. Keep your medium-term and short-term goals foremost in your mind. But project into a long-term perspective the successful achievement of a run of medium-term goals, and then you will see the terrific progress you can make after a few years.

4.5      Focus on achieving the next 5–10% gain in all your exercises. If you apply yourself to this, and keep doing it repeatedly for a number of years, you will eventually get as big and strong as it is possible for you to become. Your short-term goal should be to take the next small step to getting to your next set of 5%- or 10%-poundage-gain medium-term goals.

4.6    Suppose you can bench press 180 pounds for eight good-form reps. Ten percent of 180 is 18 pounds; so, in the bench press, live to add 18 pounds to it. Building the strength to get the additional 18 pounds for eight good-form reps will take one or two training cycles. This is not so far in the future as to seem out of reach. But it will still be challenging.

4.7    A 10% poundage gain for beginners and intermediates is no big deal, but for an advanced man it is too lofty a goal for the medium term. Adding 10% when you can already bench press 300 pounds is usually a darn sight harder than adding 10% to a current best bench press of only 150 pounds. When 10% goals become beyond what you can gain over the short-to-medium term, switch to 5%-poundage-gain targets.

## Fantasy-land muscular girths

4.8    For drug-free typical bodybuilders the muscular girths of the competitive elite are light years removed from our reality, including our reality even after years of sound training. Draw motivation from elite-level accomplishments, but get your feet firmly back to earth when it comes to designing and implementing your own training program. If you do not do this you will tread the same road to training ruin that millions have already travelled.

4.9    The top men are astonishingly big and strong, but are notorious for exaggerating their lifts and muscular girths. And it is not just the top men who do this. Plenty of big and not-so-big men add a fictitious inch or two to each of their muscular girths, and knock off an inch or few from their waist measurements. An 18-inch arm is huge, and a 19-inch arm is enormous. But men with 18-inch arms tag on two fictitious inches to make the magic 20, and those with 19-inch arms inflate their measurements to 21 or more. A 17-inch arm is very big, but that, too, is usually added to, to stand comparison with other exaggerated measurements.

4.10    But both the actual and inflated measurements and exercise poundages are irrelevant when it comes to *you*, *your* training and *your* goals. Get real about what matters most as far as training is concerned—*you* and *your* training.

## Reality-land muscular girths

4.11    If a successful hard gainer accurately measures his contracted upper arm at say 16–16.5 inches (which is one heck of an achievement for a drug-free and lean genetically typical man) and then reads of a top liner whose arm is claimed to be 22 inches, the successful hard gainer could despair. But if the hard gainer is aware that the claimed 22-inch arms are "only" 19 inches, then the difference between one and the other, while still big, is not despairingly vast. Take most claims for huge girths with a pinch of salt unless they are verified as truthful.

4.12    Keep in mind the correlation between bodyweight and muscular girths. If someone is only 185 pounds, he is going to have a lot more trouble having a genuine 19-inch arm than if he weighs a solid 235 pounds.

4.13    The appearance differences between the physiques of the successful hard gainer and the competitive easy gainer come about only partly as a product of pure size. Hardness, definition and vascularity, together with skin color and photographic and lighting assistance, are major contributing factors. Being hard, tanned and ripped gives the appearance of bigger girths, but if you were to tape girths on such a physique you might be surprised at how relatively modest they measure.

4.14    Rather than stack yourself up against even accurate but still incredible measurements of the elite, measure yourself against very challenging but believable measurements. Over the decades, several formulae for assessing target girths of male bodybuilders have been developed.

4.15    While it is impossible to get an accurate girth assessment for everyone, a helpful guide is possible. People vary so much in genetically determined factors including height, limb lengths, body structure, muscle insertion points, and relative lengths of tendons and muscle bellies. And even easy gainers sometimes have a particular muscle group that does not respond as well as do the others. (See Chapter 2 of BRAWN for a detailed look at genetic variation and how the genetic marvels are assembled.)

---

**Get each day right, each workout right, and each week right, and then you will get the months right; and then for sure you will keep knocking off your poundage-gain goals.**

4.16    The measurement targets that follow are not for a "ripped" body, but for one that is lean enough for lines to be seen on the abdominals from a distance, i.e., about 12% bodyfat for a man. Do not try to get very defined (under about 10% bodyfat) while you build yourself up. But at the same time *do not* get fat.

4.17    The point of this exercise is to show you the sort of measurements that are within the grasp of typical drug-free people. Any formula calculated today from a random sample of well-developed bodybuilders would be heavily influenced by the role of steroids, and be out of touch with reality for drug-free people.

4.18    *Urging realistic expectations does not mean accepting mediocrity.* Far from it. If you achieve something around the goals that follow you will have developed a physique that will stand you out in almost any company. The only company you will appear "normal" in will be that of very gifted and/or drug-using bodybuilders and lifters.

4.19    What follows is a guide aimed at healthy males between the ages of 18 and 35. All healthy males between these ages, even if new to weight training, can expect a gradual metamorphosis during a few years of adherence to rational training methods. Those of you in the 35–45 age group who are already very experienced in weight training can achieve a physique along the same lines as for the younger age group. Those of you in the 35–45 age group who are new to training should, at least initially, moderate your expectations.

4.20    If you are older than 45 you can achieve a metamorphosis, though less dramatic than that of the much younger man. Relative to the condition of the typical untrained 50-year old, however, a hard training 50-year-old bodybuilder can achieve a near miracle. Age is not the limiting factor untrained people make it out to be. The limiting factor is in the mind. Expect little from your body and that is what it will deliver. Expect a lot from it and that is what it will deliver.

## John McCallum's formula

4.21    In BRAWN I reported John McCallum's formula, based on wrist measurement. This provides a challenging yet realistic guide for indicating full-size potential of male hard gainers. Here it is again:

| chest: | 6.5 x wrist |
| hips: | 85% x chest |
| waist: | 70% x chest |
| thigh: | 53% x chest |
| neck: | 37% x chest |
| upper arm: | 36% x chest |
| calf: | 34% x chest |
| forearm: | 29% x chest |

4.22    You can measure your wrist just above the bone that protrudes on the little finger side of your wrist (the styloid process of the ulna), i.e., on the elbow side, as McCallum advised, or just below (on the hand side). If taken below that styloid process, your wrist girth will likely be a little less than what it is when measured above the bone, and so produce a slightly reduced set of muscular girths. Be consistent with how you measure your wrist, and all your other girths.

4.23    Not everyone will neatly fall into the set of measurements produced by this formula because it assumes that wrist size directly correlates with bone size throughout the body. With many people this is not so. Also, many people have at least one body part that responds better than does the rest of the body, producing at least one measurement an inch or so bigger than the projected one(s) or, conversely, a measurement or a few that fall behind the projected girths.

4.24    Some people have a lower-body that has a bone structure bigger than their upper-body—ankle and knee measurements that are significantly bigger than their wrist girths, proportionately speaking. Some people are the other way around. If the difference between upper- and lower-body structure is striking, at least for an appearance-first bodybuilder, care has to be given to prevent the musculature differences from becoming exaggerated and putting the physique way out of proportion.

4.25    Using the McCallum formula, a 7-inch wrist will produce a chest of 45.5 inches, hips of 38.7, waist of 31.9, thigh of 24.1, neck of 16.8, flexed upper arm of 16.4, calf of 15.5 and a flexed forearm of 13.2. At a height of 5-9 this development will come out at around 190 pounds (solid but not ripped). Such a development, for a typical man, is terrific going.

4.26     These wrist-related targets are *not* presented as limits or
         ceilings, but as guidelines. Many of you will be able to exceed
         these targets, but before you can even think of exceeding them
         you have to get to them in the first place.

4.27     Compute your own set of girths using the McCallum formula.
         Focus on achieving *only those girths* until you have actually got
         them. Only then, assuming you still want to get bigger, should
         you look to develop the next 5% on each measurement; get
         that next 5%, and then target a further 5%, and so on. These
         numbers will get you in the real world of natural
         bodybuilding right from the start.

## More on bone structure

4.28     Bone structure varies a great deal, though the extremes—i.e.,
         smaller than a 6-inch wrist, or greater than an 8-inch one, for
         a man—are very rare. While bone structure is a major factor,
         it is not the be all and end all for determining potential
         muscular development.

4.29     David Willoughby's "optimum ideal standard," presented in
         the November 1979 issue of IRON MAN, was given "as a goal for
         youths and men of *average* muscular potentialities." There is no
         need to get carried away with measurements, but note the
         impact that bone structure variation (as seen in wrist, ankle
         and knee girths) makes to muscular girths.

4.30     Willoughby's figures show the wrist being 79% to 82% of
         ankle girth. Compare that to yours and see whether or not
         you have a noticeably heavier lower-body or upper-body
         bone structure.

4.31     Though well-trained hard gainers can quite easily exceed the
         girths that Willoughby gives, relative to height, the table
         shows relative girths for physiques that are proportionately
         developed. It also shows how bodyweight varies relative to
         changes in muscular girths throughout the body. Now you
         know why anyone who claims huge measurements at a light
         bodyweight is being dishonest.

4.32     Here is how Willoughby advised the measurements to be
         taken: Wrist below the styloid process of the ulna (i.e., on the
         hand side of it) and with the hand open; all leg girths to be
         taken with the legs straight but relaxed, including ankle at the

| Height | Weight | Neck | Biceps | Forearm | Wrist | Chest | Waist | Hips | Thigh | Knee | Calf | Ankle | Delt |
|---|---|---|---|---|---|---|---|---|---|---|---|---|---|
| 60 | 114 | 14.1 | 13.2 | 11.0 | 6.3 | 36.7 | 27.5 | 33.0 | 19.8 | 12.9 | 13.2 | 7.7 | 17.2 |
| 62 | 126 | 14.5 | 13.6 | 11.3 | 6.5 | 37.9 | 28.4 | 34.1 | 20.5 | 13.3 | 13.6 | 8.0 | 17.7 |
| 64 | 138 | 15.0 | 14.1 | 11.7 | 6.7 | 39.1 | 29.3 | 35.2 | 21.1 | 13.8 | 14.1 | 8.3 | 18.2 |
| 66 | 151 | 15.4 | 14.5 | 12.1 | 6.9 | 40.3 | 30.2 | 36.3 | 21.8 | 14.2 | 14.5 | 8.5 | 18.7 |
| 68 | 165 | 15.9 | 15.0 | 12.5 | 7.1 | 41.5 | 31.1 | 37.4 | 22.4 | 14.7 | 15.0 | 8.8 | 19.2 |
| **70** | **180** | **16.4** | **15.4** | **12.8** | **7.3** | **42.8** | **32.1** | **38.5** | **23.1** | **15.1** | **15.4** | **9.0** | **19.8** |
| 72 | 196 | 16.8 | 15.8 | 13.2 | 7.5 | 44.0 | 33.0 | 39.6 | 23.7 | 15.5 | 15.8 | 9.3 | 20.3 |
| 74 | 213 | 17.3 | 16.3 | 13.6 | 7.7 | 45.3 | 33.9 | 40.7 | 24.4 | 16.0 | 16.3 | 9.6 | 20.9 |
| 76 | 231 | 17.8 | 16.7 | 13.9 | 8.0 | 46.5 | 34.8 | 41.8 | 25.1 | 16.4 | 16.7 | 9.8 | 21.4 |
| 78 | 250 | 18.3 | 17.2 | 14.3 | 8.2 | 47.7 | 35.8 | 42.9 | 25.7 | 16.8 | 17.2 | 10.1 | 21.9 |

*David P. Willoughby's "optimum ideal standard" for men, in inches; from IRON MAN, November 1979—"delt" refers to delt width. (Table 1)*

smallest part, knee across the center of the knee cap and thighs at the largest circumference; waist at the smallest point without pulling the waist in; hips at the largest point, with feet together; chest at the level of the nipples (not expanded); upper arm flexed at the largest point; forearm at the largest point, clenched; and neck at the smallest part; height in bare feet; weight unclothed. The girths in the table are based on the average of the right and left sides of the body. Delt width (called "delt" in the table) is the bi-deltoid width, measured from the lateral head of one deltoid to the same of the other. You will need assistance to take this measurement.

## Beyond measurements

4.33    A good physique is not merely a set of measurements. Some men boast of their real 19-inch arms and 50-inch chests, but are not so keen to boast of their over 38-inch waists, and mere 15-inch calves. Your physique is the result of *all* your girths. The single measurement of the waist makes a dramatic difference to the appearance a set of girths provides.

4.34    In the example set of girths given using the McCallum formula, if the waist is a flabby 35 inches the physique will be dramatically different from if the waist is a defined 31 inches, with all other girths being about the same in both cases. Your waist could be a little more than 31 inches in this example and yet still be defined, if your obliques and lower-back muscles are very well developed.

4.35    Never pile on bodyweight by adopting a long-term very-heavy eating program. You want a muscular physique, not a soft or flabby one. Upper arms measuring 16.5 inches that are solid, accompanying a 31-inch waist, are very impressive by almost any standards. But 16.5-inch arms that go with a 35-inch waist are *far* less impressive. Keep yourself on the lean side.

4.36    If you are primarily a bodybuilder you will want balance in your body, from neck to calves. Aim to have your arms and calves the same girths give or take half an inch, and neck an inch or so larger. Regardless of your personal preference for bodybuilding or strength, you need strength and development in body parts that do not have dramatic effects upon girths— lower back, trapezius, and thickness throughout the back rather than just width.

## You do not have to be huge to be impressive

4.37    Some people consider as unimpressive any achievements less than awesome by the standards of the top liners. But in reality, achievements quite a long way behind those of the elite can still be outstanding.

4.38    Set measurements and exercise poundages aside for the moment. Just see things in terms of bodyweight and bodyfat. Never mind the 250+ pounds and below-5% bodyfat of some of the male, competitive elite. A "mere" 190 pounds with a genuine bodyfat of 10%, at a height of 5-9 and a light-to-medium bone structure, is outstanding by any standards except those of elite bodybuilding. But 190 pounds and 20% bodyfat is in a different world—a decrease of nearly 20 pounds of muscle. And at the same height, even 175 pounds at 10% bodyfat is impressive for a very light-boned man (wrist of under 6.5 inches and ankle under 8 inches).

4.39    Based on observation and an overview of other formulae, here is a bodyweight guide for males that takes into account bone structure and height. At 10% bodyfat, physiques in line with these bodyweights will be very impressive. At a lower bodyfat, the physiques will be even more impressive. Start with a base of 5-0 height and 100 pounds bodyweight. Then add 12 pounds per inch for a heavy bone structure, 10 pounds for a medium

> A physique has its biggest impact according to how it looks, not how it measures. Of course the two are related, but not so closely that you should concern yourself solely with measurements.

bone structure, and 8 pounds for a light bone structure. Above 5-9, cut the increments in half.

| Structure | Wrist (inches) |
|-----------|----------------|
| heavy     | 7.5–8.0        |
| medium    | 6.75–7.25      |
| light     | 6.0–6.5        |

4.40    With 5-9 and a wrist of 7 inches as a base, you would get 190 pounds. If 6-0 with the same wrist, you would get 205 pounds. If 5-6 with the same wrist, you would get 160 pounds.

4.41    If you have bodyfat of 15% you will need a bodyweight of 200 pounds to produce a physique with the equivalent amount of muscle as one of 190 pounds and 10% bodyfat. And if you have bodyfat of 20% you will need to be about 210 pounds. But a physique of 210 pounds and 20% bodyfat is a world apart in visual impact from one of 190 pounds and 10%, though the muscular mass under the fat is almost the same in both cases.

4.42    Hard gainers who have discovered the gaining formula often allow themselves to carry too much fat. Being leaner at the same muscular mass makes for a more impressive physique. Always remember that you do not have to be huge to be impressive. While this applies to everyone, it is particularly comforting for hard gainers.

## Strength targets

4.43    Male hard gainers who build to being able to squat 400 pounds, bench press 300 and deadlift 500 for single lifts in good form are *much more* impressive, relative to the genetic material being worked with, than are the easy-gaining elite.

4.44    The 400, 300 and 500 numbers, for a man of 5-9 and a solid 190 pounds or so, *roughly* translate to a 16-inch arm and 45-inch chest, with other girths in proportion. Percentage wise, and relative to bodyweight, these 400, 300 and 500 numbers roughly translate to 200% squatting, 150% bench pressing, and 250% deadlifting. And 100% bodyweight for overhead barbell pressing can be included too.

4.45    Once you can strictly press a barbell weighing the equivalent of your bodyweight overhead, you will be a better presser than 99% of all weight trainees (including many big bodybuilders). Generally speaking, the press is a neglected exercise. Pressing overhead *at least* your bodyweight should be one of your most prized targets.

4.46    Successful hard gainers provide down-to-earth and practical examples of how typical people with busy lives should train. Though modest when compared to the huge men, a muscular 16-inch arm, 45-inch chest and other girths to match— assuming you are lean enough to see your abdominal lines—is enough to set you apart from over 95% of the members of almost any gym anywhere in the world. That is some going, though it will not win you a Mr. Universe title. With such a development, however, you could have placed very high in national bodybuilding competition back in the pre-steroids days. Take a look at bodybuilding magazines from the forties and fifties, and see for yourself.

4.47    With the link between exercise poundages and muscular girths being so strong, here are some guidelines—but *not* definitive numbers—for the sort of weights you need to be lifting if you aim to get to 16-inch arms and corresponding girths. But the strength-to-girths relationship is not uniform among all individuals. Some people need to get considerably stronger than others to develop the same muscular girths. The following *guidelines* assume a *controlled* (no cheating!) training style, and no use of powerlifting support gear. They include a *short* pause for a breath or few between reps, especially during the final stage of a set. But this group of mostly core exercises is not suitable for a *single* training routine for a hard gainer—there are too many exercises here for productive use in any single routine.

| | |
|---|---|
| Regular squat *to parallel*: | 300 lbs x 20 (and 400 x 1) |
| Bent-legged deadlift: | 385 x 15 (and 500 x 1) |
| Stiff-legged deadlift *from the floor*: | 300 x 10 |
| Bench press: | 260 x 6 (and 300 x 1) |
| Parallel bar dip: | (bodyweight plus 100) x 6 |
| Overhead press: | 175 x 6 |
| Pulldown: | 240 x 6 |
| Chin: | (bodyweight plus 50–60) x 6 |
| One-arm dumbbell row: | 110 x 6 |
| Barbell curl: | 120 x 6 |
| Shoulder-width bench press: | 220 x 6 |
| Single-leg calf raise: | 20 reps with a 60-lb 'bell |

4.48      When you make it to these strength levels, focus on the next
          5%, and then the next 5%, and then the next—for as long as
          you want to keep growing.

4.49      Some of you will get to the target girths without having to get
          as strong as the performances just given, but others will need
          to get stronger. Either way the connection between muscular
          size and strength will be clear.

4.50      The given poundages will seem modest relative to the mighty
          weights that some of the elite men can lift. But do not knock
          this "modest" strength level. How many drug-free men where
          you train can move these poundages?

## Refining the 300–400–500

4.51      Few people slot neatly into the 300–400–500 threesome that is
          specifically targeted at the male, experienced, very-well-trained
          and successful hard gainer who is about 5-9 and 190 pounds.
          Height, bodyweight, age, gender, limb lengths relative to torso
          length, knee-to-ankle (tibia and fibula) length relative to knee-to-
          pelvis (femur) length, elbow-to-wrist (radius and ulna) length
          relative to elbow-to-shoulder (humerus) length, muscle
          composition and belly lengths, type of training, posture and
          neurological efficiency, among other factors, influence how one
          body will respond relative to another, even if all variables that
          can be controlled are kept constant.

4.52      As an example, while the 300–400–500 trio is a proportionate
          representation of many well-trained men's strength, some body
          structures produce different proportions. A long-limbed person
          will likely have a deadlift proportionately ahead of the squat
          and bench. A short-limbed person would likely have deadlift
          strength proportionately weaker than the bench and squat, even
          assuming the same level of application to the three exercises.

4.53      Next time you are in a crowd of people, scrutinize the great
          variety of interpretations of the human form. We are all
          basically the same, but the range of variation is vast.

4.54      To give you poundage targets that take into account age and
          bodyweight, and thus to some degree height, here are more
          figures, again based on the squat, bench press and deadlift
          threesome. The three powerlifts are used because there are lots
          of published figures on them.

4.55    The figures are loosely based on sampling from powerlifting meets that had at least some threat of limited drug testing. The highest level of performance was ignored because such performance necessitates exceptional genetics or serious drug assistance. The figures were further modified because they are based on contest lifting.

4.56    The figures are based on competition powerlifting, e.g., bench pressing with a pause at the chest and with buttocks touching the bench throughout the lift, and squatting to parallel. Compare yourself based on the *same* technique criteria.

4.57    Powerlifting contests permit the use of support gear (belt, squat suit, squat briefs, knee wraps, and bench shirt) which inflate the squat and bench press poundages. The deadlift does not usually benefit heavily from assistance gear used in powerlifting meets (though it can for some lifters, especially the sumo style).

4.58    You should always train without support gear—other than perhaps a belt for squatting, deadlifting and overhead pressing, and *possibly* very *prudent* use of wrist straps *if* you are performing very heavy partial pulling exercises. The exception is if you are a powerlifter getting ready for a contest, when you must get used to using support gear.

4.59    With no support gear other than a belt, most people who train the deadlift and squat equally seriously will deadlift more than they squat. But in meet conditions and using squat support gear, some of them will squat about the same as they deadlift, or even squat more. A contributing factor here is that the squat is done first and the deadlift last. This favors the squat performance.

4.60    Different lifters benefit to varying degrees from support gear, according to the size of lifters, quality of paraphernalia, and how well it is used. Typically, 20–40 pounds on the bench press and 60–100 on the squat is the sort of help the gear can provide. The figures that follow assume no support gear other than a belt, and have been adjusted to a multiple of 25 pounds.

4.61    These figures are totals that do not specify the three individual component lifts. Breaking the totals into individual lifts is something you can do yourself. Consider the 300–400–500 threesome. The total is 1,200 pounds and the proportion for the bench press is 25%. For the squat, it comes to 33.33%, and the deadlift gets the balance of 41.66%. Make it a threesome of 25%, 35% and 40% for round figures.

4.62    This composition breakdown may or may not tally with your relative strength levels. Assuming you have trained each exercise equally seriously, consistently and intensively (which very few people do, usually because they prefer the bench press to the other two movements) you can calculate your own relative strength proportions. If you have not trained each of the exercises with equal seriousness and application for a number of years, then you must do this before you can accurately work out your relative strength levels.

4.63    Taking the proportions that reflect your actual relative strengths for each lift, or using the 25%–35%–40% estimation if you have no precise figures for yourself, you can calculate the breakdown of the three lifts for whichever bodyweight and age category you are considering, or targeting.

## Classification for hard-gaining men aged 25–35

| 4.64 | Bodyweight: | 120 lbs | 150 lbs | 180 lbs | 210 lbs |
|---|---|---|---|---|---|
| | Very good | 700 lbs | 850 lbs | 1,025 lbs | 1,200 lbs |
| | Terrific | 775 lbs | 950 lbs | 1,150 lbs | 1,325 lbs |
| | Outstanding | 875 lbs | 1,075 lbs | 1,300 lbs | 1,500 lbs |

4.65    Remember that these poundages are totals of three single/one-rep lifts—squat, bench press and deadlift—done with no support gear other than a belt. *But you do not have to actually perform maximum singles to compare yourself with these figures.* Using the appropriate chart you can "translate" a multiple-rep maximum-effort set into a projected maximum single, as explained later in this chapter.

4.66    The degree of attainment of each category has been divided into three levels—very good, terrific and outstanding. These category titles describe *drug-free and genetically typical people*. They are *not* to be confused with how the same adjectives are used with regard to the competitive elite who, of course, have much higher criteria.

4.67    For our purposes, "very good" means you are closing in on the 300–400–500 standard *relative to bodyweight*. "Terrific" means you have reached the 300–400–500 standard *relative to bodyweight*, and will be starting to stand out in almost any gym if you ignore the drug users. (The 300–400–500 figures are based on the prototypical, experienced and successful hard gainer who weighs about 190 pounds and is around age 30, at about 5-9 height.) "Outstanding" means you have significantly exceeded the 300–400–500 standard *relative to bodyweight*.

4.68    For a genetically typical and drug-free person not limited by health, to get to the "very good" level (relative to bodyweight, age and gender) is very challenging, but realistic; to get to the "terrific" level is harder but a definite possibility for the highly motivated and well trained, though rare; but to make it to the "outstanding" level is extraordinarily rare.

4.69    For a drug-free and genetically disadvantaged person to get to the "very good" level is even more challenging than it is for a genetically typical bodybuilder; to get to the "terrific" level is extraordinarily rare indeed; but to get to the "outstanding" level is miraculous.

4.70    The leaner you are, the better you will compare with the figures. If you are 200 pounds with 25% bodyfat you will be far weaker than if you were 200 pounds but only 10% bodyfat. Bodyweight alone is not an accurate indicator of potential strength. Lean bodyweight would be much better. The given figures are based on male physiques with about 12% bodyfat.

### Adjustment for easy gainers
4.71    The significant minority of people who are neither typical hard gainers nor phenomenally gifted will find the above "outstanding" categories to be relatively modest. This considers similar levels of effort, time and dedication among the hard gainers and relatively easy gainers being compared. The easy gainers need to increase the given "outstanding" poundages by 20–25%. This will provide more realistic "outstanding" target poundages for the easy gainers, and produce similar levels of achievement among the two groups, relatively speaking. Genetic phenomena can aspire even higher.

> **Generally speaking, the press is a neglected exercise. Pressing overhead *at least* your bodyweight should be one of your most prized targets.**

## Classifying other hard gainers

4.72     For the total of the three lifts as shown in the classification table, women get *approximately* 55–70% of what a man of the *same* age *and* bodyweight lifts. The higher percentages apply to the comparison of the lightest bodyweight categories. The relative proportions of the three lifts are not the same for women as for men. Women are weak at the bench press relative to the squat and deadlift.

4.73     For trainees in age brackets older than 35 when *starting* their training, i.e., not already strong and well developed before entering those age groups, here is a guideline for modifying the classification table. If aged 36–40, deduct 8–10% from the 25–35 figures; for those aged 41–45, deduct another 8–10%; and then make another 8–10% reduction for the 46–50 age bracket. Thus, a trainee starting in his or her early fifties needs about 25–30% less strength to produce the same relative degree of achievement as in the 25–35 age bracket. As an example, what is "very good" for a person aged 25–35 would be more like "outstanding" for an older person of the same gender, bodyweight *and* training experience.

4.74     This does *not* mean that if you started training in your teens or twenties you will get weaker as you move into your thirties, and weaker still as you work through your forties. If you train properly you will continue to get stronger so long as you are not very close to your maximum potential. And if you are close to or even at your full potential, you can maintain your strength and development until you are over 50 *if you train properly.*

4.75     What I am doing is providing a range of figures that will enable almost everyone to find something appropriate relative to age, bodyweight and gender. Aim for the "very good" category for your age, bodyweight and training experience, or initially just a proportion of it if it is very far from where you are currently. Get that and then aim for the "terrific" category. Get that, and then look higher. As your muscles grow, unless you have a corresponding loss of bodyfat, you will move into a different bodyweight category and thus your target totals will change.

## Milestones on your way

4.76     Pairings of big plates have special interest. For example, bench pressing 225 pounds for the first time (two 45-pound plates on each end of an Olympic bar) is much more satisfying than 220 pounds, even though the difference is a mere 5 pounds. Pairings of 45-pound or 20-kilogram plates produce the poundages below, assuming the use of a 45-pound or 20-kilo Olympic bar. Use of an exercise bar (which weighs less than 45 pounds) would reduce each total.

> One pair of 45-lb or 20-kg plates: 135 lbs or 60 kgs
> Two pairs: 225 lbs or 100 kgs
> Three pairs: 315 lbs or 140 kgs
> Four pairs: 405 lbs or 180 kgs
> Five pairs: 495 lbs or 220 kgs

4.77    Spring-release collars would add about a pound or half a kilogram to each total. Using large traditional collars would add 10 pounds or 5 kilograms to the totals.

## Rate of progress

4.78    What sort of time frame is needed for going from ground zero to the "terrific" marks? There are many factors involved, but if pressed here is what I would estimate. For the average, healthy, drug-free and injury-free hard gainer who sticks religiously to abbreviated and basics-first training, trains consistently, and conscientiously attends to fully satisfying recovery needs, I would say he or she can get to the "terrific" level (relative to age, gender and bodyweight) in 3–5 years.

4.79    While one very responsive person may go from ground zero to the "terrific" level in under three years, someone else may need three years to go from a nearly "very good" level to the "terrific" mark. Some of you, due to age, physical limitations or other reasons will never get to the "terrific" mark.

4.80    What matters the most to you is *your* progress, and comparing *yourself* with *yourself*. Everything you study and apply related to training should be geared to this.

## Beyond "terrific"

4.81    Once you have reached the "terrific" poundages and measurements that classify you as an advanced bodybuilder or lifter *by drug-free criteria*, you can explore avenues of advanced training that were previously out-of-bounds. But progress in size, age permitting, will still boil down to getting stronger and then stronger still—then your muscles will keep on growing. It *is* that simple. The routines that made you big and strong will make you bigger and stronger, so long as you deliver the required hard work, persistence and patience, and fully satisfy recovery needs.

4.82    At this advanced level you may not have a strong desire to get bigger and stronger, or to target "outstanding" as defined by the given poundages. If you are primarily a bodybuilder you may opt to focus on muscular detail, symmetry and definition, to produce the full outstanding aesthetic package. As far as muscle shape is concerned, the best way to improve it is to develop bigger muscles. Never forget this, especially if you start getting so carried away with details that you forget about substance.

4.83    Alternatively you may prefer to settle with the size and strength you have, and maintain it while focusing on developing a higher level of aerobic fitness at a leaner bodyweight.

4.84    Long-term trainees cannot continue to get bigger and stronger muscles indefinitely. If you only started training in middle age then of course you can get bigger and stronger for quite a few years before Nature takes its toll and things start to reverse. But if you have trained consistently since you were 20, you cannot expect to keep making progress in muscle and might into your sixties, fifties or even forties, though you may find you can continue to progress in a few exercises even while most regress. Nature takes its course and toll.

## Individualism

4.85    Working on specific weaknesses is an important part of bodybuilding, but if you get too carried away with it—which would include undertraining your strengths—you will fail to make the most of your natural advantages.

4.86    Probably all people have an exercise or two, and a body part or two, that are more responsive to training than the rest of the package. To realize your full potential you need to exploit to the fullest whatever natural bias(es) you have.

4.87    You may be short-limbed, long-trunked, wide waisted, squat and thick. Or you may be longer-limbed, narrow-waisted, well-proportioned and classically aesthetic. The former is never going to develop a "body beautiful," but he can become a powerhouse. The aesthetic cannot become a powerhouse, but he can become a "body beautiful." The first can probably become a terrific squatter and bench presser, but always remain—relatively speaking—poor at the deadlift. The aesthetic may have a terrific potential for deadlifting, but be far weaker, relatively speaking, in the squat and bench press.

4.88     Satisfaction from weight training comes from getting good results. Hard gainers have a difficult time gaining as it is, but if you swim against the tide of your own body you will make the job far more difficult. Make sure you discover what your natural biases are, and exploit them.

4.89     On top of the personal satisfaction that exploiting a natural advantage produces, there is, at least to some extent, a carry-over and knock-on effect throughout the body, especially if the natural advantage is in a major exercise.

4.90     There are not just the three powerlifts to consider as exercises to focus on. There are other core exercises that are worthy of being focused on. These include the Trap Bar deadlift, stiff-legged deadlift, overhead press, parallel bar dip, and pullup. This may mean exaggerating the differences between your strong and weak areas, but by doing so you may develop an exercise or two that is/are exceptional. *Recognize your individualism and then exploit it to the full.*

## One man's meat

4.91     Weight training has a number of forms—bodybuilding, strength training, powerlifting, Olympic weightlifting, and all-round lifting. Each has its ardent followers, with some of them having absolutely no interest in the other forms of training. Of course there is overlap and many trainees belong to more than one category.

4.92     There is nothing wrong with being 100% into bodybuilding, 100% into strength training or 100% into any other weight-training activity. All can be very rewarding.

4.93     The same pivotal principles of productive training apply to all categories of lifting—a focus on basic exercises, hard work, and progressive poundages in good form.

4.94     Never feel pressured if someone is critical of the specific category of training that most appeals to you. Instead, look closely at the other categories and methods being promoted and try to find aspects that you can apply to your own training. Each training contingent can learn from the others.

4.95    Different people have different values and preferences. What one person may dislike, another may admire. Some people are appearance-first bodybuilders not much interested in raw strength and power. There are function-first strength trainees who *apparently* have little concern with the aesthetics of their physiques, or their bodyfat percentage. But even some of the latter enjoy throwing arm and chest poses in front of a mirror.

4.96    Some trainers are adamant about the supposed superiority of their preferred method. Each method will work well for some people, and perhaps work very well for the advocates, but this does not mean that the same will hold true for everyone.

4.97    What matters most to you is what works best for you. An eclectic approach to training is the best way. Keep an open mind, be riveted to the basic tenets of rational training, and be super alert and discriminating when you hear of anything that sounds too good to be true. Then critically select and apply what you think will be helpful to you.

4.98    Training preferences are influenced by genetic factors. Some people cannot satisfy the aesthetic qualities needed for pure bodybuilding, so they move towards raw strength activities where they can shine. Some people are not purely power-orientated because they do not have the body structure that is well-suited to it; so they gravitate towards bodybuilding, where appearance has priority over function.

4.99    You must have a great passion for what you are doing if you are to be successful at it. If you try to achieve at something that your heart is not really into, and that your body does not respond to, you will not get far.

> Exercise is not only about size and strength, though they are the biggest factors for most weight trainees for many years. There is much more to the exercise lifestyle. As you get older you will see this more clearly, and modify targets, expectations and values so you always have challenging and exciting goals.

4.100    If you love single-rep training, can consistently perform it
         safely, and gain well on it, why do high reps? But if your body
         structure cannot tolerate singles no matter how carefully and
         progressively you work into using them, do not use them. If
         you enjoy high reps and respond well to them, stick with them.
         If you enjoy very slow reps and they work for you, use them.
         But if you hate very slow reps, then never mind that someone
         else can gain well on them.

4.101    Find what *you* like, find the exercises that work best for *you*,
         find what *you* can do safely, and find what *you* gain on. Then
         with those factors in order, *pour in the effort.*

## Your specific poundage goals

4.102    If you are a beginner, or barely into the intermediate stage of
         training, you may want to use the poundages given earlier in
         this chapter as your long-term goals. But unless you have a
         natural gift for strength and development that is well above
         average, those targets are going to appear a very long way off.
         It may be better to set your sights on only a proportion of the
         full "very good" figures (say 75%), get there, and then work on
         the next 5–10% for each exercise, etc. Do this until you get to
         the "very good" targets, and then target the "terrific" ones, but
         work on getting there by focusing on 5% gains at a time.

4.103    If you are not a relative beginner, then go straight into goal
         setting based on the figures I have already given, but target the
         "very good" category first.

## Converting singles to multiple reps, and vice versa

4.104    Here is a method for converting one-rep maximum lifts
         (singles) to repetition lifts, and vice versa. For example,
         without actually having to do singles you can compare your
         current lifting for reps with the one-rep-maximum totals given
         in the classification table provided earlier in this chapter. You
         can also compare your current lifting with that in an earlier
         cycle that had you focusing on a different rep number. For
         example, maybe you are in a cycle of 10-rep squats and want
         to compare yourself with your best one-rep maximum, but do
         not want to disrupt your cycle in order to spend a period
         adapting to singles. Or perhaps you are performing low-rep
         work and want to compare it with the much higher rep work
         you were using in an earlier cycle, but without spending the
         time needed to adapt to higher reps.

## Upper-body exercises

| Desired ⇨ | 1 | 2 | 3 | 4 | 5 | 6 | 7 | 8 | 9 | 10 | 12 | 15 |
|---|---|---|---|---|---|---|---|---|---|---|---|---|
| ⇩ Current | | | | | | | | | | | | |
| 1 | 1.00 | 0.97 | 0.94 | 0.91 | 0.89 | 0.86 | 0.83 | 0.81 | 0.78 | 0.76 | 0.72 | 0.65 |
| 2 | 1.03 | 1.00 | 0.97 | 0.94 | 0.91 | 0.89 | 0.86 | 0.83 | 0.81 | 0.78 | 0.74 | 0.67 |
| 3 | 1.06 | 1.03 | 1.00 | 0.97 | 0.94 | 0.91 | 0.89 | 0.86 | 0.83 | 0.81 | 0.76 | 0.69 |
| 4 | 1.10 | 1.06 | 1.03 | 1.00 | 0.97 | 0.94 | 0.91 | 0.89 | 0.86 | 0.83 | 0.78 | 0.72 |
| 5 | 1.13 | 1.10 | 1.06 | 1.03 | 1.00 | 0.97 | 0.94 | 0.91 | 0.89 | 0.86 | 0.81 | 0.74 |
| 6 | 1.16 | 1.12 | 1.10 | 1.06 | 1.03 | 1.00 | 0.97 | 0.94 | 0.91 | 0.89 | 0.83 | 0.76 |
| 7 | **1.20** | **1.16** | **1.13** | **1.10** | **1.06** | **1.03** | **1.00** | **0.97** | **0.94** | **0.91** | **0.86** | **0.78** |
| 8 | 1.24 | 1.20 | 1.16 | 1.13 | 1.10 | 1.06 | 1.03 | 1.00 | 0.97 | 0.94 | 0.89 | 0.81 |
| 9 | 1.28 | 1.24 | 1.20 | 1.16 | 1.13 | 1.10 | 1.06 | 1.03 | 1.00 | 0.97 | 0.91 | 0.83 |
| 10 | 1.32 | 1.28 | 1.24 | 1.20 | 1.16 | 1.13 | 1.10 | 1.06 | 1.03 | 1.00 | 0.94 | 0.86 |
| 12 | 1.40 | 1.36 | 1.32 | 1.28 | 1.24 | 1.20 | 1.16 | 1.13 | 1.10 | 1.06 | 1.00 | 0.91 |
| 15 | 1.53 | 1.49 | 1.44 | 1.40 | 1.36 | 1.32 | 1.28 | 1.24 | 1.20 | 1.16 | 1.10 | 1.00 |

*Repetition-conversion tables for upper-body exercises, based on the formulae of Maurice and Rydin. See text for an explanation. (Table 2)*

## Lower-body exercises

| Desired ⇨ | 1 | 2 | 3 | 4 | 5 | 6 | 7 | 8 | 9 | 10 | 12 | 15 | 20 |
|---|---|---|---|---|---|---|---|---|---|---|---|---|---|
| ⇩ Current | | | | | | | | | | | | | |
| 1 | 1.00 | 0.99 | 0.97 | 0.96 | 0.94 | 0.93 | 0.91 | 0.90 | 0.89 | 0.87 | 0.85 | 0.81 | 0.75 |
| 2 | 1.02 | 1.00 | 0.99 | 0.97 | 0.96 | 0.94 | 0.93 | 0.91 | 0.90 | 0.89 | 0.86 | 0.82 | 0.76 |
| 3 | 1.03 | 1.02 | 1.00 | 0.99 | 0.97 | 0.96 | 0.94 | 0.93 | 0.91 | 0.90 | 0.87 | 0.83 | 0.77 |
| 4 | 1.05 | 1.03 | 1.02 | 1.00 | 0.99 | 0.97 | 0.96 | 0.94 | 0.93 | 0.91 | 0.89 | 0.85 | 0.79 |
| 5 | 1.06 | 1.05 | 1.03 | 1.02 | 1.00 | 0.99 | 0.97 | 0.96 | 0.94 | 0.93 | 0.90 | 0.86 | 0.80 |
| 6 | 1.08 | 1.06 | 1.05 | 1.03 | 1.02 | 1.00 | 0.99 | 0.97 | 0.96 | 0.94 | 0.91 | 0.87 | 0.81 |
| 7 | **1.09** | **1.08** | **1.06** | **1.05** | **1.03** | **1.02** | **1.00** | **0.99** | **0.97** | **0.96** | **0.93** | **0.89** | **0.82** |
| 8 | 1.11 | 1.09 | 1.08 | 1.06 | 1.05 | 1.03 | 1.02 | 1.00 | 0.99 | 0.97 | 0.94 | 0.90 | 0.83 |
| 9 | 1.13 | 1.11 | 1.09 | 1.08 | 1.06 | 1.05 | 1.03 | 1.02 | 1.00 | 0.99 | 0.96 | 0.91 | 0.85 |
| 10 | 1.15 | 1.13 | 1.11 | 1.09 | 1.08 | 1.06 | 1.05 | 1.03 | 1.02 | 1.00 | 0.97 | 0.93 | 0.86 |
| 12 | 1.18 | 1.16 | 1.15 | 1.13 | 1.11 | 1.09 | 1.08 | 1.06 | 1.05 | 1.03 | 1.00 | 0.96 | 0.89 |
| 15 | 1.24 | 1.22 | 1.20 | 1.18 | 1.16 | 1.15 | 1.13 | 1.11 | 1.09 | 1.08 | 1.05 | 1.00 | 0.93 |
| 20 | 1.33 | 1.31 | 1.29 | 1.27 | 1.25 | 1.24 | 1.22 | 1.20 | 1.18 | 1.16 | 1.13 | 1.08 | 1.00 |

*Repetition-conversion tables for lower-body exercises, based on the formulae of Maurice and Rydin. See text for an explanation. (Table 3)*

## The Maurice and Rydin method

4.105     In the September 1992 issue of HARDGAINER (issue #20) Dave Maurice and Rich Rydin presented two formulae for converting poundages between different rep numbers. They are presented here in much more convenient chart form.

4.106    To convert from one poundage and rep combination to another,
         using the Maurice-Rydin formulae, see the tables accompanying
         this segment. Here is the relevant explanation from Maurice and
         Rydin, in HARDGAINER issue #34:

> To use one of the charts, look in the left column to find
> the rep number you have been performing (i.e., your
> current reps). Move across the row until you are under
> the rep number to which you wish to project your
> performance (i.e., your desired reps).
>
> For example, if you have been bench pressing for 10
> reps, and want to try 6 reps, you would multiply your
> best 10-rep poundage by 1.13 to estimate your best 6-rep
> poundage. Similarly, if you have been squatting for 6
> reps and now wish to try 20 reps, you would multiply
> your best 6-rep poundage by 0.81 to estimate your best
> 20-rep poundage.

4.107    These tables are not presented as valid for everyone. A
         minority of trainees, at least in some exercises, are terrible at
         high reps relative to their low-rep achievements. Conversely,
         some people are excellent at high reps but cannot produce the
         corresponding low-rep poundages that would be expected.
         Despite this shortcoming the tables can still be useful once you
         become familiar with using them in the best way for you.

## Comparison of rep and poundage progression

4.108    It might be thought that one more rep, or one more pound on
         the bar, are similar increases in load on the body. In fact, these
         two progressive increases are very different. According to the
         Maurice and Rydin chart for upper-body exercises, an increase
         of one rep corresponds to about a 3% decrease in resistance. If
         you are overhead pressing 180 pounds for 5 reps, to increase
         your rep count by a mere one, to 6, is comparable to adding 5.5
         pounds while keeping the rep count at 5. This is a big increase if
         the 180-pound 5-rep set is already very demanding. So adding
         very small increments, while using a constant rep count, is a
         better trick (mentally and physically) for progressing
         sufficiently gradually that gains can be steady and consistent.

4.109    Even when you cannot increase your rep count you can
         probably perform the same number of reps but with a very
         small increment on the bar. Do that several times and, using
         the above illustration, you will creep to the 5.5 pounds that is

equivalent to a one-rep gain. And you can do this without perceiving any increase in training difficulty. Then keep doing that, again and again. A lot of little increments add up to a substantial gain. [BB]

> Focus on achieving the next 5–10% gain in all your exercises, and a tad more on each of your muscular girths—these are your medium-term goals. If you apply yourself to this approach, and keep doing it repeatedly for a number of years, you will eventually get as big and strong as it is possible for you to become. Your immediate short-term target should be to take the next small step towards your next set of medium-term goals.
>
> As much as is practically possible, gear every aspect of your life to create the conditions needed to add iron to each exercise every week or two, be that increment a pound or two, for example, or just a few ounces. Poundage progression *in good form* is what building muscle and might is primarily about, though *some* specific forms of training yield strength gains but little or no accompanying muscle growth. The possible differences between strength-focus and strength-*and*-size focus training methods will be explained later in this book. *Never lose sight of the pivotal importance of progression.* Organize your training program, workout frequency, nutrition, sleep and rest habits so that you make progression a reality.

To realize your potential, you need to become an achievement-orientated, goal-driven and success-attaining individual.

Achievement comes in small steps, but LOTS of them. Lots of little bits add up to huge achievement. Weight training exemplifies this bit-by-bit process. Strive to get each rep right, each set right, each workout right, each day's nutrition right, each night's sleep right, and then keep doing that, again and again and again and again...

# 5. How to Plan Your Growth

5.1      Success is rarely an accident in any endeavor. Success in the gym is *never* a hit or miss activity. It is planned. If you put together an intelligent program, tailor it according to your own individual recuperative abilities and possible physical limitations, follow it diligently and conscientiously for long enough, and fully satisfy your rest, sleep and nutritional needs, then you *will* get much bigger and stronger muscles. *Sensible* weight-training programs work. But too few people know what sensible programs are, and too few trainees are targeted at specific goals by a specific time.

## A. Strategies for the Long Term

5.2      The need to focus on the *now*—today—is the building block for long-term success. Not living in the past, and not living in the future, but riveting most of your attention on the present is the only way to make sure you get most if not all of your "todays" in good order. If you do not get the daily units right, you do not have a hope of long-term success.

5.3      There is a strong connection between the daily units and your long-term goals. Getting the latter in good order provides the overall strategy into which the daily units slot. Regular reminders of the long-term programming keep you on track for getting the daily units right.

5.4      Competitive athletes have a major advantage over non-competitive ones. That is the motivating, focusing, pressurizing and concrete-goals-creating effect of competition. The need to be your best at a certain date and place will dramatically focus your attention, and force you to be more efficient with your time. Without a definite where and when to be at your best, human nature makes most people casual with their time. You may take years to get to where you could have gotten in just six months had you been nailed down to a rigorous schedule to get things done on time.

5.5     Deadlines are imperative for making people take action, in all areas of life. Consider how many things you need to do but have been procrastinating for weeks because you do not have a fixed deadline to do them by. But give something a deadline and urgency, and it usually gets done.

5.6     Nail yourself to long-term deadlines. Make your goals specific by writing down numbers and deadlines, for example. Then nail yourself to the daily must-dos in order to keep on schedule for reaching the long-term goals.

5.7     There is nothing like the urgency of concentrating on a specific goal by a specific deadline to focus attention, application and resolve. Without something specific to rally attention and resources, people tend to drift along and never get even close to realizing their potential. As the months go by there is little or no improvement.

5.8     Set the goal(s), make your plans, focus your application, dedicate yourself, and then start making month-by-month improvement a reality. And then when you have achieved your medium or long-term goal(s), do it all over again, and then again, and again. Then you will set yourself up to achieve more over the next twelve months than perhaps you achieved over the previous few years. And whatever you learn from the value of nailing yourself to targets and deadlines in the physique and strength spheres, apply it to the rest of your life.

5.9     There are deadline situations that can rivet attention just as well as formal bodybuilding or lifting competition. Some of them may seem too simple, or even trite, but they work if you work.

# TACTIC #1
## Small, specific targets
5.10    Do not just agree that nailing yourself to specific targets is the way to go, nod your head, and read on. Stop, grab a sheet of paper and a pencil, and write down some specific training-related goals you want to achieve three months from today. Perhaps you want to drop 10 pounds of bodyfat; perhaps you want to add 10 pounds to your bench press poundage; perhaps you want to work three-times-weekly aerobic activity into your exercise program; perhaps you are finally going to apply yourself with a vengeance to a very abbreviated training program. Really put in some thought here. Finalize some

challenging but *realistic* goals. Chew them over; and then carefully select the *one* or *two* that you are going to dedicate the next three months of your training life to.

5.11    Break the target(s) down into a series of weekly goals, and produce a three-month program. Get down in black and white what you need to do with your training, rest and sleep schedule, and nutrition. Then knock off the weekly installments of success. Like a competitive athlete closing in on a big meet, deliver the goods every day, every week, every month.

## TACTIC #2
### Before-and-after shots

5.12    Have your photos taken this week, to display all your physique in a given number of well-lighted poses. No matter how happy or unhappy you are with how you look, get the job done so that you have a photographic record of your current condition. If you are too embarrassed to have a professional do it, get your spouse or boyfriend/girlfriend or sympathetic relative to do it. But have it done seriously and as well as possible.

5.13    Set a six-month target, and give your all to improving your physique as much as possible, with the litmus test being the next photo session. Then with proof in photographic print you can see what you did with the previous six months of your life.

5.14    It is easy in bodybuilding and strength training to mull away time, go through the motions, and lose track of the passage of time. Working in six-month slots gives tremendous focus, and you will have a photographic record of what you achieved over each six-month stretch. After each photographic session, set another six-month deadline with an even more determined effort to make the next six months your most productive training period ever.

5.15    Be meticulously consistent about the conditions used for each photo session. Consider if you have poor lighting, a hairy and untanned body, unkempt long hair, long baggy shorts, and poorly focused photos of amateurish and clumsy poses for one session. Then, next time, after a hair cut, you have excellent lighting and sharp photography, and a shaven and tanned physique posed professionally in a well-fitting swim suit. You will look dramatically better in the second batch of photos even if your physique is unchanged.

5.16     Keep an album of your photographs. Refer to the album regularly. Be dissatisfied with what you see but recognize the visible improvement you have made, when you have made it. Resolve to do better, to improve the physique that currently is not good enough.

5.17     Put the resolve into practice. Do not quit on the final rep of each hard work set. Add an extra bit of iron to the bar when possible. Tighten up on loose form. Resist the bit of food you know is in excess of your daily caloric allocation. Substitute first-class food for second-rate fare. Spend the time performing aerobic work when you know you need it. Be disciplined at all times.

5.18     The added spark of the possibility of getting yourself in print should motivate you to take everything even more seriously than you already are. When you are in the gym, at the dining table, or doing anything else connected with your progress, think of the improvement you *must* make. Then be sure to do whatever you know has to be done, *every* day. No loafing, no stalling, no weakening of resolve. Do it—*now!*—and become the best you can for the "after" shots.

5.19     When the deadline arrives, reflect on what you did over the last six months that was good, and resolve to do that again, or better. Then reflect on what you did that was a hindrance over the last six months, and resolve not to do that again.

## TACTIC #3
### Video tape your physique
5.20     Having yourself on photographic prints or slides is one thing. To see yourself strutting your stuff on video is another. Once you have done a couple or more photographic sessions as in *Tactic #2*, upgrade the seriousness to video taping (and photos, too, if you prefer to have both formats). If you feel embarrassed about the taping, get your spouse or a close friend or relative to do the recording. Fix the six-month taping sessions so that your training is geared around them, just as if they were public competitions you were preparing for.

## TACTIC #4
### Video tape your lifting
5.21     Rather than a pure-appearance focus, spend a long while focusing purely on getting stronger. Get yourself on video tape while performing your best sets. Then schedule yourself to be

recorded performing the same exercises six months later. Gear the next six months of your life to increasing your strength as much as you can.

5.22    Assemble a good routine, keep the focus on progressive poundages in good form, keep remembering the video recording to come, raise the intensity of your work, become possessed in the gym, and get plenty of rest between workouts.

5.23    Come deadline time you will have a good bit more on the bar for each exercise, for the same reps you used six months earlier. Get a straight comparison on video tape. See the improvement. Then apply yourself to getting stronger still, and come back for another recording session after a further six months.

## TACTIC #5
### Landmark years

5.24    Once you are over 30 years old, you may come to see certain birthdays as landmark points—35, 40, 45 and 50, for example. Set each of these birthdays as video taping days for physique and lifting. And of course each one of these landmark recordings should see improvement relative to the previous one. Gear the in-between years for keeping you on track to becoming better as you get older.

5.25    Bodybuilding and strength training are wonderful activities for many reasons, one of them being their potential for enabling you to improve with age, even well into your middle years. (The older you are when you start, the older you can be and still make progress in strength.) And when you start to regress due to aging, work hard to hold onto as much strength as possible. Then, because your peers will deteriorate much faster than you will, you will continue to get better, relatively speaking, as the years go by. Exercise keeps you young.

5.26    Rise to the challenge of proving all this. Get yourself down on video tape on each of your landmark birthdays. Remind yourself daily of the importance of doing your utmost every day to be better next time around.

5.27    Break each five-year period into six-month slots, and make visible and measurable improvement over each of those periods. Add up those six-month stretches of improvement over five years and you will produce dramatic change.

5.28     Never settle for anything other than your finest effort to be
         your best on your six-month deadline days. And never settle
         for doing anything other than your very best each day of the
         journey. You have to get the individual days in good order if
         you are to achieve your long-term goals.

5.29     What you concentrate on for a given landmark year will reflect
         changing values as you age. At ages up to 35 or so your training
         focus may be solely on size and strength. As you approach 40 or
         45 you might place more emphasis on flexibility and a low
         percentage of bodyfat. Around age 40 you may be overhauling
         the goals to target. Maybe getting to 8% bodyfat will be more
         important than making a 300-pound bench press. Perhaps
         having a resting heart rate under 55 will be more important
         than deadlifting 500 pounds. Perhaps at 50 you will want to hit
         250, 350 and 400 in the big three at say 175 pounds bodyweight,
         but simultaneously have a resting heart rate of 55. At age 35
         you may have wanted 350, 450 and 550 at 210 pounds, but paid
         no attention to your resting pulse. (Though a low resting heart
         rate is usually an indicator of a healthy and efficient heart, it can
         be a symptom of some health problems.)

5.30     Whatever interests you for the time being, set specific goals for
         it—say 10% bodyfat, not just "to get lean"; to have a resting
         heart rate of 60, not just "to be fit," etc. Then nail yourself to a
         specific time deadline—e.g., six months from today, not "quite
         soon"—and devise the strategy to reach your target.

## TACTIC #6
### Competition

5.31     While competitive bodybuilding and powerlifting act as terrific
         deadline creators, do not enter without expecting competition
         from drug users. Testing is either non-existent or such a joke
         that some of the most prominent "naturals" are well-juiced.

5.32     A much more realistic and fair type of competition is to set up
         something informal with a training partner, friend or pen pal.

> There is a world of exercise-related goals to target and
> achieve. Avoid getting locked into tunnel vision that
> keeps you looking at the same sort of targets
> throughout your training life.

Make it bodyweight related for maximum reps for each exercise, e.g., squat 150% bodyweight, bench press bodyweight, and barbell curl 50% bodyweight. Set the date of the competition a few months away, structure a training cycle to peak on the meet day, gear yourself up for it, apply yourself with zeal to the preparatory training, and then give forth of your very best on the big day.

5.33    Alternatively, compete with yourself. Add an *end-of-cycle* test day to each of your programs. On the test day perform a fixed challenge workout radically different from how you normally train. Each time you do it, give your all to bettering what you did the previous time. Take a few days rest from your previous workout prior to the test session. Here are some *suggestions*:

> Maximum reps in the squat with 100, 135 or 185 pounds.
> Maximum reps in the bench press with 135 pounds.
> Maximum reps in the deadlift with 150 or 200 pounds.

5.34    You could impose a time limit if the reps will be very high, e.g., maximum reps within 15 minutes; and you could use percentages of bodyweight rather than fixed weights. You could even get away from regular weight-training exercises for competition days, or use a mixture. Use your imagination and find some movements you would enjoy performing. For example, you could perform your maximum number of floor pushups (perhaps put a time limit on it), walk with a given pair of heavy objects for time, hold a 2-inch bar loaded to 100 pounds for time, etc.

5.35    Do not choose exercises you have no recent experience of. For example, do not go for maximum reps in the squat if you have not squatted for a few months.

5.36    Keep accurate records of your poundages and reps. Keep the exercises and weights or percentages constant from one competition day to another. Be sure to keep *all* conditions of the competition days constant (including the order of the exercises used, and rest periods), so that you are comparing yourself under the same conditions.

5.37    Weight training can be much more interesting than most people make it. Competition days are just one way to make your training more challenging, productive *and* enjoyable.

## How to make each tactic work

5.38    All the determination in the world counts for nothing if you do
        not know how to train effectively. But having an extraordinary
        level of determination speeds up the learning process.

5.39    Treat each self-imposed deadline as a major part of your life. If
        you treat the deadlines casually you might as well not bother
        going through the process of aiming to be your best by a given
        date. As with everything in training you have to take what you
        are doing *very* seriously. Hard gainers have little room for error,
        whereas easy gainers can make many errors and yet still gain.

5.40    Give your 100% best to a good overall plan broken down into
        daily units, and you will amaze yourself with how much you
        can achieve. Compare the sort of attention you have given your
        training over the last year, with the sort of application I am
        suggesting here, and you will probably find a big difference.

5.41    If you want to be successful in achieving your potential you
        need to program that success. Stop leaving life to chance.
        Forget about the indifference and disorderly state of others,
        and do not let any negativity rub onto you.

5.42    It does not matter a whit what other people are doing with
        their training. Your own life is what matters the most to you.
        Get in charge and make the most of it.

# B. Daily Units of Training and Living

5.43    Building big muscles, and then bigger muscles still, depends on
        an organized plan of action—broken down into daily units—
        coupled with a great will to achieve. Achievement in any
        sphere of life depends on getting the individual moments right,
        at least most of the time.

5.44    By getting today right, and by getting every today right, you
        will get the weeks and months right too. Then you will get the
        years right and start to get close to realizing your potential. The
        secret of life is getting today right. Everyone can get today
        right, and if you can do it once you can do it repeatedly.

5.45    Success in any walk of life comes through goal-directed action
        broken down into small daily units where each item connected
        with your long-term goals is focused upon and executed to the
        best of your ability.

5.46       You cannot make sudden and huge jumps in achievement. Achievement comes in small steps, but *lots* of them. Lots of little bits add up to huge achievement. Weight training exemplifies this bit-by-bit process. Strive to get each rep right, each set right, each workout right, each day's nutrition right, each night's sleep right, and then keep doing that, again and again and again. Then you will get somewhere.

5.47       You will not get everything right each time, but by keeping your attention where it should be for most of the time—on the *now*—then you can get most things right most of the time, and that is enough for you to do one heck of a good job, so long as you do it for enough *years*.

## Training diary

5.48       An essential part of the organization needed to get each workout day right is a training diary. At its most basic minimum this is a written record of reps and poundage for every work set you do, *and* an evaluation of each workout so that you can stay alert to warning signs of overtraining. After each workout, reflect on your evaluation and, when necessary, make adjustments to avoid falling foul of overtraining.

5.49       A training diary or journal is indispensable for keeping you on track for training success. No matter where you are now— 180-pound squat or 500, 13-inch arms or 17, 135-pound bench press or 350—the systematic organization and focus upon achieving goals that a training journal enforces will help you to get bigger and stronger.

5.50       As simple as it is to use a training log, do not underestimate the critical role this can play in maximizing your training efficiency and productivity. Most trainees are aware that they should record their workouts in a permanent way, but few actually do it. And even those trainees who keep some sort of training log usually fail to exploit its full potential benefits. This is one of the major reasons why most trainees get minimal results from their training.

5.51       Keeping a skimpy record of your training on loose sheets of paper, backs of envelopes, or scraps of paper—all of which are likely to be lost—will not do. Your journal should hold at least twelve months of detailed workout records, be durably bound and robust enough to withstand heavy use, and be capable of being opened flat. And you should be able to see many workout records on each pair of log pages, for ease of entering data and analyzing it.

5.52    When used properly, a training journal enforces the organization needed to get each workout right, for week after week, month after month, and year after year. By recording your poundages and reps, your training journal logs your entire training program, and the week-by-week breakdown of how you work through the routine(s) of each training cycle.

5.53    A training log eliminates reliance upon memory. There will be no, "Did I squat 8 reps with 330 pounds last squat workout, or was it 7?" Refer to your journal and you will see precisely what you did last time—i.e., what you need to improve on if you are to make your next workout a step forward. While a small error of memory in the very early part of a cycle may not be critical, it could be later on in a cycle when you are in new poundage territory—a mistake of just a few pounds at this stage could destroy a set and possibly ruin a workout.

5.54    With a first-class training journal that is meticulously kept up to date you will never wonder, for example, when it was that you broke the 300-pound bench press barrier, or first squatted with 400 pounds. A journal will keep your memory accurate.

5.55    You must be 100% honest when entering data. Record the quality of your reps. If you did five good ones but the sixth needed a tad of help from a training partner, do not record all six as if they were done under your own steam. Record the ones you did alone, but note the assisted rep as only a half rep.

5.56    It is not enough just to train hard. You need to train hard with a target to beat in every work set you do. The targets to beat in any given workout are your achievements the previous time you performed that same routine/workout.

5.57    If you train hard but with no rigorous concern over reps and poundages, you cannot be sure you are training progressively. Unless you have accurate records of the achievements to be bettered, you cannot be sure that you really are giving your all. But for accurate records of sets, reps and poundages to have meaning, your training conditions must be consistent. If one workout you rush between sets, then next workout you take your time, you cannot fairly compare those two sessions. If one week the deadlift is your first exercise, and the following week you deadlift at the end of the workout, you cannot fairly compare those two workouts. And the form you use for each exercise must be consistent and flawless every time you train.

5.58    Get all the details of your training in black and white, refer to them when appropriate, and get in control of your training. You will then have a detailed record of the evolution of each training program, and of your training as a whole from year to year. In addition to control over the short term, this permanent record will give you a wealth of data to analyze and draw upon when designing your future training programs.

5.59    Keep accurate records of each workout, each day's caloric and protein intake, how much sleep you get, muscular girths, and your body composition. Then you will remove all guesswork and disorder from your training program. But if you only track one or two of the components you will not have the full story. Even an exaggerated attention to one or two components will not compensate for neglect of the remaining elements.

5.60    But all of this is just a bunch of words. You have to make the theory and rationale come alive with your conscientious and methodical practical application. Do exactly that, now, and take charge of your training!

5.61    Most trainees have neither the organization needed for success, nor the will and desire to push themselves very hard when they need to. But these are the very demanding essentials for successful bodybuilding and strength training-satisfy them, now, and then get on with achieving your potential for muscle and might.

## Training partner
5.62    Getting your daily units right means getting each workout right. How can you help yourself to get each workout right? Get yourself hands-on supervision.

> **CS Publishing's** THE MUSCLE & MIGHT TRAINING TRACKER **is a tailor-made week-by-week journal for recording your training and daily nutritional data.**

5.63    Armed with the will to get the job done, and the basic
        knowledge of what to do, most trainees should be able to get a
        good training partner or supervisor.

5.64    Fine physiques and super-strong bodies have been built
        without training partners or supervisors. Do not be discouraged
        if it is impossible for you to get hands-on help. But the
        assistance of a serious and like-minded training partner or
        supervisor is nearly always a tremendous advantage. But
        anyone with anything less than a 100% commitment is a
        negative influence, and should not be tolerated.

5.65    Few people can consistently train at their *very* best without
        hands-on supervision. And even most of those who do train
        alone successfully may gain even better if they had good
        supervision at least some of the time.

5.66    While recognizing the value of good supervision, it is pivotal
        that you can train well *by yourself.* If you can only train well
        when supervised, you are dependent on supervision and will
        never be able to train well over the long haul. Even if you have
        a reliable training partner there will be times when your
        schedules do not coincide and you have to train alone. Never
        become dependent on another person to get in a good workout.

## Some of the advantages of being well supervised

5.67    Effective training has to be intensive, and intensive training is
        very difficult to deliver on a consistent basis without a
        demanding taskmaster to urge you to deliver. Most trainees
        have experienced the occasional workout when, unexpectedly
        and only for the one workout, someone got involved during
        part or all of a training session. Someone might have spotted
        you on an exercise; or someone you wanted to impress was
        watching you; or someone might have worked in with you on
        a few exercises. As a result you found yourself doing more reps
        than you normally would, or doing the same reps with a bit
        more weight than you had planned. You really produced for
        that workout, while previously you had been loafing. Quality
        supervision can get this degree of effort out of you on a regular
        basis, and can speed up your progress dramatically.

5.68    Remember that successful training is not about effort per se. It
        is about how you apply the effort. A sloppy set of an exercise
        worked very hard is not going to do you as much good as will

a good-form set of an exercise worked very hard. But the sloppy form may lead to injury. The sharp eye and words of a good supervisor will help to keep your form tight.

5.69     While a good training partner or supervisor pushes you all the way, alerts you to form imperfections that start to creep in (and which you must cut out), he is also there to spot you. This will give you the confidence and security to keep pushing when the reps get tough.

## Getting supervision

5.70     A training partner, someone who trains with you, is likely to be your most practical option. Either alternate sets (especially if your training programs are identical or very similar), with each of you taking turns at supervising as you go along, or, one of you completes the workout with the other supervising, and then you reverse roles. The second alternative usually takes much longer for both of you to get your workouts done. It also may be hard to supervise someone well while feeling wiped out as a result of having just completed your own workout.

5.71     If you train at a commercial gym, getting a training partner is likely to be much easier than if you train at home. As you get to know gym members you may find someone you could work with. Publicize your search for a training partner using the gym's notice board, or newsletter if there is one. If possible, also put up a notice in other gyms in your town. You could even extend your search to any colleges that might be in your area. Even if you train at home you can use the same channels for your search for a training partner.

5.72     It is not necessary that you have approximately the same level of strength, or are using the exact same sequence of exercises. What matters most is having a similar training philosophy and degree of seriousness, and that you get along with each other and are both punctual for workouts. You also need to have similar recovery abilities so that you can agree on a mutually suitable and productive training frequency.

5.73     Regardless of if your supervisor is a training partner or a non-training one, he needs to understand that your training is a very serious matter, and has to be treated as such. It is not difficult to keep your attention on training if you have set the rules beforehand. There will be:

a.  No non-constructive criticism or advice from either of you.

b.  No defensiveness to constructive input. Each of you must learn from the input of the other and be open to criticism.

c.  No socializing chit chat until after training has finished.

d.  No personal discussions until after training has finished.

e.  No fooling around and taking things lightly.

5.74    If you can afford to employ a personal trainer, be sure to check out his competence first. Despite the "qualifications" tagged on their calling cards, many personal trainers have major deficiencies in their knowledge of training.

5.75    To help determine whether someone can help you in the gym, critically watch the trainer at work with a client, with this checklist in mind:

a.  Is the form he teaches like that explained in THE INSIDER'S TELL-ALL HANDBOOK ON WEIGHT-TRAINING TECHNIQUE?

b.  Does he remind his charge of key points of form before a set starts, and even in the course of a set when necessary?

c.  Has he modified his client's exercise selection and form according to any limitations the trainee may have? Has the trainer avoided a "one size fits all" training program?

d.  Does he keep accurate records of weight and reps for each work set performed?

e.  Does he consult his client's training log before each set, to ensure that the correct weight is selected? And does he carefully load the bar?

---

**If you cannot find a compatible and reliable regular training partner, and assuming that you use a public gym, at least work in with someone on each of your major exercises—for the safety that spotting should provide, and the extra motivation too.**

  f. Is he supportive, serious and respectful?

  g. Does he keep his charge's mind totally focused on the work at hand?

5.76 If he does not score positively on all these points, look elsewhere. If he scores well on these points but the deadlift, squat and some other major movements were not done in the workout you inspected, ask the trainer to demonstrate how he teaches those movements. Compare his instruction with what is described in THE INSIDER'S TELL-ALL HANDBOOK ON WEIGHT-TRAINING TECHNIQUE. If there are more than just minor differences, then look elsewhere for hands-on help with your lifting technique, though the trainer in question may be valuable in other areas.

## While training with a partner

5.77 Either of you could do the record keeping (poundages, sets and reps—in a training log) during the workout. Check the poundages you need set by set, and then verify that the resistance has been loaded correctly before performing any set. If there is a mistake you want to discover it before the set starts, not during it. Miscalculations can ruin sets and perhaps cause injuries; and regular errors will strain the relationship between you and your training partner or supervisor.

5.78 Treat your workouts as very serious working time. Get down to business and keep your training partner or supervisor at a distance. Keep your mind focused rigidly on your training.

## Some caveats

5.79 Do not let anyone push you to train before you have fully recovered from your previous session. Do not let anyone push you to perform exercises in ways that do not suit you. Do not let anyone add unplanned exercises to your program. Do not let anyone push you to abuse forced reps and negatives. If you allow a training partner or supervisor to do any of these things, then he is going to mar your progress, and possibly injure you and stymie your gains.

5.80 Work together in an intelligent way so you do what is best for *both* of you. You must avoid pushing each other to do things that are reckless. A training partner or supervisor can be invaluable for pointing out form errors, making suggestions, and helping you to improve your exercise technique. But that is different from pushing you to do something that will hurt you.

5.81    One of the potential problems from having a training partner is that his specific needs, limitations, strengths and weaknesses are different from yours. Be sure that your training program suits *you*, and that your training partner's program suits *him*. While your programs may be very similar, they are unlikely to be exactly the same. Never allow a training partner to oblige you to do something in your training that is not appropriate for you.

5.82    Remember that you must not become dependent on supervision. Always be able to train well by yourself. Have spells where you intentionally train by yourself, to be sure you can still deliver the goods alone.

## Daily review

5.83    For a few minutes every evening, review your day. Be sure you have a specific time you do this review. If you just leave it for when you can fit it in, you will end up not fitting it in.

5.84    Find out how you did in trying to make today another step towards achieving your next set of short-term goals. Have all of today's actions—training (if a training day), diet and rest— met or exceeded the goals for the day? If not, why not?

5.85    A daily critical analysis of what you did and did not do to take another step forward will help you to be more alert to improving tomorrow. Some days will be ruined by mini crises that destroy your good planning. When this happens, learn from how you coped—or did not, as the case may be—so that when something similar happens again, you are prepared for dealing with it.

5.86    Never miss this daily appointment with yourself. This will help to ensure—calamities excluded—that you always keep to your plan for training success. If you extend this daily review to other aspects of your life—especially work or business—you will find that it will help you there too.

5.87    Take as much control over your life as you can. Learn from your mistakes. Capitalize on the good things you have done. Do more of the positive things you are already doing, and fewer of the negative things.

## Putting it all together

5.88     The combination of a training diary, training partner or
         supervisor, and the daily review can bring about a huge
         increase in your training application. It can move you into
         another sphere of seriousness and organization.

5.89     But all of this is academic. You must supply the determination,
         hard work and persistence needed to make the organization
         deliver the goods. Most trainees have neither the organization
         needed for success, nor the will to push themselves very hard
         when they need to. These are demanding essentials—satisfy
         them, *now*, and then get on with achieving your potential. [BB]

---

### How to be a better spotter

The primary importance of spotting is the prevention
of injury. Good spotting also provides the security to
push yourself harder, because you know there is
someone to help if you get stuck. Acting as a spotter is
one of the major roles of a training partner. To get your
training partner's trust you must be a competent and
dependable spotter. Here are five tips:

a. Be honest with yourself, and respect your limitations.
   If you cannot spot adequately by yourself, get help.

b. Do not injure yourself! While spotting, keep an
   arched back, feet planted in a symmetrical way, and
   stand as close to the lifter as possible.

c. Know your partner's intentions prior to each set, e.g.,
   does he need help getting into the starting position?

d. Focus totally on what your partner is doing during
   each set. Cut yourself off from everything else.

e. Keep your hands close to the bar but without
   interfering with the exercise; and when needed, apply
   assistance with *both* hands in a *symmetrical* way.

*This book's companion text,* THE INSIDER'S TELL-ALL
HANDBOOK ON WEIGHT-TRAINING TECHNIQUE, *provides
specific tips on how to spot individual exercises.*

*At its basic minimum a good home gym takes up surprisingly little space and is less expensive than you may anticipate. Though an initial investment is involved, consider the gym fees you will not be paying, and the traveling time and expenses you will not have.*

# 6. Where to Train, and the Equipment You Need

6.1    A good barometer of an effective gym is its *sparsity* of equipment, and its insistence on basics, basics and nothing but basics for nearly all of a member's training. While some machines do offer good and safe alternatives to barbells and dumbbells, most gyms do not have this type of machinery.

6.2    If you train at a commercial gym you have no control over the equipment there unless you can influence the owner. But you do have control over what equipment you use, and how you use it. If you have a home gym you have control over the equipment stock and how you use it.

6.3    The information on equipment given later in this chapter is especially aimed at home gym users, to help with purchasing decisions. But if you use a commercial gym, the information still has value because it will teach you about equipment priorities, proper use, and safety.

6.4    If you cannot get well on the way to being Herculean using just a regular barbell, plates, flat bench, power rack, and maybe a Trap Bar, too (whether in a commercial gym or anywhere else), then even a gym equipped with every different piece of leading-brand training machinery would be unlikely to help you to build the physique and strength you want.

## Commercial and institutional gyms

6.5    Here are ten factors you need to avoid if you are to progress well in a commercial gym, or an institutional one such as a college gym. Only a *minority* of gyms are guilty of all of these shortcomings. But nearly all gyms are guilty of some of them. You may not be able to improve equipment deficiencies there, or correct attitude shortcomings of others; but by being well informed and applying yourself to your training with discipline, *all the other defects need not affect you*. It is even possible to turn a gym's shortcomings to your advantage. If the power rack and other basic equipment usually stand vacant, because an abundance of inferior gear distracts most members, then you will have little waiting time while you train.

### 1. A mainstream mentality

6.6    If the norm is to use lots of isolation exercises and standard split routines, and give supplements excessive attention, then sooner or later you are going to be pulled into the same way of thinking. This applies even though nearly all the drug-free advocates of this system never make much progress.

6.7    A related point is that it is in the financial interest of the gym owners to have you training many times each week. Consider that the more frequently you are in the gym the more drinks and other products you are likely to buy, and the more you will pay if fees are proportional to gym usage.

### 2. Gyms where there are resident awesome physiques

6.8    Awesome physiques—"awesome" as in 240+ pounds and under 5% bodyfat—can inspire discouragement because they are so far away from what a typical hard gainer can ever build. They may also motivate some of the dissatisfied to use drugs to try to compensate, to some degree, for genetic shortcomings.

6.9    Of those who do not get into drugs, many will be so disgusted with the mess of chemicals in bodybuilding and lifting that they will give up their training aspirations. Most of the balance of people that remains will follow the instruction received from the gym, which is usually a watered down version of the training that works for the elite. This will result in adding ever more names to the huge roll of weight-training failures.

### 3. Gyms with resident or visiting drug peddlers

6.10    Feeding on the dissatisfaction bred by the resident awesome physiques, and the general ineffectiveness of conventional training routines, drug sellers may find many customers.

### 4. Instructors who know nothing about training hard gainers

6.11    Ignore the certificates for pseudo qualifications that decorate gym walls. And be especially suspicious about instruction for typical members that comes from awesome builds. Anyone who has an awesome physique can *never* get into the shoes of a very hard gainer who may never be able to build muscular 16-inch arms. Yet these awesome physiques successfully present themselves as instructors for the masses.

## 5. Gyms full of distractions

6.12    What with music blaring, social gatherings in the gym, and too many sensual sights to catch people's attention, it is almost impossible to keep one's mind on where it needs to be for serious training. Ideally you need an environment free of distractions. Squeezing out the final few reps in a set is darned hard work. What you do not need are distractions that prevent you from pushing yourself through to the end of a set.

## 6. Equipment shortcomings

6.13    Any equipment other than the basics nearly always serves to divert attention from where most application should be given (for typical hard gainers, that is). Put pec deck, cable crossover, leg extension and hack squat machines in a gym, for example, and all the most underdeveloped members will be eager to use the gear, "like the big guys do." Overwhelmed with so many different pieces of equipment, not only do members lose sight of training priorities, but so do gym owners and instructors. Spoil trainees for choice, and you spoil their progress too.

6.14    Having inferior equipment as well as well-maintained basic training gear gives you a choice. But if there is no squat rack or power rack, and the free-weights equipment is poorly maintained, you do not have a choice at that gym and need to look elsewhere.

6.15    The great advantage of a very well-equipped gym is that it is likely to have a power rack, squat rack and other important basic items, and maybe some of the better pieces of high-tech machinery. Ironically, the gym with the greatest source of potential distractions may actually be your best bet because among its abundance of gear is what you really need. But you need to be very knowledgeable and highly disciplined to be able to train there without getting distracted and confused.

## 7. Self-consciousness

6.16    If you are training in an unusual way relative to regular conventions, as you must be if you are to pack muscle on a hard-gaining body, you are going to feel self-conscious if you are the only one in the gym training that way. This is especially so if you are a beginner or intermediate. This will likely make you uncomfortable and weaken your resolve to stay the course.

## 8. Excessive focus on food supplements

6.17    Selling food supplements offers a very lucrative sideline for a gym. Supplements are often promoted hard, and in some cases presented as cure-alls for training woes. I am not saying that all supplements offer no nutritional value. Many do have nutritional value, but that does not mean they will necessarily improve your training progress.

6.18    Supplements will never be the answer to training problems. But because supplements are promoted by some people, either implicitly or explicitly, as being quick fixes, then of course gym members' attention is going to be diverted from the things that matter most.

6.19    Until you can get the basic package of training, food and rest to deliver good steady gains in muscle and might, forget about any fine-tuning with supplements.

## 9. Short-term vested interests of gym owners

6.20    So many gyms are ruled by short-term income at the expense of their members' long-term progress. Personalized and quality instruction is non-existent. Members are encouraged to buy worthless products. The gyms are unable to deliver good results for most of their members. Stress is given to getting new members to fill the gaps left by dissatisfied former members. This further encourages a rapid turnover in membership, and the neglect of the long-term interests of each member.

## 10. Bullies and show-offs

6.21    Unsympathetic and disrespectful people who hog equipment, do not allow beginners to have their turns on time, and pass

> Do you really have some progress in muscle and might to show for your efforts in the gym over the last few months? If not, your training is not working and it is time to make major changes—time to try the advice given in this book. Time is pressing!

belittling comments about others' lesser builds, only serve to alienate people. Some gyms have plenty of this kind, often drug fed, which reinforces the belief that a commercial gym can be a very poor place to go to if you want to build a good physique. Steroids enhance the aggressive anti-social attitude.

## The two sides of weight training

6.22    On the one side weight training is a marvelous activity in which you compare yourself only with bettering yourself. It is a potentially healthy and long-term activity, a joy to train, and so satisfying to see strength gains and physique improvement. On the other hand you have the egotistical, look-at-me, short-term, drug-infested, all-appearance-and-no-substance destructive side of weight training. It is theoretically possible to get into the former in any gym setting. But to be able to do it in a potentially destructive commercial setting demands that you are extremely well informed and disciplined.

6.23    If you are serious about training in the best possible way for you, and putting aside all distractions and mischief makers, you have three choices:

   a.  Find a good commercial gym. Though good commercial gyms exist, they are in short supply and probably cannot be found in your locality.

   b.  Train in a home gym or small multi-user facility.

   c.  Go to whatever gym is available and make the best of it.

### How to make a commercial gym work for you

6.24    It is not practical for many people to set up a home gym or a small multi-user gym. They have to make do with what is available. And perhaps some people cannot motivate themselves to train alone at home, in which case they probably cannot motivate themselves to train hard anywhere on a long-term basis.

6.25    If you have to make do with whatever gym is available, here is how to make it work for you:

   a.  Try to train at the quietest time.

   b.  Take your own little discs and chalk if the gym has none.

    c. Keep your mind on your training and stay clear of distractions.

    d. Learn from this book how to train, and then get on with applying what you have learned.

    e. Never forget that you are there to train yourself using an abbreviated and basics-first approach. You are not there to copy others in order to feel at ease through conformity.

    f. Avoid arguments to defend your style of training.

    g. Never use any equipment just because it is there. Only use what is best for you.

    h. Ignore anything and anyone that will hinder your progress. *You* are in charge of your training. Never surrender that authority to others.

    i. Persuade the gym's management to buy a Trap Bar and a cambered squat bar, and a power rack if it does not already have one. Both bars are inexpensive relative to machines, and will add greatly to the gym's functional value for all members. If the management is not open minded, offer to buy one of the bars in return for a discount on membership. Win the management over on one bar, and perhaps it will get the other.

## Setting up a home gym

6.26    For those who have the means—location and funding—the home gym is a great way to go. Even if you have always thought a home gym to be out of the question, reconsider. The advantages you get from a home gym are so profuse and profound that, if you are serious about training, you should do your utmost to get one.

6.27    At its basic minimum a good home gym takes up surprisingly little space and is less expensive than you may anticipate. Though an initial investment is involved, consider the gym fees you will not be paying, and the traveling time and expenses you will not have. Also keep in mind that you can use the gear for the rest of your life and may pass it onto your offspring. It is a long-term investment that does not wear out. Unless you get into buying equipment you do not really need, your home

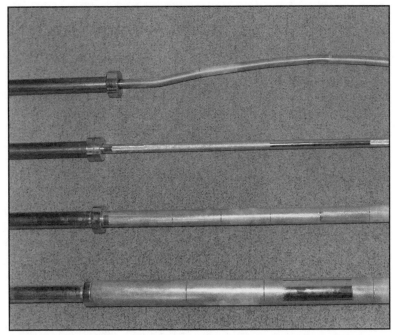

*A comparison of four different long bars. From the top: cambered squat bar, standard Olympic bar, 2-inch diameter bar, and 3-inch diameter bar.*

gym will pay for itself after a few years, or perhaps less time, depending also on the cost of where you currently train.

6.28    If you pool your resources with those of a few other like-minded trainees, you can all have access to a terrific training den with very little money outlay from any one of you. You need to agree on the location of the gym. Put it in someone's spare room, basement or garage, so you have no rent to cover.

6.29    Being oversupplied with equipment in commercial gyms colors people's minds to think that a lot of equipment is needed to get big and strong. In a mere 7-foot x 10-foot space you can get enough equipment to get you about as big and strong as you are ever going to get. You do not need a whole room for your home gym—a portion of a room you use for something else can be adequate. I have trained in a 7-foot x 10-foot space and managed to include a full-size power rack, an Olympic bar, a bench, a weight tree, and a few small accessories. Two people could train in such a space, alternating sets, and three could fit in, though it would be cramped.

6.30    The minimum equipment investment for providing a great
        variety of productive training opportunities is:

        a.  A bar and plates, including little discs.

        b.  A reliable method of self-spotting and securely setting up
            a barbell in some sort of stands, e.g., a four-post power
            rack, a half rack, or sturdy and stable squat stands
            together with spotter/safety racks or bars.

        c.  A sturdy and stable bench.

6.31    As time goes by, add a Trap Bar, an overhead pulley and/or an
        overhead bar, a pair of adjustable dumbbells, parallel bars for
        dips, a cambered squat bar, a few specialized items for grip
        work, a *heavy-duty* adjustable bench, and a 2-inch thick bar.
        Then you will have a gem of a gym.

## A bare minimum

6.32    You can train very effectively even without a rack, safety bars,
        straight bar or bench, if you do not do squats or bench presses.
        Trap Bar bent-legged deadlifts, plus chins and dips, cover most
        of the body's musculature. (The Trap Bar, comparing equal
        strength of bars, is cheaper than an Olympic bar. The Trap Bar
        has no revolving sleeves.) Just those three exercises, if worked
        progressively and for enough months, can produce a lot of
        muscle. Overhead presses with the Trap Bar could be done too.
        Some method of getting the Trap Bar into the starting position
        would be necessary, though, because the rhombus-shaped bar
        cannot be cleaned to the shoulders like a straight bar can.

6.33    This equipment bare minimum could be the perfect starting
        point for a very productive home gym where economy is the
        priority, and space is very tight.

## Bars and plates

6.34    Bars come in different varieties, qualities and prices. There are
        Olympic bars, power bars, exercise bars, cambered bars, and the
        Trap Bar. Of course all of them are used for exercising, but the
        "exercise" bars are for use with "exercise" plates, i.e., the ones
        that have small-diameter holes (usually about 1.125 inches) and
        thus the bars have ends a little smaller, at 1–1.0625 inches, to fit
        in the plates. Olympic and power bars manufactured according
        to the specifications of the International Weightlifting

Federation are 220 centimeters long, with a sleeve diameter of 50 millimeters. They have revolving sleeves and large-diameter ends to take plates bored with holes 2 inches in diameter (or slightly bigger, depending on the manufacturer).

6.35    Because of inconsistencies between manufacturers of bars and plates, you may get plates (and collars) that are a tad too tight for your bar. Take your plates (and perhaps collars too) to a local machine shop and get the holes bored a little bigger.

6.36    At the most expensive end of the market are the elite Olympic bars, including Eleiko® and Ivanko®. But most of the Olympic-size bars around today are poor and weak imitations, so as to be much cheaper. If a bar bends as you are lifting, it could cause a serious loss of form, and injury. You would also end up with a useless bar.

6.37    For big poundages you need a good quality bar. You do not have to jump to an elite bar to get a good quality one, but you need to get something a lot better than the cheapest bar you can find. Several manufacturers, e.g., York®, produce quality bars that are moderately priced. For serious Olympic lifting even the moderately priced bars may be unsuitable because they do not flex during lifting under load, as Olympic weightlifters want a bar to. A bar that flexes must, however, return to being perfectly straight after use. *Flexion does not mean that the bar stays bent.*

6.38    For the squat, center knurling on the bar will help greatly to keep the bar from slipping while on your traps.

6.39    Plates come with large- and small-diameter holes, and either in plain metal, with rubber coating (bumper plates), or in total rubber. The cheap plates in particular are notoriously off weight. The rubber plates are cheaper than the bumper plates, a lot thicker (a York solid rubber 45-pound plate is 5 inches in width), but will not damage the plates, bar or floor if the loaded barbell is dropped. They also make for quieter training. To get the advantages of rubber plates not damaging the floor, and making less noise than metal ones, you may only need one pair of rubber plates per bar. This only applies so long as the metal plates on the bar are of smaller diameter than the rubber ones. Alternatively, use solid-metal plates and do your lifting on some thick rubber matting, for shock absorption. But if you are using good form and controlling the bar properly, and not using the Olympic lifts, you should not be dropping the bar anyway, though you should be prepared in case you do.

6.40    Take care of your bars. If you regularly wipe an oily rag over the sleeves, this will help reduce the wear on the chrome from the friction between bar and plates. Also regularly check that the sleeves are securely fastened.

## Bench, rack and stands

6.41    If a flat bench weighs about 50 pounds, or more, then it is probably a fine bench. You want weight, stability and comfort (i.e., not too much width). For very heavy use, a flat bench of 70 pounds or more would be a wise choice. If you get an adjustable bench—for incline work, and back support while performing seated presses—get a heavy-duty one with an adjustable seat. There are many flimsy adjustable benches, often coming with attachments that distract from the exercises that really matter.

6.42    A power rack is perfect for self-spotting and safety. You can even do all your long-bar exercises inside the rack. If you set the pins/rods just below the lowest point of each exercise, the rack will catch the bar should you fail on a bench press or squat, for example. Do not touch the bar to the pins unless you are intentionally doing each rep from a stationary start at the bottom, or if you fail on a rep and have to set the bar down.

6.43    Using a tape measure, work out exactly where your bench needs to rest to be perfectly centered in the rack. Mark the base of the rack accordingly, so you never need to fiddle around getting the bench centered when it is time to bench press.

6.44    Number the holes in all the rack's uprights (either directly on the rack, or using masking tape), so it is easy to put a pin through holes at the same height. You also need to have the holes numbered so that you can keep notes of which setting(s) you need to use for a given exercise.

6.45    The power rack can be used for pullups/chins, by setting the saddles high enough so that a bar in position can function as a chinning bar. (A rack, because of its width, requires a full-length bar—e.g., an Olympic bar.) Some power racks have an integral chinning bar. Even a lat-machine pulley can be built into a power rack.

6.46    There are alternatives to a power rack. You can use a half or
        open power rack, or a pair of heavy, stable and adjustable
        squat racks or stands (which are not only for squats) together
        with a pair of adjustable and robust spotter racks. A power
        rack and half rack are the more versatile options. The power
        rack might be considered safer, as it offers horizontal obstacles
        to bar movement should you lose control.

6.47    Consider having a power rack made locally—see the design on
        page 169. Box section of 60 x 60 x 5 mm would be perfect.

## Other equipment

6.48    A weight tree/plate holder is convenient for storing your
        plates when they are not in use, but is not a necessity. You can
        always rest plates against a wall (first protecting the wall and
        floor against damage, unless you have bumper plates or rubber
        ones). If you have the option, get a weight tree with a chalk
        dish built into it on its highest point.

6.49    An adjustable dumbbell is a valuable addition, at least for side
        bends (though a barbell can be used), one-legged calf work,
        and external rotator work for the shoulders, all of which are
        important exercises. If you have an Olympic bar and plates,
        the regular dumbbell rod will be too narrow for your plates.
        You will need to buy narrow-holed plates for the dumbbell
        bars (smooth-sided plates take up the least amount of space),
        or get a local metal worker to weld a tube around the
        dumbbell bars' ends to fit the Olympic plates. If you are
        feeling flush, you could buy dumbbell rods especially for
        Olympic plates. Another option is buying spiral-lock dumbbell
        rods. These make plate changing easy. Whatever option you
        use, be sure to use secure collars so that the dumbbells do not
        come apart during use.

6.50    There are two basic types of collars. One type has some
        mechanism that needs to be tightened before the collars are
        secured in place. These collars come in different sizes and
        variations. The other basic variety is the spring type where
        nothing has to be screwed into place. Instead, the handles are
        squeezed together while the collar is slipped into place, and
        then the tension on the handles is released to secure the
        collars. The latter are easier to use, but have only a limited
        use. For dumbbells, and for barbell exercises where a lot of
        weight is used and/or there is a lot of movement of the

plates (e.g., when the plates touch the floor on each rep), the heavy-duty collars that lock the plates firmly together are a necessity for safety.

6.51    For calf work you will need a raised platform or box to stand on for full extension, or use a staircase or other improvisation.

6.52    A Trap Bar is essential in my view, and a lat-machine is very valuable. Some other equipment will help over the long term, especially a cambered bar and thick bar. But most other gear is usually a distraction that will only hinder your progress.

## High-tech equipment

6.53    On the high-tech side there are several possible additions, money permitting and once you have already acquired the essentials of a good home gym. A leg press and a pullover machine can be fine additions. Hammer Strength® makes some very good machines as do Southern Xercise®, MedX® and Nautilus®. The Tru-Squat® from Southern Xercise is an especially good machine, particularly if you cannot squat safely with a barbell. But it is also an excellent machine for trainees who *can* squat safely with a barbell. The Tru-Squat can be much more valuable than a leg press, because the former involves more musculature and produces a greater overall anabolic effect.

6.54    If you are considering purchasing a high-tech machine, test it first, preferably at a gym where you can use it regularly for a while. Testing it once, unless the machine obviously does not fit you, is unlikely to teach you much about its potential for causing chronic irritation, or even injury over the longer term. Ideally, and if possible, try several models/brands before you make a purchase. A machine that may be great for one person may be harmful for another.

## Gym table

6.55    Place a small table in a corner of your home gym, primarily to use for entering data into your training log. Alternatively, use a sturdy shelf. Your training log is a very important item and as such should have a special location reserved for it.

6.56    Keep the table or shelf tidy, and use the space alongside the training log for your chalk (in a bowl of some sort), and any reference material you need to keep at hand. Keep a large bottle of pure water there for ready access between sets.

6.57    The table or shelf could also be where you keep the tools you need to have at hand, for tightening nuts and bolts on a power rack, collars on dumbbells, or whatever else that needs regular adjustment. These tools may include an adjustable wrench, and Allen/hex wrenches of the appropriate sizes. Further, and not just for home gym use, keep a tape measure handy for when you may need to check, for example, if you have a bench or bar centered correctly in a rack.

## Accessory items

6.58    Have a specific location for storing each accessory piece of training gear, be it a lifting belt, clean towel, specialized grip item (wrist roller, deadlift handle, pinch block), weight holder for dips and chins, etc. A number of pegs on a board fixed to a wall is ideal for hanging a number of small and lightweight items on. A clock on the wall is a good idea.

6.59    A full-length mirror can help you to master exercise form, at least in some exercises, because you can see what you are doing.

## Key purchasing decisions

6.60    For exercises where you are not going to be handling more than around 200 pounds, even a cheap Olympic or power bar (or exercise bar) will be adequate. There is nothing magical about an Olympic bar. It just has revolving sleeves that make for smoother and easier handling, relative to the plain one-piece exercise bar. But for heavier exercises you *must* have a quality bar that is not going to bend.

6.61    Rather than start with a shoddy bar and later move to a quality bar, start with a good bar. While you can manage well with one good bar, you will find a second bar useful—to spare you from having to keep stripping the same bar down.

6.62    If money is tight, rather than get a second regular-diameter straight bar, you would be better served by getting a Trap Bar.

6.63    If you are into Olympic weightlifting, you will need a bar that has the necessary flexibility, together with the smoother revolving sleeves of the higher priced Olympic bars. But if you are not into the very quick lifts—and you are unlikely to be if you are reading this book—then a good quality power bar (or a one-piece exercise bar) will do fine. You will not want the bar to flex much as you lift.

6.64     Shop around for a barbell set, or buy bar and plates separately. Get enough plates—appropriate for the diameter of the bar(s) you choose—to cover your immediate needs, and add to them as required. Hunt around for a robust power rack (or half rack, or squat stands and a pair of self-spotting stands) and a heavy-duty bench. Examine what you are considering buying, or buy from a reputable mail-order function-and-durability-first supplier. Never buy flimsy, lightweight gear. Prices vary and so does quality. Price tends to go with quality, but not necessarily so. Compare different brands for quality and price.

6.65     Do not consider buying something so shoddy that it could let you down and cause an accident. And if you buy something as a temporary measure, but plan to buy something of better quality later on, that is probably going to be false economy.

## Home gym location

6.66     If possible, choose a place that has good ventilation. You may need a fan in the summer, if you live in a warm climate, and some form of heating to take the chill off the room during the winter. If the lighting is poor, e.g., in a basement, then invest in some good lighting, for practicality and safety. Whatever space you use, work on it to make it really look like a small gym. Fix the floor, walls and ceiling. You will come to love the little place, so fix it up right from the start.

6.67     A room of its own is best, and more space is better than less. But a home gym does not have to have a room entirely for itself. As noted earlier, productive training quarters can occupy as little as 7-foot x 10-foot.

6.68     If the floor is wooden, pay attention to where you put your heavy gear. Away from the center of the room and next to walls will be best, and a smaller room will be an advantage as far as the strength of the wooden floor is concerned.

## Horizontal training area

6.69     Hardly anyone checks to see that they are training on a horizontal surface. Go to the trouble of checking it. While a concrete floor should be horizontal, a wooden floor or lifting platform may not be. If you are squatting or deadlifting on a floor or platform that is slightly higher on one side than the other, you are going to be applying skewed stress on your body. It could be enough to throw your form and cause an injury if you are used to a perfectly horizontal surface. Over the long term it could even cause a chronic condition.

6.70    If you use a machine, e.g., a leg press, then its base needs to be positioned perfectly horizontally; otherwise, you will distort the stresses of the movement and invite trouble.

## Surface to train on

6.71    It is very important you stand on a non-slip surface that "gives" while you train, especially for exercises where you have weights overhead or over your shoulders. This spares your joints from having to do all the giving. Do not train directly on concrete.

6.72    If you plan to train on a carpeted and/or wooden floor, or a concrete one, cover at least part of it with a sturdy shallow wooden platform (or thick rubber flooring) for performing your standing exercises on. This will spare your joints, floor, carpet and weights from damage, spread the load from the weights when they contact the floor (very important if you train on a wooden floor), and also reduce the noise you make in your gym.

6.73    For deadlifts, especially rest-pause ones, the plates easily roll on a smooth floor, and necessitate that you reposition for every rep. Of course you should always check that your feet are in the right position relative to the bar before performing a deadlift rep (whether with a straight bar or Trap Bar), and adjust them if need be. This rolling of the plates can be minimized by deadlifting on some hard-wearing carpet or rubber fixed to a wooden surface. Two squares of plywood with a carpet or rubber surface would serve you well. Place the squares so the plates contact them between reps. Because of the give in the carpet or rubber, the plates stay somewhat stuck to the floor during the pause between reps, so long as form is good when the bar is set down.

6.74    If you do all your barbell exercises inside a power rack (other than Trap Bar deadlifts, which cannot be done in a rack), you need never set a loaded straight barbell on the floor. Instead, position the rack pins so that you can put your bar down on the pins between sets, and even between reps during rest-pause work. This teaches good form and controlled reps, and prevents the barbell from being dropped on the floor.

6.75    Keeping the plates off the floor also makes plate changing easy because you do not have to lift the end of the bar in order to unload or load the largest diameter plates.

6.76    If you have to load or unload a heavy barbell that rests on the floor, lift the end up and slip a disc underneath the inside plate. The raised end will make plate changing much easier. A better way, if available, is to use a device that levers the bar off the floor, and holds it in position while you load or unload plates. When loading a vertical bar—e.g., for a plate-loading lat machine—put plates on with the smallest at the bottom, or alternate a large diameter plate with a smaller diameter one. This makes it easier to unload the plates.

## Satisfaction

6.77    Having your own gym will be a source of pride and pleasure. Look after the place, as simple as it may be. Keep it tidy and clean. That little or not-so-little training den will become very precious, and over the years you will spend a sizeable chunk of your life there. It will become a sanctuary from the trials and tribulations of life. Time spent there will be valued much more than time spent at a commercial gym. The convenience is terrific, and no longer will you have to put up with the elements that bothered you in a commercial gym.

6.78    Be careful that you do not get so overwhelmed with the convenience aspect that you lose your regularity of training. Because you can always train tomorrow does not mean that you should become a procrastinator. If it is training day today, and so long as you feel well recovered from your previous workout, then train today.

6.79    This is where a home gym offers great convenience. It simplifies how you fix your training days. For example, it becomes easy to train every fourth day, which may be impossible to coordinate with the schedule required by your work and the hours of a commercial gym.

6.80    Be careful that you do not do extra work on your planned rest days. Because you will always have the training equipment at hand, it may be tempting to visit your home gym and get in some extra training. This is a road to ruin. Devise a first-class training program of workout days and rest days, and stick to it.

6.81    A home gym makes practical some types of training programs that would be impractical if you had to depend on a gym away from home. For example, an advanced interpretation of rest-pause training could have you performing a near-limit single every hour for say ten consecutive hours. That would be your day's workout, spread over most of the waking day. Time it for a day you spend at home. As another example you may want to train each exercise apart from the others in your program. To spread your training out over the course of a single day is not practical at a commercial gym, but it is practical at a home gym so long as you are home all day on the days concerned.

6.82    Training should always be a joy, though darn hard work. But when you train in your own private gym, and can do what you want to without interruptions from others, it should become a greater joy. And it may be the most productive training you ever do, so long as you apply the heightened focus to good routines.

6.83    With your own gear you can venture outdoors for some variety when the weather is suitable. Do not try to take your power rack outdoors, but getting your bar and some plates out to do your deadlifts, curls and rows under sunshine and a blue sky may help motivate you to pull out a corker of a workout.

## Equipment control

6.84    If you want to use the Trap Bar, cambered bar and thick bar, and perform feats of grip strength, then a membership-gym will cramp your training. While you can take your own small plates to a commercial gym, taking your own Trap Bar, cambered bar, thick bar and various grip devices is not practical. (But you may be able to persuade the gym's management to improve its equipment line.) Many large training facilities do not even have a power rack, so to use that great piece of equipment you may need to get your own.

6.85    Once you have your own home gym, get acquainted with a local competent metal worker. You can then have simple pieces of training gear produced conveniently, economically and to your own design.

6.86    A home gym opens new avenues of training because some of the best equipment you can get is, paradoxically, not available in public gyms, e.g., the Trap Bar. Your own gym enables you to use the gear you want, rather than be limited by a commercial gym's equipment. A home gym gives *you* control over *your* training.

6.87    An aspect of this control is that you determine how you perform a given exercise, not the commercial gym or its traditions. For example, suppose you have discovered you cannot safely squat to parallel. If you train at a gym where anyone who does not go to below parallel is considered a wimp, you may be pressured into squatting too deep and suffering a serious injury. In your home gym, you train as you know you should, not as others think you should.

## Domestic delight

6.88    With a home gym you are set up for getting family members involved in training, though not all at the same time. This is perhaps the best way to win people over to your preoccupation with training—get them training themselves. With the convenience of a home gym there is little or none of the self-consciousness an untrained person feels in a commercial setting. You will therefore find more potential trainees than if the commercial gym route was the only option.

6.89    For family people, a home gym keeps you at home for your training, eliminates travelling time, and gives you more time for family matters. While you need to avoid being disturbed while you train, other than for emergencies, your family will probably appreciate having you home more of the time.

## Support gear

6.90    Regardless of where you train, the use of support gear is a possibility. If used it can easily become a crutch that is difficult to rid yourself of.

6.91    You may be able to add about 100 pounds to the *total* of your best squat and bench press singles, but without building any strength or adding any muscle. Just become an expert with the use of a squat suit, knee wraps, a thick belt, and a bench shirt. This serves no function other than removing an advantage your competitors would have should you be lifting in powerlifting contests. As they prepare for a contest, powerlifters must use all the support gear that is legal. At other times, though, and for all non-competitive powerlifters, train without support gear other than perhaps a belt.

6.92    A belt can help to prevent injuries to the lower back, especially if you have previously had problems there. But it cannot help you much unless it is very tight. A tight belt is uncomfortable, so cannot be used for high-rep work. Strong torso musculature, especially the midsection, is your own natural belt. Be sure to train your midsection seriously and progressively.

6.93    A belt, if used, should not be on for every exercise or every set. It should not be worn as part of the trainee's "uniform." Use it selectively—for low-rep squats and deadlifts, and overhead presses—or not at all. Otherwise, you will become dependent on it to generate the necessary intra-abdominal pressure you need to protect your spinal column during heavy lifting; and without that armor you will be a shadow of your usual self.

6.94    If you are used to wearing a belt for all your heaviest lifting, do not lift heavily without it. Start a new cycle with reduced poundages, and no belt, and build back your poundages over time. Then you can safely condition your belt-free body to lift increasingly heavier weights. Eventually, and belt-free, you can return to your belt-assisted poundages, but you will need a few months to do it.

6.95    Wrist straps and hooks, though illegal for competition lifting, are used by many people in their regular training. These are temptations that are best avoided or else you will become dependent on them for some exercises. Instead, invest the time and effort needed to build a grip to hold the bar with no assistance other than the use of lifters' chalk, which is a recommended support aid.

6.96    Using straps and hooks to tie yourself to bigger weights than you could otherwise handle, can be dangerous. There is a risk of injury because of a large weight increase without the necessary strength having been built up in the involved joints and connective tissue. For example, you need extra strength in your elbows and shoulders when performing the deadlift and pulldown with substantially more weight. If you add 50 pounds and 25 pounds respectively, in one jump each, you are asking for injury. Never impose a sudden big increase in load. ▪▪

*Please pause for a couple of minutes to ponder upon the following two paragraphs, and let their message sink in so deep so that you will never forget it.*

*Never bemoan the discipline that must accompany serious training. Never bemoan the discipline that must be applied to your diet and other components of recovery. To have the opportunity to apply all this discipline is a blessing. Appreciate it, and savor every moment of implementing that discipline.*

*You will not be able to train forever. Eventually you will not be able to apply dedication and determination to anything, let alone your training, diet and recovery. So be sure you make the absolute most of the present!*

# Section 2

## How to train

No matter what your individuality, there is so much to learn from this book on how to make the most of your training.

This book can save you years if not decades of wasted training toil. It will propel you into the practical know-how needed to turn even a novice into a tremendously informed bodybuilder or strength trainee. Then apply it and you will develop a degree of muscle and might that will make a mockery of what you would have realized had you stayed with conventional training methods.

Put what this book teaches into disciplined, diligent and persistent practice. Please do not just study this book, grasp why conventional training is useless for most people, learn how to train properly, but then not apply what you have discovered. Time is pressing!

# 7. How to Set Up Your Training Cycles for Big Returns

7.1    While there are many effective interpretations of a training cycle, there are fundamental components common to each. The better your grasp of these components the better equipped you will be to fine-tune the routines in this book to fit your individual needs and limitations.

7.2    Successful weight training in its various forms is about progressive resistance. Despite this being so obviously central to training, its implications so often go ignored or only barely noticed. Successful training is about making lots of small bits of progress, with all the bits adding up to huge improvement. To achieve this you must have persistence galore, patience in abundance, and revel in knocking off each little bit of accumulation. Concentrate on knocking off one little bit at a time, and long-term success almost takes care of itself.

7.3    While dramatic progress in a short period of time can happen even to typical hard gainers, it is not how most progress is made. If you are new to a very effective mode of training, and are a good way from realizing your ultimate potential, then you *can* greatly increase your muscle and might over 4–6 months. Striking examples include raw beginners in general, first uses of abbreviated training following years of stagnation on conventional training schedules, and first encounters with the correct use of a power rack. For most intermediate and advanced trainees, however, think over the long term for making substantial gains—slow but steady progress.

7.4    Slowly, steadily, safely and surely enforces productive behavior, both when training and when out of the gym. Keep to the rules and you will keep making progress year after year. Break the rules and you invite stagnation, frustration, regression, injury, and failure. This is the lot of most typical gym members who, in their hurry to make short-term metamorphoses, turn short-term failure into long-term failure, and add more names to the endless roll of those who have trained but yet got little or nothing to show for it.

7.5     Here is memorable advice from Peary Rader, founder of IRON MAN magazine back in the thirties. It came during an interview late in his life, published in IRON MAN, November 1986, page 37. Rader was asked, "But, what do you consider the single most important rule to remember during a workout?"

> Always err on the side of conservatism. Even if you know you can do better, drop back to the point where you are using just a bit less weight or doing one or two reps less than you had planned to do. Then, every week or two, gradually increase your sets, reps or weight.

7.6     Later in the interview he returned to the theme of conservatism:

> Yes, you have to work very hard but you do have to work within your ability and capacity to recover before your next workout...People who promise shortcuts in time and effort are among the worst abusers of the interest of weight training.

7.7     The fastest progress is made by having the longest possible stretch of consecutive full-bore workouts, greatest possible frequency of training, and largest possible weight increments. But in practice the "fastest possible" is usually very slow.

7.8     Full-bore workouts are no good if you are not increasing your poundages regularly. Progressive poundages are the barometer of progress, not effort per se. It is possible to work yourself into the ground but not train progressively. It is also possible to keep poundages progressive without working yourself into the ground every workout. Properly applied effort is what is needed, not effort pure and simple.

7.9     The greatest number of consecutive full-bore workouts is no good if you are not recovering fully from each of them. You need to adapt your training intensity and frequency so that you are getting stronger on a consistent basis, albeit slowly. If you push too hard and too quickly, not only will you not go forward, but you may regress. You need to cycle your training intensity to some degree.

## Criticism of cycling

7.10    The practice of cycling training intensity involves "down time" when no effort is made to produce new gains in muscular size and strength. There is some detraining because, by cutting back, you get a little weaker than your previous best, before pushing again to go into new (for you) poundage territory.

7.11    Taken to its extreme, i.e., if you cut back too much and for too long, cycling is a disaster. *Do not abuse cycling.* A six-month "perfectly" organized stretch that brings you to a peak for just two new-ground workouts is a perversion of cycling. You need to train very hard for a darn sight more than a few weeks out of every twenty-six—for most of your workouts, in fact.

7.12    Some people see intensity cycling as a waste of time because they think that the more hard workouts they have, the better. They are so eager to get training flat-out, or very near to it, that they never develop the gaining momentum needed for long-term progress. Also, by dropping right into full-bore work, how are exercise form and mental concentration going to be learned or reviewed, and then perfected?

7.13    While you should push yourself to the limit for most of your workouts, "most" does not mean "all." Learn *not* to push yourself to the limit during some periods. This is difficult to do if you have been locked into the "hard all the time" philosophy.

7.14    Those who try to train full-bore all of the time have a built-in natural cycling format, whether they like it or not. Is there any typical working and family person who can train full-bore two or three times each week for fifty-two weeks of the year while being 100% healthy, 100% motivated for every single session, and not having work or family circumstances disrupt training? The disruptions and constraints of life force people to have ups and downs in their training, giving it a natural cycling format.

7.15    The typical adult—i.e., someone who is none of the following: very young, genetically better-than-average, superbly supervised, free of demanding work and family obligations—is best off slotting into a formal but not-too-rigid cycling format along the lines described in this book. It gives a structure that almost guarantees training success.

7.16    Never mind that in some circles cycling is all about drug dosage. In other words the most intensive training and heaviest drug use coincide, and the low-intensity phase coincides with the period off drugs. Some abusers, however, even take drugs when they are "off," because they lose so much size otherwise.

## Cycle breakdown

7.17    Focusing on the single-progression scheme—fixed target reps for each exercise, though not necessarily the same rep target for each exercise—here is a breakdown of a cycle. The breakdown applies to the double-progression scheme, too, but instead of frequently adding a little weight you add larger amounts much less frequently. In the weeks between the poundage increments in the double-progression method, you build up your reps from the low end of your rep range to the upper end.

### a. Preparation, and form consolidation

7.18    The first stage of a training cycle, following a layoff for 7–10 days in order to get fully rested and recovered from your previous cycle, has you using weights 10–15% lighter than your most recent best working poundages. This gives you a running start. With the stress at this stage not being on squeezing out all possible reps, you can focus on developing (or consolidating, if your form is already good) perfect exercise technique and rep grooves, and excellent concentration. In addition, your mind and body get a break from full-bore training.

7.19    One of the many snags of jumping straight into full-bore work for a new program is that exercise form is not well learned or consolidated, and it quickly breaks down to some degree, inviting injury. This especially applies to people who train without hands-on expert coaching—i.e., nearly all trainees.

7.20    Your training volume, unless you are a rank beginner, may be at its greatest during the first few weeks of a cycle, though still modest relative to the norms of conventional training. As the severity of training increases over the course of the cycle, the volume of work may be reduced in terms of the number of work sets you do for each exercise, the number of exercises you perform, and perhaps the frequency of training.

## b. Second stage

7.21    Over the first stage of a cycle the poundages are quite quickly built back to about 95% of your previous best working weights. Then during the next stage you take a few weeks to creep back to your previous best working poundages. Taking your time like this, using little discs, enables you to return to your best weights without feeling that you are at the limit of your abilities. This sets the scene for many weeks of venturing into new poundage territory.

7.22    As always, your barometer of progress is poundage progression. If the poundage gains are not coming, then cut back your training volume by reducing total sets and/or exercises, and perhaps by training less frequently. Less work but harder work, and less total demand upon your recuperative abilities, will usually get the poundage progression back on track.

7.23    During the early stage of a cycle you may find that one exercise (or more than one) is (or are) out of step with what you had planned. If so, reduce the weight on the exercise(s) that is (or are) too difficult for that part of the cycle, to get all your exercises moving along at a similar degree of difficulty.

## c. Growth stage

7.24    This is the most important stage of each cycle, and what you have been preparing for during the other stages. Prepare well, and then give your absolute all to ensure that you extend the growth stage for as long as possible and milk it dry of gains. The preparatory first and second stages are easy relative to the rigors of the growth stage.

7.25    Each training program has its core exercises. Here are five sets of examples, one with just two core exercises, and the rest with three:

> **The fastest possible rate of progress can be made by having the longest possible stretch of consecutive full-bore workouts, the greatest possible frequency of training, and the largest possible poundage increments. But in practice the "fastest possible" is usually very slow.**

          a.  Trap Bar (bent-legged) deadlift and parallel bar dip
          b.  Trap Bar (bent-legged) deadlift, incline press and pullup
          c.  squat, bench press and partial deadlift
          d.  squat, prone row and parallel bar dip
          e.  squat, incline press and pullup

7.26     If you are gaining in your core exercises for a given cycle, you will be gaining in size and strength generally. The core movements are what you need to focus on as the cycle gets ever more heavier and demanding, and closes in on its end.

7.27     The secondary exercises should not restrict progress in the core movements when you are focusing on building mass. Ideally you will progress in a cycle at the same relative rate in all your exercises, until progress ceases across the board. But in practice, to maximize gains on your core exercises, you may need to phase out some of the secondary movements as you approach the end of a cycle, or reduce their training frequency. Ideally you should not phase out any exercises unless you have made some gains on them relative to your pre-cycle bests. But phasing out of secondary exercises could be done earlier if progress in the primary exercises is being hurt by the secondary movements. If, however, you are an extreme hard gainer you may not, at least temporarily, be using any secondary movements even at the start of a cycle.

7.28     One core exercise may peak before the others. Do not stop a cycle because you have come to a halt in only one core exercise. But do not risk terminating progress everywhere by banging your head against the wall in the stuck exercise. Do maintenance work in the stuck core exercise, drop it, or substitute it, and then get a few weeks of additional gains out of the other core movement(s). Then stop the cycle.

## An example of a cycle

7.29     The exact length of any cycle should not be predetermined unless you are locked into a deadline that cannot be extended, e.g., a competition, vacation or some travelling. Generally speaking, stretch each cycle out for as long as you can keep adding a little poundage to each of your core exercises. When you get stuck for three or at most four weeks at the same poundages and reps in most of your core movements, despite using all possible cycle-extending tactics, you are temporarily at the end of your training tether, and that is time to stop.

7.30     Do not be so stubborn that you continue battling with a body
         that has had enough (for now). If you continue to battle on,
         you may pay for it—mentally and physically—by needing to
         take longer than you should need to, to get back in the flow of
         productive training in your next cycle.

7.31     A medium-to-long duration cycle could run in these four phases:

         a.  Start with three or four weeks of form and concentration
             consolidation. But do not ease back mentally. Still attack
             the weights with controlled aggression. During this phase
             the poundages are built back from 85–90% of your
             previous best weights, to 95%.

         b.  Next are a few weeks of creeping back to your previous
             best weights.

         c.  Then comes the start of the growth phase—the first few
             weeks of moving into new poundage territory. Reduce the
             number of sets you do, and even reduce the training
             frequency of some of your secondary exercises, *if* the total
             demand feels excessive.

         d.  Keep the growth phase going for as long as possible. If
             necessary cut back on your secondary work to give greater
             focus to the core exercises. Notch up a pound or two a week
             on each of your core exercises. Keep the secondary exercises
             progressing, too, if they are not inhibiting the core ones.

7.32     The net gain from an entire cycle lasting 15–26 weeks could be
         10–20 pounds on your best working poundages in the core
         exercises. While this underestimates what a beginner or early
         intermediate can gain, it is terrific for anyone else.

7.33     Some people sneer at this rate of gain, thinking and advocating
         that almost everyone, regardless of age and lifestyle, can add
         lots of poundage to any exercise in a mere month or two. Had
         these people added just 10 pounds to their squat each 4–6
         months for the last few years, they would be much bigger and
         stronger than they are now, even though such a rate of gain,
         when looked at as a per-week gain, is tiny.

7.34     How much did you add to your 6-rep bench press over the last
         4–6 months? Would you have been happy with a 10–20 pound

gain, and then another over the next 4–6 months, and then another over the next 4–6 months? Add up these small per-cycle gains and they become large increases. Remember, for typical people who have demanding jobs and family responsibilities, and who have little time in which to work out, successful training is about the long term.

7.35    Some people prefer long cycles, others prefer shorter ones, and some prefer a mix of the two. To each his own. A short cycle could be a five-week stretch in which you cut back 5–10% and take three weeks to get back to where you were and then in the fourth and fifth weeks go into new territory. With the gain made, cut back and start another five-week cycle. Such a short cycle is easily disturbed by the ups and downs of life, whereas the long cycle can accommodate more of the ups and downs. An 8–10 week stretch for a short cycle is a better length of time to get some gaining momentum going, and gives more leeway for accommodating the trials and tribulations of life.

## Cycle disruptions

7.36    No matter which interpretation of cycling you adopt, you have to be flexible enough to cope with the ups and downs of life, and still keep on track.

7.37    If you get a cold or other minor sickness, skip a workout or two. You may need to cut your weights back 10–20 pounds when you get back in the gym. Then take a couple of weeks to return to where you were before getting sick. This will take about three weeks out of the overall gaining momentum, but will keep you firmly on track. You may not, however, need to cut back your poundages after skipping just a workout or two. You may be able to return to your usual poundages, and continue to progress. You will learn through experience when you need to cut back a bit, and when you do not need to.

7.38    Suppose you have a hectic working week, or a domestic crisis, and have to miss a workout or two and exist on half your usual amount of sleep, and skip meals. Then you may need to cut back a little once you have returned to the gym, and take a couple of weeks to get back to where you were before the crisis.

7.39    This is how life is for typical people. Flow with it and adjust your short-term training to keep you on track for the medium and long term.

7.40    This back-pedaling in the course of a long or not-so-long cycle may even be advantageous. It provides a break that can set you up for a better shot at going deeper into new poundage territory than if you had not had that break.

## Gaining momentum

7.41    Do not judge the potential outcome of a cycle by how it feels in its early stages. Laying off training for 7–10 days, reducing the poundages initially, becoming *slightly* detrained, finding the groove in new exercises (or relearning ones not done for a while), and adjusting to a new or different set and rep scheme, can and probably will unsettle you for a few weeks. This is normal, so do not let it bother you.

7.42    As you settle into the new program, and fine-tune it in terms of exercise choice, order of exercises, and training frequency, you will get into the groove of the cycle and feel better about it. But still the going will likely feel tougher than you may have thought it would, considering you are using poundages less than your best for whatever reps you are performing. Again, do not be alarmed.

7.43    As you slowly and progressively increase the poundages, your conditioning and strength will progress too. Your exercise technique should improve which may make the weights feel less heavy. This especially applies to low-rep work where just a slight loss of the groove can greatly increase the perception of how heavy the weight is. Gradually your workouts will feel smoother and less uncomfortable than they were earlier with lighter weights.

7.44    Now you are into the gaining momentum, and progress is looking good. Continue with the slow poundage increments, and progress will continue to feel smooth, good and strong. When back at your previous best poundages you should not feel at your limit. You should be confident that there are many small increments to go before you terminate the cycle. This is great training and can continue for quite a long while.

7.45    You may even find that when a cycle starts out feeling too easy, that is a bad sign. It may encourage you to add weight too quickly and not look closely at possible fine-tuning. As a result you will rush and hit a short-lived peak. Conversely, when the going is difficult to begin with, you analyze your routine more, make better judgements in fine-tuning, add weight more carefully, pay more attention to getting form perfected, focus your concentration more, and find the right training frequency for you. As a result your conditioning builds up and the gaining momentum gets well established. Then you are set for a long and very productive cycle.

## Annual planning

7.46    If you can anticipate your annual schedule, plan your training accordingly. If you are vacationing in the wilderness for a couple of months in the summer, make sure you plan your pre-vacation cycle so that you have your peak just before you leave. Do not leave yourself short of time and unable to get well into new poundage ground. If your wife is expecting a child to be born in November, then plan your training so that you will have voluntarily ended a cycle just before the baby arrives (because the first weeks of having a newborn at home is likely to devastate your sleeping habits). If you are relocating in February, and know well in advance, plan things so that you will be in the first few weeks of a new cycle at the time—so your hard and most important training is not destroyed by the commotion that can accompany a major move.

7.47    By intelligently thinking ahead you can design your annual training schedule and the timing of your full-bore stretches so that your working out is not ruined by some out-of-the-gym factors over which you have no control. This is real-life training, and something you need to get to grips with, or else it will cause no end of frustration.

## Poundage increments and progression slavery

7.48    While it is essential to add poundage to the bar as often as possible, it is imperative not to be enslaved by it. If you get so besotted with poundage progression, even when using tiny discs and making only very small weekly increments, you may find yourself getting lenient with your exercise form. You

> The greatest number of consecutive full-bore workouts is no good if you are not recovering fully from each of them. In practice, you need to adapt your training intensity and frequency so that you are getting stronger and stronger, albeit it very slowly.

may find yourself ignoring aches and pains in order to be able to persist with increasing the load too often.

7.49    Make each increment as soon as you can, but only if you have made your full quota of target reps in good form, and thus have truly earned the increment.

7.50    If you are not feeling well enough to push yourself very hard, then do not push yourself so hard. With experience you will be able to distinguish between the times when you need a kick in the seat of your pants, and the times when you are just not up for training hard. Do not be foolhardy, or else you may regret it later. Back off and come back next week for a hard workout when you are ready. This aspect of conservatism especially applies once you are in your thirties, and older.

7.51    Remember, safety first, at all times. Patience, conservatism, and training longevity will serve you best over the long term. Haste and short cuts invariably backfire.

## Little gems

7.52    Most trainees try to increase their training poundages too quickly. This is almost inevitable because most gyms do not have very small discs. Here is what commonly happens. Say your recent best barbell curling is 6 reps with 110 pounds, and that was darn hard work. You felt exhilarated but burned out at the end of the cycle, and now decide to target 120 pounds.

7.53    If you are headstrong and impatient you may decide to keep the cycle going another two weeks, adding 5 pounds to the bar each week. What will happen is that the 115 will feel like a ton and you will have trouble getting 2 or 3 reps out in good form. You will relax your form, cheat and throw the weights to get all 6 reps out. You may do that without hurting yourself; so next week, on goes another 5 pounds—to 120. That feels like a boulder has been added to the bar and you cannot get even one good rep out. So you cheat right from the start and give your lower back, elbows and deltoids a real battle. A shoulder starts aching, an elbow bothers you and there is something not quite right in your lower back. You now need to recover from injury before starting another training cycle.

7.54    As an alternative way of coping with the excessive poundage increments you may go the forced rep route—you get someone to assist, and you perform a set almost entirely of forced reps. This pseudo progress may fire you on for another week or few. This type of training is hard work, though how hard depends on how much of the work your partner does. The forced set may wipe you out and exceed your ability to recuperate. This sets you up for overtraining and injury as you exceed what your connective tissue can tolerate. Forget that way.

7.55    Get your own set of little discs, or make improvisations, and then you will be able to make very small poundage increments, and thus slowly, safely and surely accumulate success.

7.56    Little discs are those lighter than the standard 1.25-kilogram and 2.5-pound plates that are usually the smallest ones available in most gyms. (See *Resources* for suppliers of little discs.) While these little gems are a great help for male trainees, they are even more useful for female trainees.

7.57    With the little discs you are perfectly set for adding very small increments, especially to the smaller exercises such as barbell overhead presses, curls, grip work, and basic dumbbell work. If you use fixed-weight dumbbells, which usually go up in 5-pound increments, securely tape the little discs to the actual dumbbells when you need to add just a little weight. (If you use adjustable dumbbells, then you will load the little discs as normal, inside the collars.) Bigger exercises such as the powerlifts do not demand the lightest discs as much as the smaller basic movements do. But at the end of a cycle you can eke out more growth weeks *if not months* on the biggest exercises by using very small discs. Once you start using them you will quickly appreciate their huge value.

7.58    Exercises that have the potential for the biggest poundages, e.g., short-range pulling movements, especially if done for singles (by advanced lifters), can progress over the long term without little discs having to be used. Increments of 5 pounds or perhaps even more can happen weekly, for months on end, in those specialized exercises. Those are not, however, the exercises being considered here.

7.59    Ideally, get yourself a set of discs that enables you to cover a 5-pound "distance" in 1-pound jumps, or 2.5 kilos in 0.5-kilo increments. To do this you need more than just one pair of small discs. You will need, for example, two pairs of 1-pound

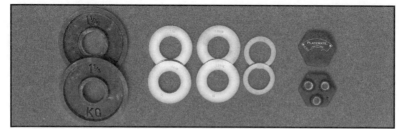

*Comparison of a 1.25-kilo plate with four "little gems," i.e., 0.5-kilo, 0.25-kilo and 0.1-kilo plates for Olympic bars, and a 1.25-pound magnetic PlateMate® which can be attached to larger plates, fixed-weight dumbbells and barbells, and weight stacks.*

discs and a pair of half-pound ones. With metric plates, two pairs of half-kilo ones, and one pair of quarter-kilo ones will do the job. If you are performing leverage bar work for your forearms, you will also appreciate a quarter-pound disc or a 100-gram plate.

7.60    You may get small discs with small holes in them when you really need discs with the large holes for use on Olympic bars, or vice versa. Olympic plates can be used on an exercise bar, but jam them between much larger plates to reduce their rattling while exercising. The small exercise-bar discs will suffice for an Olympic bar, but you will have to tape them *securely* onto the bigger plates loaded on your bar, or *securely* tie/hang them onto the bar itself. It might seem weird to attach the discs in this way, but if that is what is needed to get the job done, do it. You may cause smiles in the gym, but after a few months you will have gained while most in the gym will have continued to stagnate.

7.61    There are even small "plates" which are magnetic, so that you can easily stick them to barbells, dumbbells or weight stacks.

7.62    If you cannot find any small discs, or do not want to buy them, visit a hardware store, a metal workshop or supplier, and get some metal washers, preferably with holes the right size to fit the bar(s) you use. Get enough to total 4 pounds. Then you can add them in 1-pound increments to take you, for example, from 280 to 284 in the bench press and then be ready to use regular plates to make the full 285. Then you would use the washers to build to 289, and so on. If the washers do not fit your bar(s), tape them onto your loaded barbell as needed.

7.63    To discover the weight of each washer, ask a post office worker
to weigh one on the calibrated scale there; or use a kitchen
scale. You could weigh several washers if they are of identical
size, and then divide the total weight by the number of
washers, to get the weight of just one.

7.64    As an alternative to the washers, tape bits of metal of known
weight onto your large plates, or fix ankle or wrist weights
onto your bar. You can use a combination of imperial and
metric plates to produce an increment of about 1 pound, if both
types of discs are available, or use bars of slightly different
weights. Use your imagination and you will manage.

7.65    You do not need your little discs or substitutions during the
early stage of a training cycle when you are having a mental
and physical rest before hitting the full-bore training stage once
more. For the early part of a cycle, after having *cut back* your
poundages by 10–15%, you may be able to add 5–10 pounds a
week in a *big* exercise. Then as you get very near to your
former best poundages, get out the 1-pound discs and nudge
yourself up to your former best, then continue with the 1-
pound discs as you go into new poundage territory. Perhaps
later on you will need to use the *very* little discs.

7.66    Doing it this way, assuming you are continuously healthy and
well rested, and well short of your ultimate strength potential,
this week's full-bore 256 pounds in the bench press, for
example, should feel as difficult as last week's 255, and as
difficult as next week's 257, and the following week's 258. Once
you have found the volume, frequency and intensity of
training, along with your optimum nutritional and rest
schedule, that enables *you* to progress like this, you can
maintain it for long periods—this is the "slow cooking" way to
gain. *Then you will have found the Golden Fleece of bodybuilding
and strength training—linear progress for long periods.* It will not
be a pound a week on every exercise, but it can be for the
biggest movements. And it could even be two pounds a week
in the deadlift and squat, for a long period; then later on
dropping to a single pound a week. In smaller exercises the
progression could be half a pound every week or two.

7.67    You could argue that this method takes months to build up
substantial poundage gains whereas just a couple of weeks at
a bigger weekly increment will get you there, thus saving you

weeks or even months. If you can keep the bigger increments coming, *in good form*, then you will make more progress. But if you try to increase the weights faster than you can build strength, your form will break down, the momentum of your training cycle will be killed, and you may not even make it back to your former best poundages, let alone exceed them. Much better to take the long and sure route rather than try the supposedly fast way but only end up short-circuiting the cycle and killing your progress.

7.68    Work at the rate of 1 pound each week to get from 255 pounds to 265, for example, and you will have a good chance of doing it. And after the ten weeks you would need, maybe you could keep going for another ten weeks at half a pound a week, thus adding a total of 15 pounds to your best bench press work set. Though a beginner can progress at a faster rate than this, this is a fine rate of progress for any other category of trainee.

7.69    There are hundreds of thousands of people training with weights who stay roughly at the same poundages for year after year. Break out of the common rut of stagnation.

7.70    Get yourself some little gems—get your name engraved on them, treasure them, and exploit the magic they possess to add loads of muscle to you *over the long term*. Slowly, steadily, safely and surely is the "slow cooking" successful way to go— it is not spectacular over the short term, but it *is* spectacular over the long term. Successful hard-gainer training, except for raw beginners, is about the long term—forget the claims for safe quick fixes.

7.71    Suppose your bench press is currently 225 pounds for 6 reps. Compute adding a mere half pound to your bench press each week. Too little to matter? Baby stuff? You are in a hurry to gain and cannot afford to waste time on such tiny increments? Progress at that rate for ten years and you will add 260 pounds to your bench press, taking you to 485. Impossible you say, and

> **Get your own set of little discs, or make improvisations, and then you will be able to make very small poundage increments, and thus slowly, safely and surely accumulate success.**

it is unless you are blessed with a phenomenal genetic inheritance for building muscle and might. Okay then, progress at that rate for only five years and you would add a "mere" 130 pounds to your bench press. I bet there are few trainees beyond novice status who would not settle for adding 130 pounds to their bench press over the next five or even ten years.

7.72    Many people want gains fast, and their efforts to get them fast end up leaving them behind the person who settles on progressing in the slow and sure way. Of course, if you could add 5 pounds alternate weeks while maintaining good form, and keep it up for a year, that would be magnificent. You would make the 130 pounds gain in a single year. But progress does not happen that way for genetically typical and drug-free people who are beyond the novice level.

7.73    Poundage progression cannot be linear indefinitely, even at a mere half pound a week. If progress could be linear indefinitely, there would be lots of people who would eventually end up bench pressing 600+ pounds. There are limits, though precisely what they are for you, only you can discover.

## Conservatism

7.74    Now to build on the conservatism that Peary Rader urged early in this chapter. Here are some "rules" for applying conservatism to your training, and thus helping you to gain slowly and surely for year after year after year. Some people will think that the rules are too conservative. Without doubt, some people—especially the very young, competitive and genetically better-than-average—can break these rules and still gain. But I am primarily aiming my advice at working, married, non-competitive and genetically average people who are in their late twenties or older. Of course, less-stressed and less-limited people will benefit *even more* from applying abbreviated and basics-first training.

7.75    Conservatism, with few exceptions, is the way to go for most people who lift weights. Erring on the side of greater conservatism rather than less, is the best choice.

7.76    While you do not have all the time in the world in which to make progress, do not reduce your most productive years by forcing yourself to go where you are not ready to go just now. Haste nearly always makes waste. Make haste slowly.

## Some rules for effective cycling

7.77    When planning your training routines, allow for more weeks and longer cycles rather than fewer weeks and shorter cycles.

7.78    When building back to your previous best weights, in readiness for the journey into new poundage territory, take an extra week, or two, or three. Build the springboard necessary for the big push into new poundage territory.

7.79    When adding poundage to the bar, use smaller rather than larger increments.

7.80    When you have made your last perfect rep and know there is only a partial rep left in you, keep it in and wait the extra workout or two until you can perform that rep perfectly. Do not drive yourself to exhaustion and stagnation by forcing out (with help) reps you cannot currently do. Save that energy and effort, and combine them with a bit more time and patience.

7.81    When in the final stages of a training cycle, get an extra hour of sleep each night.

7.82    Take an extra day or two between workouts when you do not feel 100% recovered.

7.83    Take the extra breath, or two, between reps—do not rush your reps. But if you are performing continuous reps, then this rule does not apply.

7.84    Take more rest between sets, not less (unless you are experimenting with a faster pace of training).

7.85    When you are struggling to keep up with pre-determined poundage increments, delay the next planned increment and stay with the old weight until you have adapted to it.

7.86    Take the extra week or longer to add the next 0.5 kilo or 1 pound on the bar. Give your body time to build strength. Try to rush your progress and all you will get is sloppy form and, eventually, an injury. Once in new poundage territory, unless you are a beginner, adding 5 pounds to the bar in small doses over a few weeks using small discs will enable you to adapt and keep growing. But put the 5 pounds on in a single jump and you may bring on a sticking point.

7.87    Note: I am not saying that 0.5 kilogram equals 1 pound. More accurately, 0.5 kilogram equals 1.1025 pounds. In this book I often simultaneously refer to nearly equivalent weight plates to cater for metric and imperial discs. To quickly convert kilograms to pounds, double the kilos and add 10% of it. For example, 80 kilos equals 80 x 2 (or 160) plus 10% of 160, i.e., 16, for a total of 176 pounds.

7.88    Lots of little bits over half a year add up to far more than a couple of much bigger jumps over less than a month. This is especially true when, as so often happens, the latter is followed by stagnation, mental fatigue and physical injury, and having to start all over again.

7.89    Do not ruin the potential magic of abbreviated routines by adding poundage too quickly, in too large jumps, or by training too frequently.

7.90    To paraphrase a cliché, Rome was not built in a few months or a year or two, and neither will you be.

7.91    Take more time to learn perfect form before piling on the weight.

7.92    Make time to study more about sensible training methods.

7.93    Find the time to develop a flexible body and then maintain it.

7.94    If in doubt, perform extra warmup work, but keep the reps low.

7.95    Do less training, but do it perfectly. Less done properly is always better than more done improperly.

7.96    Learn from your mistakes and unproductive training practices. Do not keep repeating the same errors in the hope that more of the same will eventually work.

7.97    Conserve your energy, and focus your effort. Always focus on the big basic exercises—the builders, not the refiners.

7.98    If in doubt, consume more food rather than less, but without getting fat, and rest more rather than less.

7.99    Do not ignore signs of protest from your body—aches and pains. If you push too much, your body will stop you, eventually.

7.100    When you are feeling especially energetic, *resist* the temptation
         to add more than your usual small poundage increment.
         Otherwise you will be unlikely to be able to cope with that
         weight the following workout. The important exception to this
         rule—and to rules 7.79, 7.86 and 7.105—is if you are nearing
         the peak workout of a cycle on almost-maximum singles and
         you feel "ready for the big one." In this case, it is not only okay
         to add a little more weight than planned, but it is imperative.
         You may never feel that strong for a long time, and perhaps
         never again if you are very close to realizing your strength
         potential and are "on a roll."

7.101    Haste truly makes waste, and encourages the use of steroids
         because of the hurry to have big results immediately.

7.102    The names of the game are effort *and* progressive poundages,
         but the effort *must* manifest itself in terms of progressive
         poundages. If you are driving yourself very hard in the gym,
         but continue to use the same poundages, then the effort is
         being wasted. Judge the effectiveness of your training by the
         poundages you are moving, in good form, not by effort per se.

7.103    At the end of a cycle you are better off training "very hard"
         (but not to total failure) for week after week, rather than
         training mega hard for one week, exhausting yourself
         mentally and physically, and hitting a wall. Progressive
         training means being able to do a little more next week or the
         one after, and a little bit more again another week or two later,
         and on and on. If you take yourself to the absolute limit this
         week, then you will have trouble doing the same next week,
         let alone handling a little more weight or performing a rep
         more in each movement.

7.104    Keep just *a little* left in you so that you know there is always
         something there for next time (unless you are training to total
         failure in line with the cautions given later in this book). By
         always keeping just a little left in you, by adding weight very
         slowly, and by training in cycles, then you can nearly always
         do the "more." But this is absolutely not a justification for
         loafing. While there should be a slack period at the beginning
         of every cycle, the rest of each cycle must involve hard work
         and then very hard work. For most people, however, "hard"
         does not mean "killing" yourself and being unable to come
         back for more.

7.105   A qualifying note here: If you can "kill" yourself, *and* keep
        coming back for more, again and again, and your poundages
        are going up, then you *are* training within your capabilities
        and doing fine. Few people can do this, however, because they
        do not have the recovery ability to cope with it, and do not
        have the training supervision needed to push themselves so
        hard and often while maintaining good exercise form.
        Remember to judge the effectiveness of your training by your
        training poundages. So long as they keep inching farther and
        farther into new territory over the final stretch of every cycle,
        you are doing fine.

7.106   In the very final stretch of a cycle, when you are pushing to the
        hilt, cut back or even eliminate as much as possible every
        demand upon your energy and recovery reserves. This
        includes any little exercises you may be using, and any out-of-
        the-gym physical work and aerobic activity. This temporary
        and perhaps extreme conservation of energy, together with
        extra sleep and food, should enable you to put more additional
        pounds on each of your core exercises.

## Other interpretations of intensity cycling

7.107   A compromise some people may want to pursue is to have
        two cycles running concurrently. Half of your exercises could
        be in the intensive stage while the others are only just starting
        on a new cycle. An advantage of this is that only half your
        exercises would get full-bore treatment at one time, so your
        recovery system would get less of a beating than it would if
        all exercises were to the hilt at the same time.

7.108   An extension of this approach is to have each exercise running
        in its own cycle independent of the other movements. Rich
        Rydin and Dave Maurice recommended an interpretation of
        this approach in their article in HARDGAINER issue #34:

            Eventually you will reach the point where no progress is
            being made, or is forthcoming. This represents the end of

> **Conservatism, with few exceptions, is the way to go for
> most people who lift weights. Erring on the side of
> greater conservatism rather than less, is the best choice.
> Haste nearly always makes waste. Make haste slowly.**

the cycle *for that exercise*. As a general rule, the "smaller" the exercise the earlier this will occur. As an example, we would expect a trainee to peak on curls well before peaking on deadlifts. When this happens, drop the exercise you have reached a plateau on. Select another movement which works the same muscle functions, though perhaps in a different way, and start it at an 80–90% effort level.

Let's look at some likely examples...When progress is halted on overhead presses, our trainee should, on his next [press workout], simply perform another pressing movement of his choice. This might be another variant of overhead pressing, or a dumbbell bench exercise, for example. If he feels that his progress is nearing an end on his larger exercises, he can of course continue his program without the presses. Likewise, if he stalls on pullups, he might try some dumbbell rows, or some shrugs, or again, drop the exercise.

What if he stalls on a "big" exercise? It really shouldn't change the procedure. If squats stall and progress is still being made on deadlifts, he should do front squats in place of squats, or "restart" his squat cycle, perhaps with a different rep target. As long as progress is being made on just one major movement, then a lack of progress on the other movements should not be considered indicative of anything more profound than just that—a lack of progress on those movements. If you are still progressing on either squats or deadlifts, then gross overtraining should not be a concern. If you think about this philosophy, you will see that it is quite conceivable to finish a cycle performing an entirely different set of exercises than those used at the start of the cycle.

7.109    A possible advantage of these interpretations of intensity cycling is that every workout is likely to have some challenge in it but not necessarily from a core movement. New-ground challenges every workout are necessary to keep some people motivated.

7.110    The drawback with these variations of intensity cycling is that you may never have a break because you will always be pushing very hard in at least one exercise. Thus both your body and mind may never get the chance to restore themselves. If you apply one of these interpretations you need to take a precautionary measure to avoid total systemic overtraining. Take a complete break from training for at least a week when progress has ceased on both squats and deadlifts, if your original cycle included both. If it only included the squat or deadlift, take the break when progress ceases on that single movement. In either case, start a new cycle after the break.

7.111　　How practical these variations of intensity cycling are will depend a great deal on the circumstances of your life, how much stress you have out of the gym, and how successfully you are able to meet the out-of-the-gym contributions to training success. In other words, one approach may be perfect for you during some stages of your life, but be useless at other stages when your circumstances are radically different.

## An independent cycle within an "orthodox" cycle

7.112　　There are times when specific exercises can run in their own cycle independently of the overall cycle. Grip work is a clear example. Most trainees have so much untapped potential there. This is because so few people do specific grip work, and are used to using straps for deadlifts and shrugs. Intermediates and even some advanced trainees can, if they set about it properly—i.e., by progressing *gradually*—gain continuously in two or three grip exercises for over a year. Their regular exercises cannot progress linearly for so long, and thus need to fall into several cycles over the same period.

7.113　　Another example of an independent cycle within an overall orthodox cycle is with an exercise that necessitates special care in progression, perhaps following recovery from an injury. Starting very light, and adding only a small increment each week, would mean that the cycle for that specific exercise could continue unbroken for over a year before reaching the point when a more orthodox cycling approach should be adopted.

## Double-progression method

7.114　　There is an alternative to the use of little discs, to be used either for training variety or for trainees who do not want to invest in little discs. This is the system of repetition *and* poundage progression—the double-progression method. Here you perform your work sets in a rep range, sticking with the same weight for as many weeks as you need until you make the top number of the rep range, in good form. Then add a few pounds to the bar next time you train the exercise concerned, and drop the reps to the low count of the range.

7.115     For example, you could use a 12–20 rep range in the squat
          rather than stick to a steady diet of 20 reps. With the steady-
          reps method, at least once the sets become intensive, you
          cannot increase the poundage much each week and still get
          your full 20. In the double-progression method you build up
          over a few weeks from 12 to 20 reps, add 5 or 10 pounds for
          the next workout and drop the reps to 12. You will make all 12
          with the new poundage, and with it exacting less from you
          than did the previous week's set of 20 reps with 5 or 10 pounds
          less. Then over the following weeks you build up the reps.
          Once you hit 20, and perhaps do it for two or three consecutive
          weeks—to adapt thoroughly to its demands—add another 5 or
          10 pounds and drop back down to 12 reps.

7.116     This is a good way of adding variety to your training without
          getting into excessive exercise variation. A steady diet of 20-
          rep squats is brutal, and few people can stick to it. Switching
          to a 12–20 scheme for a cycle will provide a change of pace but
          still enable you to work into the high reps.

7.117     The bigger the rep range and the bigger the exercise, the
          greater the poundage jump you can make and yet still get the
          full lower end number of reps with the new weight. The
          12–20 squatting or deadlifting scheme, for example, gives
          you more potential for adding over 5 pounds per increment
          each time you make the full rep count than does using a 6–8
          rep range. Building up from 6 to 8 reps is easier than from 12
          to 20. Because you build less strength while progressing
          through the 6–8 range, you should add 5 pounds *maximum*,
          with less weight than that being a better idea. When working
          with short rep ranges you need little discs for the optimum
          rate of progression.

7.118     Be patient when building up the reps. If you are working on
          an 8–12 range, for example, aim to go 8, 9, 10, 11, 12. To try to
          go 8, 10, 12 or, worse, 8, 12, is akin to trying to add weight too
          quickly in the single-progression system. For a rep range with
          a large difference, e.g., 10–20, increasing by 2 reps at a time
          may be possible, at least early on in the progression.

7.119     Some rep schemes you may want to try are 4–6, 5–8, 6–10, 8–12,
          8–15, 10–15, 12–15, 12–20, and 15–20. According to how you
          "connect" with different rep counts, some ranges will be more
          productive for you on a given exercise than others.

7.120    Some people are better "reppers" than are others. Some people will find it much easier, at least in some exercises, to add a little weight next time, and still get their regular fixed rep target, than they would trying to get more reps with the old weight.

7.121    Perhaps in the bench press you are a low-rep person who, using 4-rep sets, can, once in new poundage territory, add half a kilo to the bar each week for a few months, but may struggle for weeks to build up from 4 to 6 reps with the same poundage. If you are not a good repper, like in this example, stick with a fixed rep target and concentrate on poundage progression, i.e., single progression. If you are a good repper, then at least for some spells use the double-progression method.

## Comparison of rep and weight progression

7.122    Relative to the choice of adding reps or weight, recall what was said in Chapter 4:

> According to the Maurice and Rydin chart for upper-body exercises, an increase of one rep corresponds to about a 3% decrease in resistance. If you are overhead pressing 180 pounds for 5 reps, to increase your rep count by a mere one, to 6, is comparable to adding 5.5 pounds while keeping the rep count at 5. This is a big increase if the 180-pound 5-rep set is already very demanding. So adding very small increments, while using a constant rep count, is a better trick (mentally and physically) for progressing sufficiently gradually that gains can be steady and consistent.
>
> Even when you cannot increase your rep count you can probably perform the same number of reps but with a very small increment on the bar.

## Constant working poundages

7.123    As John McKean explained to me, some of today's old timers, when they were in their prime, used constant "working poundages" for most of their training. (McKean has extensive experience in competitive Olympic weightlifting, powerlifting and all-round lifting, with the latter being his current focus.) A constant poundage means a fixed weight for each exercise, not the same poundage for all exercises.

7.124    This approach ties in with what was explained towards the end of the segment *Little Gems*, earlier in this chapter. Poundage progression on a weekly or monthly basis cannot continue indefinitely. Once a drug-free trainee reaches very advanced status, poundage progression slows down dramatically, though it does not have to cease for quite a long while. Now is the time to consider intentionally using a fixed poundage for the working sets of each exercise.

7.125    To clarify, the use of fixed poundages for relatively long periods by the old timers came *after* they had already become very strong. Prior to that stage, and over a period of many years, they had focused on making small but regular increases in strength. Once at the very advanced stage, however, they would only rarely increase the poundages in their regular training. For months at a time they would continue to knock out their usual three or so work sets of however many reps they chose for a given exercise. The poundages would tax them but never push them to the limit.

7.126    A few times a year though, when they felt good, and perhaps motivated by competition (formal or informal), they would pull out the stops and try for new personal bests with limit weights. Then they would increase their regular working weights a little for the next stretch of their training lives. They would still keep the poundages less than their limit weights for the reps they were doing, but hold them until they started to feel not-quite-so-taxing. Then another record day would be lined up, and, if records were made, some new working poundages (just a few pounds heavier than before) would be used for the next few months, or longer.

7.127    The use of constant working poundages for long periods, even for a super-advanced trainee, would not apply to a new

> **In the very final stretch of a cycle, when you are pushing to the hilt, cut back or even eliminate as much as possible every demand upon your energy and recovery reserves. This includes any little exercises you may be using, and any out-of-the-gym physical work and aerobic activity. This temporary and perhaps extreme conservation of energy, together with extra sleep and food, should enable you to put more additional pounds on each of your core exercises.**

exercise, or to a movement that was being reintroduced after a long period away from it. In these cases, even the super-advanced trainee would start comfortably. Time would be needed to learn/review form, and build up the poundages in the regular bit-by-bit manner. Only once very near the hilt of the individual's potential in that new exercise would it be an option to move to constant working poundages.

7.128     Here are some of McKean's comments on this approach:

> If one of the old timers was a local, national or world record holder, he knew that one more year's uninterrupted, constant-poundage training might yield a mere 5-pound gain. Not much, but a new record, and all that could be reasonably expected for such a super-advanced trainee. Many of my present very-advanced all-round buddies are happy to increase their records by 5 pounds at each annual national contest.
>
> Many wise old trainees liked to keep their workouts simple and enjoyable. Most of them still laugh at the so-called scientific formulae and other numbers which the younger generation seem to pull out of thin air. But in performing an invigorating workout with a familiar, comfortable yet strength-stimulating poundage, these more down-to-earth guys always left the gym with a confident smile on their faces. None who I ever knew tortured themselves to failure on a set, or spent any workout time barfing into a bucket.
>
> A final note pertains to the importance which most old timers devoted to perfect form on all lifts. Fixed-poundage sets allowed the security that the lift would always go, so even more attention was devoted to ideal positioning, and perfect angles of push. They never went to the wall (or even wanted to think in terms of any failure) on these sets, where serious breakdown of form could occur, and thus develop bad habits or injury.

7.129     The use of constant working poundages is an advanced training technique you might want to experiment with. Remember that you must first already be very strong, and closing in on realizing your strength potential. If you do try constant working poundages, you would need a few weeks of experimentation in order to discover the ideal working weight for each exercise. It should be taxing, remember, but not draining. You should be able to do it twice every 7–10 days per exercise, though some of the gifted old timers did this three times a week, and keep it up for several months at a stretch. If you do not feel your conditioning and strength increasing as the months go by, you will probably be using weights that are too heavy for you, or using too much training volume and/or frequency.

## Fixed rep target vs. a rep range

7.130   I have a preference for fixed-rep target training rather than using a rep range. Perhaps you do not, and that is fine so long as what you use is something you can consistently do well on.

7.131   There is something comforting, controlled and measured about always performing (for a given exercise, for a given training cycle) a particular number of reps, be it 5, 6, 8, 10 or whatever. If you are using multiple work sets, you would have fixed reps for each set, e.g., 6 and 4, or 5, 5 and 5, or 5, 5, and 4, or 7, 6 and 5, or 10 and 8, or (more conservatively) even 5 and 6, or 7 and 8, or 5, 5, and 6, etc. You establish in advance the reps you are comfortable with, and that are realistic for the style of training you are using. Then you adhere yourself to them and *only* increase poundage when you satisfactorily achieve your rep target(s) for a given exercise.

7.132   Suppose you are performing 2 work sets of bench presses, of 6 and 4 reps. You would never do more than 6 and 4, even if you could. Occasionally you may not get the 6 and 4 but you stick with it until the workout you do get them, and then nudge up the poundage for the next time.

7.133   With fixed-rep training you only concern yourself with increasing poundage. By using very small increments you can sustain the fixed-rep training for long periods. You get into a rep groove, mentally and physically, that is comforting and comfortable. But from cycle to cycle you can change the specific rep target for a given exercise.

7.134   It is not necessarily a case of fixed reps *or* a rep range. Both approaches can be used in the same cycle, with some exercises using fixed reps, and other movements using the double-progression method. It depends on which style seems to be best suited to a given exercise for each individual. [BB]

*This book can guide you to get much bigger and stronger. It can motivate and inspire you. It can remove the guesswork from your training.* BUT IT CANNOT DO YOUR TRAINING FOR YOU. *The practical application of what this book teaches demands great resolve, dedication, effort and persistence. The book can give you the advice, but it cannot give you the resolve, dedication, effort and persistence. Where it matters most, you are on your own.*

*The better you rest and attend to nutrition between workouts, the better you will recuperate. The better you recuperate, the more able you will be to progress at your next workout. Between workouts, remind yourself of this fact and be sure you deliver what needs to be delivered. Get to bed earlier. Spend the time needed to prepare good meals. Find the time to consume the regular feeds you need.*

# 8. How to Achieve Your Fastest Gains

8.1      Having just read of the conservative approach to training, in the previous chapter, you may be wondering how some people make very fast gains. In the modern era the very fastest gains are experienced by formerly very well developed men who are rebuilding their former development while assisted by steroids. And genetic superiors can build a lot of muscle very quickly, even drug-free.

8.2      But in the pre-steroids era some people were making very fast gains over two months or so. This can still be done today. You may be able to do it occasionally in your own training life *if* you can satisfy all the requirements. But it cannot be a long-term strategy. While I will not say that you must be in your teens or early twenties to make this fastest rate of gain a possibility, it is almost a necessity.

## The requirements

8.3      To make your fastest rate of gain you need to satisfy the following requirements:

     a. To be quite a long way from reaching your full potential for muscle and might.

     b. To have a body free of any serious physiological problem that would hamper growth, e.g., digestion and assimilation problems.

     c. To focus exclusively on a handful of the biggest exercises— e.g., squat, deadlift, bench press or dip, pullup or a torso-supported row, and an overhead press. And it is a given that you know what excellent exercise form is, and that you practice it.

d.   To have already done the preliminary work that builds up to the full-bore stage of the cycle.

e.   To pour your absolute all into every workout during the quick-gain period, using a training frequency for each exercise that enables you to add weight to the bar every workout. If you cannot add *at least* 5 pounds each week to what are already your best-ever poundages for your top sets of squats and deadlifts, you are not building strength quickly enough to gain a lot of muscle quickly.

f.   To have no back pedaling, back cycling or maintenance workouts.

g.   To feed substantially every three hours *every day* on a high-quality diet composed of easily digested meals that are rich in protein and adequate in *healthful* fats. You are unlikely to be able to gain well on a very low-fat diet.

h.   To get 9–10 hours of quality sleep every single day.

i.   To have a forceful training partner or supervisor push you to produce the most intensive, brutal, progressive, sleep- and food-rich period of your life.

j.   To do nothing physically demanding outside of your weight training.

k.   To be free of distractions, sickness, injuries and hitches.

l.   To be so motivated that your training and everything related to it become the reason you live. Almost all other responsibilities and commitments need to be shelved for the quick-gain period. There is absolutely no room during this period for corner cutting and compromises in anything related to your training and recovery.

m.   To be willing to accept a pound or so of fat for every 2–3 of pounds of muscle.

n.   To be willing to live with the stretch marks that may accompany very rapid gains. (A diet adequate in essential fatty acids will help to keep your skin supple and resistant to stretch marks.)

# Rate of gain

8.4      While packing on 20–40 pounds of *muscle* drug-free in 6–8 weeks is just promotional hype, 10–20 pounds of muscle in three months or so is possible *if* you satisfy all the requirements just listed. This rate of gain cannot be sustained, though, and is only for short-term occasional application. But few people can realistically implement the full package. Most people are far better off sticking with the slow and steady method of gaining because it is much more practical and realistic. If, however, you *can* satisfy the full package for speedy gains, do it for 2–3 months on an occasional basis and you will accelerate your progress to realizing your potential. **BB**

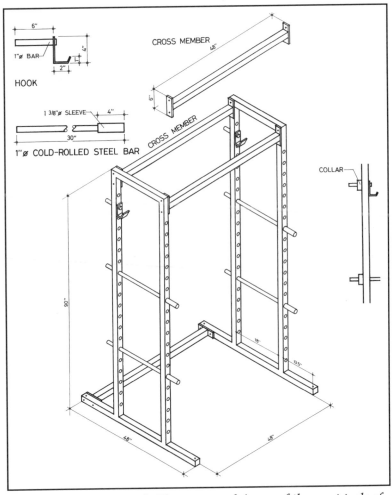

*A design for a power rack. The power rack is one of the great tools of weight training.*

Millions of gym members have got buried under relatively marginal details of workout and meal planning, while neglecting the omnipotent combination—hard work and progressive poundages.

So long as you increase your exercise poundages slowly and steadily, using consistently good form, then whatever training intensity and volume you are delivering, is working (at least for strength training, and probably but not necessarily for muscle building too). Do not feel that you have to train to the point of exhaustion to realize poundage progression.

# 9. Hard Work—the Biggest Test of Training Character

9.1      Once you are in the new ground stretch of a cycle you will find out whether you really want bigger muscles or only think you want them. You will find out how much control you have over a protesting body, how much willpower and self-discipline you have, how much tolerance of exercise-induced discomfort you possess, how much you enjoy post-workout muscle soreness, and how much hard-gainer grit and character you have.

9.2      You have got to want muscle and might so much that you cannot live without them. You must relish driving yourself to deliver what it takes. You have to be a hard-training junkie.

9.3      When you are battling into new ground you will discover one of the principal reasons why there are so few well-built hard gainers around—because intensive training is such hard work, and so few people deliver it on a consistent basis.

9.4      No matter how good your program design is, and no matter how well you attend to recovery factors, it will all go to waste if you do not have the *ferocious* passion needed to train hard on a consistent basis.

9.5      Delivering effort demands guts, will power and determination in abundance. It is about pushing your body to go further, then a bit further still, and a bit further again, always done safely and with good exercise form. It is the slow but steady accumulation of the "bit more" that adds up to substantial gains.

9.6      It demands enormous determination to keep pushing yourself hard time after time. No supplement, routine, gym, equipment, diet, writer, personality, course, book, seminar, video or whatever else exists to get you to drive yourself hard in the gym on a regular basis. The buck stops with you. Only you can push yourself through the discomfort of hard training—again and again. A good training partner or supervisor can be a great help for extracting the growth-stimulating extra effort from you, but you need to have the ability to be able to train that hard by yourself.

9.7    As a caveat, getting the intensity side of matters in order is not good enough in itself, though it is the most difficult component to satisfy. No matter how determined you are to train intensively, if between workouts you do not supply all the factors for recuperation, you will not be able to respond to the growth stimulus arising from the intensive work. And if you cannot respond to the stimulus, your body will not produce the muscle growth and strength gain you want.

9.8    Remember, you stimulate growth and then you rest, recuperate and grow; then you stimulate again and follow it with sufficient rest and recuperation in order to respond and grow again. If you train an exercise before you have fully recuperated and overcompensated from the previous time you worked it—i.e., built some "reserve"—how are you going to use a slightly bigger poundage, or perform a rep more?

9.9    Ensure that you can meet all out-of-the-gym recuperation factors *before* you go training very hard in the gym. If you do not ensure this, quality effort in the gym will be wasted and only wear you down. Hard gainers have to be much more particular about this than easy gainers.

9.10   The harder your training becomes, the greater care you need to give to being well rested during the day, having lots of sleep every night, and following as good a diet as possible. Absolutely no corner cutting! And if your life is full of stress and turmoil from work, personal relationships and any other source that runs you ragged, then that will ruin your progress. Your body can only cope with so much before it stops being able to respond to intensive training.

## Three types of muscular failure

9.11   Consider these three types of conditions—concentric (lifting), isometric (holding) and eccentric (lowering). They are directly related to three types of muscular failure. Using simplified terminology, concentric strength is less than isometric strength which, in turn, is less than eccentric strength. In other words, when your concentric strength is exhausted you still have isometric strength left. And when your isometric strength is exhausted you still have eccentric strength left. To be able to exercise what eccentric strength you have left you would need assistance to get the resistance through the concentric phase of a rep. When your eccentric strength is exhausted—i.e., when the resistance cannot be controlled in its downward descent—the involved musculature will be temporarily paralyzed.

    a.  Concentric (or positive) failure occurs when you can no longer lift the weight through a full range of motion under your own steam, i.e., when the resistance gets stuck before the normal end point of a rep.

    b.  Isometric failure occurs when you can no longer hold the weight statically, and the resistance starts descending despite your very best efforts to hold it still.

    c.  Eccentric (or negative) failure occurs when you can no longer lower the weight under control. Control can be defined as the ability to keep the descent time to *at least* four seconds for a single eccentric phase.

9.12    Total and absolute muscular failure occurs only once eccentric failure has been reached.

9.13    Training to eccentric failure is potentially very dangerous, especially in exercises where the resistance is overhead or bearing down on you, e.g., bench press and squat. There is a risk of losing control to such a degree that you get crushed, or the involved musculature and connective tissue are overstretched. It is also not a practical way to train because, at least in the big exercises, it necessitates the use of at least two strong spotters to help you raise the weight through the concentric phase. If the assistance is not provided properly, your risk of injury is considerable. On top of this, to train to eccentric failure in the biggest exercises is likely to devastate you systemically, and produce overtraining.

9.14    A situation where working to eccentric failure on a regular basis can be a good idea is the pullup/chin when the trainee is not strong enough to perform full reps. To build the strength to perform a set of successive full-range concentric chins, stick to a set of slow eccentrics. A bench or box should be used to get into the starting position for each rep, with the clavicles or upper chest touching the overhead bar, and then the pull of gravity should be resisted as much as possible. The set should be terminated when the eccentric cannot be controlled. (An alternative way to build the strength needed to perform full chins is to use the pulldown until about 5% over bodyweight can be used in good form for reps.)

## Three categories of effort

9.15    To help you understand the practical application of hard work, here are three categories of effort. All of them can be productive, depending on the application.

> a.  *First category of effort:* Here, a set is continued till one or two reps short of the absolute last rep you could do in good form. This is "hard" training. Of course, if you have never trained to failure consistently, you will not know where one or two reps short of failure is. Still, so long as you keep adding weight to the bar, you will progress.

> b.  *Second category of effort:* Here, a set is continued until no further full rep can be done in good form, i.e., to one or two reps more than in the first category. This is "very hard" training, and hardly anyone does it on a consistent basis. It takes quite some experience to know when another rep is truly impossible.

> c.  *Third category of effort:* Here, a set does not stop merely because no additional full rep can be performed. It continues into the next rep during which you will become stuck. Once you get stuck mid-rep you hold the isometric (or static) contraction as long as you can and then resist the negative phase as much as possible. This prolongs the set and leaves the muscles concerned almost totally spent. This is "brutally hard" training.

9.16    There is a fourth category of effort—to eccentric failure, i.e., "paralytic" training. This is not recommended other than in exceptional circumstances for very robust trainees. The shortcomings of paralytic training (discussed earlier) are considerable, and this level of effort takes training intensity to overkill for most people.

9.17    The harder you train, the less training (volume *and* frequency) you need to stimulate strength increase and muscular growth.

9.18    As you gain experience of training hard you will learn to tolerate more discomfort. What you may perceive as being full-bore now may appear relatively comfortable in a year's time. And with experience you should develop the discipline to maintain good form at a higher level of intensity. Then you will be able to go deeper into each set without your form breaking down.

9.19    There is a relative difference in how training is perceived in different exercises. Taken to the same degree of failure, a set of squats is hugely more demanding than a set of curls. The biggest exercises have a severe systemic effect in addition to causing local muscular fatigue. The other exercises are felt mostly locally. It is *much* less difficult to train hard in a small exercise than a big one.

## The dangerous reps

9.20    The first rep of a set can be dangerous if you do not move the weight in proper form. This danger is exaggerated in low-rep work and is a major reason why adequate warmup work is needed prior to work sets. The first rep or few of even a medium-rep set can also be dangerous if you apply a lot more force than is needed to complete each rep.

9.21    During the final reps of a set you need even more caution and discipline. If you are using singles or very low reps, then all your reps are in the final reps category. Even if you are training in a slow cadence with no momentum, the need for caution still stands true. Suppose you are bench pressing and the sixth rep grinds to a halt but you keep pushing because you want to make that rep. As you push, the bar tilts slightly to one side, you lose the groove a little, you push slightly asymmetrically, and one shoulder lifts a bit from the bench. Those few small deviations from perfect form can be enough to injure a shoulder.

> Good exercise form is critically important *no matter what training intensity you use.* But the harder you train, the greater the importance. Whenever you take intensity to the extreme you increase the chance of injury because the body is working at its limit.

9.22    In exercises where you can be pinned you must use safety bars
or alert spotters. This is not optional. During brutally hard
bench pressing, for example, you would continue until the bar
is at your chest and you cannot get it up unassisted.

9.23    At the end of each work set, when reps become hard to eke
out, resist the tendency to rush or jerk them. It is at the end of a
set that your control and discipline are most severely tested.

9.24    Good exercise form is critically important *no matter what
training intensity you use.* But the harder you train, the greater
the importance. Whenever you take intensity to the extreme
you increase the chance of injury because the body is working
at its limit. At this level of intensity you can easily lose an
exercise's groove, and potential weak links are seriously
exposed. Hold back a bit when you are training an area you
know is not 100%. Better to do a bit more work at a hard level,
and perhaps do it a little more often, than go to a more
intensive level and get an injury. You cannot make any
progress if you are injured. Be sure not to do things that invite
injury in your own individual case.

9.25    How can perfect form be guaranteed on the final rep when the
focus is on effort? It cannot, so if you know you have a weak
link, do not push that weakness to the hilt. Better to hold back
on the very final full or partial rep; or, if when performing a
rep and you know it is not going to go, hold it and fight the
negative rather than risk breaking form to get the full rep out.
Keep a little in you and come back next time and try to get the
rep properly. Push too far this time and you may get injured
and then be unable to train hard for a few weeks.

9.26    Single-rep work, if done with a maximum lift, may be
dangerous more for the fact that it is a final rep of a set (albeit a
one-rep set) rather than it being a maximum poundage. Many
trainees have gained very well on single-rep work, but they *did
not use absolute maximum singles.* Since they were not straining
at their absolute maximum with a rep that *might* not make it,
they were able to maintain good form.

9.27    Though brutally hard training may be the fastest way to gain,
at least for some people, it will only be so if it is done without
injury. Training at that level demands extreme discipline and
control. If you feel that you cannot maintain your form

discipline at the end of a set, then do not use brutally hard training. The danger factor is much more evident in some exercises than others. An isometric followed by a slow negative to wrap up a set is much safer in a pullup than it is in a squat or deadlift. Do not take any chances—do not go all the way in any exercise where you fear you may lose control.

## Intensifiers

9.28     There are several intensifiers that can be employed after failure has been reached in a set. These include forced reps, negatives and drop sets. Forced reps occur when someone helps you to get reps you could not do by yourself. Negatives happen when training partners lift the weight, because it is too heavy for you to lift on your own, and you concentrate on a slow lowering or negative phase. For drop sets, some of the weight is stripped off the bar immediately after you fail with the initial weight, so that you can continue the set.

9.29     A major problem with using intensifiers like these is that you are likely to become distracted from the priority of getting the most out of the initial set. "Straight" sets without any intensifiers are the mainstay of effective training. If trainees focused on getting each straight set done perfectly, they would be better off than complicating things with additional techniques. Forced reps, negatives or a drop set added onto an initial set that was not well done will not make a bad or even a so-so set into a good one.

9.30     For trainees who go to the limit on the initial set, adding the intensifiers may be counterproductive because they are likely to produce overkill. The point is to stimulate strength gains, not traumatize your muscles and overtrain through training too hard. That some huge men pulverize themselves with intensity heightening techniques, and grow, is irrelevant for drug-free typical people.

9.31     Forced reps should be distinguished from having a training partner give you a touch of help to get out the final rep that would otherwise not go. This sort of assistance is important for helping to prevent injury from a rep that gets stuck or falls out of the groove. If you are bench pressing or squatting *without* safety bars or rack pins correctly set in place, which is a very risky practice, then having a couple of alert training partners standing by to help you through the final rep is essential.

9.32    While for most people for most of the time these intensifiers are going to do more harm than good, occasional and very cautious use of them can give your training a jolt that may help to keep your poundages progressive, and growth happening. But if they do not help in at least one of these areas, they are not assisting you. If in doubt, do not use them.

### Pre-exhaustion

9.33    In pre-exhaustion, an isolation exercise is immediately followed by a compound movement for the same target muscle. This is supposed to intensify the stress on the muscle concerned and increase the growth stimulus. For example, leg extensions would be followed immediately by squats or leg presses. Some people promote this method with vigor, but it has serious theoretical and practical shortcomings. Probably the most obvious theoretical shortcoming is that the maximum tension on the target muscle is *reduced.*

9.34    Pushing any single set hard takes great effort and focus. To do two exercises back to back with a high degree of effort is *much* harder to do. What happens, even with strongly motivated trainees, is that consciously or subconsciously the isolation exercise is stopped short of being worked very hard. Or, more likely, the compound exercise becomes a joke because the trainee is wiped out from training hard on the isolation exercise and cannot push hard on the multi-joint movement. A typical hard gainer will never get big and strong from working hard on just isolation exercises, so it makes little sense to perform pre-exhaustion sets when they result in the major exercises being done with diminished intensity and poundages.

9.35    Rather than trying to do the near impossible of consistently training hard on pre-exhaustion, concentrate on the more practical option of straight sets. Getting straight sets done properly is difficult enough, without complicating things.

> Training intensity is a means to an end, not the end in itself. Too many people have got wrapped up in intensity per se, to the detriment of the real bottom line. Training intensity is a fundamental and irreplaceable *component* of making muscle growth and progressive poundages a reality, but that is all.

9.36    And the irony in this (as with forced reps, negatives and drop sets) is that, even if you can deliver the extreme level of intensity, it may not be necessary to train like that in order to make gains. So even if you could deliver this sort of intensity on a consistent basis, you could be knocking yourself out for no benefit. Not only that, but you would be risking overtraining through training too hard.

9.37    There is, however, an important use of pre-exhaustion set aside for *super-strong* trainees. A steady diet of extremely heavy weights imposes enormous stress on the body. To pre-exhaust will reduce the size of the poundage needed in the compound movement to deliver a good training effect.

## Warning!

9.38    Do not treat all exercises equally when training to failure. Do not push all the way to total momentary failure in deadlifts or stiff-legged deadlifts. Do not go all the way in an area where you know you have a slight weak link. Be in tune with your body and keep a little in reserve if you know that you cannot go all the way in full safety.

9.39    Some very experienced trainers adamantly caution against going all the way in any exercise—train hard, even very hard, they say, but not quite to total momentary failure. You have to travel the road yourself, and see what works best for you. Take comfort from the fact that it is not a necessity to train with gut-wrenching intensity, to gain. Some people train successfully using extreme intensity, because it suits them physically and mentally, they can do it safely, and they can provide the necessary recovery factors; but extreme intensity is absolutely not the only way to train.

## Why go "brutally hard" when "very hard" & "hard" work?

9.40    If you can make steady gains from hard and very hard training, why train even harder? Because you might make faster gains, and perhaps the fastest gains you can possibly make. It is a big reward if you can do it, but the price in terms of effort is extraordinarily heavy, and one that very few people can deliver. If you can do this all the time, *and* recuperate properly, you are going to realize your ultimate potential for muscular size and strength as quickly as possible. If you can only train that way for short spells, but actually gain faster during those periods, then use that sporadic strategy.

9.41     But if you cannot deliver the brutally hard work, do not feel
         any less of a person as a result. Train as hard as *you* can. If it
         means you reach your ultimate size and strength slower than
         perhaps you would if you trained harder, that does not
         matter. You will still get there, and in the process you will
         learn to train harder.

9.42     If *you*, however, cannot gain from the brutally hard approach,
         there is no value in doing it, even if others can gain well from
         it. If you can gain from brutally hard training for short spells,
         but then find yourself so wiped out (mentally *and* physically)
         that you cannot subsequently train well enough to maintain
         your gains, then the brutally hard method is not suited to you
         either. What matters most to you as far as training goes is how
         *you* are responding to *your* training, and maintaining *your*
         gains and building on them in subsequent cycles.

## Focus and mental ferocity

9.43     Weight training must be a very serious business if you want it
         to be successful. When you are in the gym you cannot afford to
         divide your attention between training and anything else. *There
         is no room for compromise.* Get all your problems and concerns
         out of your mind when it is time to train.

9.44     Your focus should peak for each work set. For the duration of
         each work set you must "become" the set. Nothing else matters
         other than the safe and intensive completion of that set. You
         cannot correct a bad set, so make sure that you give your all
         and do not produce a bad set.

9.45     High-rep sets demand the most sustained concentration
         because they take longer to perform than lower-rep sets. The
         concentration is needed not just to drive you on mentally, but
         to ensure you use good form. For high-rep work, having a
         knowledgeable person watching your form, and verbally
         reminding you of technique points, can be invaluable for
         ensuring you do not let your form break down. Concentration
         is easier to maintain for a short-duration set than a long-
         duration one. Keep this in mind if you find that your
         concentration powers diminish quite quickly in a set. In such a
         case you would be better off avoiding high-rep work.

9.46     Do not coast through the early weeks of a cycle and expect to
         turn on the mental ferocity needed for full-bore work when

you need it. Practice applying focus and mental ferocity in all your workouts. If you do not do this you will find that weights which should be relatively comfortable at the start of a cycle, actually feel heavy. If you save your training ferocity for only the final stretch of a cycle, when you get to that stage you may find that you do not know how to deliver the needed ferocity.

## Training intensity is not the bottom line

9.47   Training intensity is a means to an end, not the end in itself. But too many people have got wrapped up in intensity per se, to the detriment of the real bottom line. Training intensity is a fundamental and irreplaceable *component* of making muscle growth and progressive poundages a reality, but that is all.

9.48   It is too simple a solution to tell people that the reason why they are not gaining is because they are not training hard enough. While insufficient effort is certainly a big part of most underachievers problems, there are plenty of people who make minimal or no gains despite training hard enough to stimulate good gains.

9.49   *Before* you go making a big deal of training intensity you must get other factors in perfect order. It is an appalling situation that someone with 100% dedication to their training should get no gains from it. That was exactly what happened to me for a number of years. And plenty of people are guilty of this same mistake today. They train too much, too often, have too few days between workouts, eat too little, rest too little, and sleep too little.

9.50   I can vividly recall, in the early eighties, taking sets to failure followed by having a training partner help me to squeeze out a few forced reps, followed by a few negative-only reps. I truly crucified my muscles. Not only did they not grow fast like the intensity-zealots said they would, they did not grow one iota over that long period of intensity fixation.

9.51   So long as you increase your exercise poundages slowly and steadily, using consistently good form, then whatever training intensity and volume you are delivering, is working (at least for strength training, and probably but not necessarily for muscle building too). Do not feel you have to train to the point of exhaustion to realize poundage progression. Remember, you want the *minimum* quantity, frequency and intensity of training that will produce progressive poundages and muscle growth for you.

9.52    While delivering high-intensity training is the hardest part of the formula for training success, there are a substantial number of people who *are* delivering it but while giving short shrift to one or more of the factors of recovery. What an irony it is that some people deliver on the most difficult to satisfy area, but fail to deliver in the areas that are, relatively speaking, easy to satisfy.

9.53    If you are not gaining in the gym, do not immediately conclude that you are not training hard enough. Though insufficient training intensity *may* be part of the problem, it is more likely that the major problems are elsewhere. *But I am writing here strictly for serious trainees who have the passion to train hard and who are almost incapable of loafing in the gym.*

9.54    If you are training on an abbreviated program dominated by the big movements, with a good diet that provides a slight excess of calories, and a generous rest and sleep schedule, and you do not gain, *then* you may have a serious deficiency in training intensity (and/or some physical problem in digesting and assimilating food). *Then* is the time to apply yourself to boosting your effort levels.

9.55    I am a big advocate of training hard, because I know it is a pivotal part of training success. But I also know that intensity alone will not cut it. *All* the support factors have to be in decent order. Bodybuilding and strength-training success come about from a total package, with all the involved factors being fully satisfied. You cannot compensate for a serious deficiency in one area with an excess in another.

## Training intensity general recommendation

9.56    Recall the three categories of training intensity—hard, very hard, and brutally hard. To be practical, *the more mileage that can be gotten from hard and very hard training, the better*. The reality is that very few people have the mentality, willpower, youth or physical robustness to withstand very hard or brutally hard training on a long-term basis.

9.57    Hard training as defined under *Three Categories of Effort* is genuinely hard work, and harder than most people train. This is adequate for most of your work sets, and is the mainstay of productive training. This level of intensity is actually a rep or few more per set than most people deliver.

9.58    An occasional set in very hard mode (one set per exercise
        every 2–3 weeks), and a rare set taken to isometric failure
        (brutally hard mode, no more than once every 4–5 weeks, and
        only in exercises where it is safe) *may* provide a productive
        boost in intensity. Whenever you inject such an intensity boost,
        cut back your work sets in the exercise concerned, to reduce
        the chance of overtraining.

9.59    Whatever you try, never persist with something that does not
        help to keep *your* training poundages moving up, no matter
        how much it may be promoted by others.

9.60    In the context of intensity cycling there is the initial relatively
        easy stage for a few weeks, and then comes the hard stage. So
        long as you keep the poundage progression very slow,
        gradual and within your abilities to build strength, you can
        sustain hard training for a long time and may never need to
        go much into the two higher levels of effort. You could
        reserve the two highest categories for the final stretch of a few
        weeks at the end of a cycle. Alternatively, mix up your
        exercises, performing some at one level of intensity one week,
        and others at another level.

9.61    You can and probably should do multiple work sets of hard
        training—up to three sets—rather than the usual single work
        set of the very hard or brutally hard training. This is because, *to
        a point*, intensity can be traded for volume. But if you can do
        more than three work sets for a given exercise, you are loafing
        and need to apply more effort so that you do not want to do
        more than three sets.

9.62    Training more intensively does not necessarily produce its
        benefits only because of the increased effort. A contributing
        factor is that harder training enforces a reduced volume of
        training and thus a lesser likelihood of overtraining. Too many
        sets, even on an abbreviated program, will overtrain you.

## Cumulative-fatigue training

9.63    *Additional* to the hard, very hard and brutally hard training
        categories already described in this chapter, there is a type of
        training that can combine all three modalities in a *single* format.
        This can provide an excellent variation that may prevent your
        training getting in a rut. Abuse it, though, and you will get
        nowhere but into a mire of overtraining.

9.64    Cumulative-fatigue work is modified "volume" training—six sets of a fixed number of reps for an exercise, using a fixed weight for all six sets, and a rigid one minute rest period between sets. The short rest periods produce a fast accumulation of fatigue. A poundage should be used that lets you *just* eke out your target series of reps. The first few sets *must be* much less demanding than the last few. If you use a weight that causes you to struggle early on, you will never get your full target reps on the final sets of the series.

9.65    Six sets of six reps is a good standard to use for cumulative-fatigue work. Six sets is definitely enough, but any rep count between four and ten will work well for most people. Choose the rep count that best suits you for the particular exercise concerned. While medium reps are very demanding, high reps are brutally tough. Before you try high reps for any exercise using cumulative-fatigue work, first spend a couple of months using medium reps.

9.66    Select a weight that is approximately 70% of your current best effort for the chosen rep count. Some people may be able to use slightly more than 70%, while others will need to use less. You will learn through experience what suits you, and the percentage may vary among different exercises.

9.67    Wear a watch, stand in front of a clock while you exercise, or have an assistant be your time keeper. Using six reps as the illustration, perform a set of perfectly controlled reps. After the sixth rep, even though you could do more if you pressed on, set the weight down and note the seconds on the clock/watch. Take exactly sixty seconds rest before you perform the first rep of the second set. If you need a few seconds to get in position for a set, e.g., the squat, then start getting in position a few seconds before the full sixty is up.

9.68    Perfectly execute the second set of six reps, and then put the resistance down. The second set will feel less easy than the first, but should still be very comfortable. Again, rest exactly sixty seconds before performing the first rep of the next (third) set. Now you will start to feel some accumulation of fatigue. You should get all six reps without much struggle, but muscular congestion should be very apparent. The fourth set should be hard; and the fifth set should be very hard. Then the final set should be extremely hard. This is when your muscles will be spent and you need to marshall all your determination to keep squeezing out the reps. This final set *must* be extremely hard to complete. If it is not, you need to use a little more weight the next workout you train that exercise.

9.69    The perceived fatigue from this type of training is different from that which the other types of hard work described in this chapter produce, because of the *accumulation* of fatigue.

9.70    The first few times you do this type of training, assuming you start out training hard, you could experience extreme soreness during the days following each workout. If you get sore easily, carefully break into this type of training over a few weeks.

9.71    A single warmup set for a non-core exercise should be adequate prior to a series of six sets of six reps performed as described. Two warmup sets are probably only required in a core exercise.

9.72    Why take six sets to reach almost total muscular failure with a moderate weight when you could reach failure in just a single set using more poundage? Answer: To stimulate the muscles in a different way.

9.73    You have now been given four different ways to work your sets—hard, very hard, brutally hard, and through cumulative fatigue. (And there is a fifth way if you include training to eccentric failure.) All can work, but not equally well for all trainees. Over time you can prosper from all four formats, and use all four to keep productive variety in your training. Through experience you will find which styles work best for you. You may find that different body parts or exercises respond better than others to the same style of training.

9.74    Cumulative-fatigue training is primarily geared for short-term muscular growth rather than absolute strength gain. To translate the strength gains from cumulative-fatigue training into absolute strength increase, return to your regular training for long enough to build up to new poundage bests.

9.75    When recording sets of cumulative-fatigue training in your log book, you do not need to record each set individually as you would with other types of training. What matters is the entire series. The only set in which you should possibly be at risk of not making all the target reps, is the sixth one. If the fifth set is seriously at risk, you are using too much weight. As an example, record "130, 6 x 6" in your log. If you do not complete the final set, then record it, for example, "130, 5 x 6 + 5," i.e., five sets of six reps and a final set of five reps. Then next time give your absolute all in order to make the entire series of 6 x 6.

9.76      Whenever you get all six sets of target reps, increase the poundage *very slightly* next time. Ideally, structure the weight progression so that you have to fight like hell to get your final two sets (especially the sixth set), but nevertheless you always get the full quota of reps. The bottom line, as always, is poundage progression in good form.

9.77      Here are some practical guidelines to help you to make cumulative-fatigue training work for you:

     a.   First experiment with just one single-joint exercise, e.g., the curl, or calf raise. Take an accurate measurement of the muscular girth concerned. Then once a week, or three times every two weeks, train the given exercise exactly as described above. After two months, measure the muscular girth again. If you have grown, albeit only a little, you have a technique that works for you. If you did not grow, and assuming you trained as directed, along with fully providing all the recovery factors, then just put the experiment down to the learning process.

     b.   If the test went well, consider using cumulative-fatigue training on a maximum of two exercises per routine, but rotating which two exercises you select. As your gains dry up in any given exercise, revert to another format for that exercise and, if you wish, select another exercise for cumulative-fatigue training. The six sets per exercise of this type of training may produce a severe demand on your recovery system, which is why you should be conservative

> Training more intensively does not necessarily produce its benefits only because of the increased effort. A contributing factor is that harder training enforces a reduced volume of training and thus a lesser likelihood of overtraining. Too many sets, even on an abbreviated program, will overtrain you.

and use only one or two exercises per routine in this format. If you use cumulative-fatigue training on two exercises, make only one of them a major core movement. Applying it to two core exercises is likely to overtrain you.

c.  Use no more than 6–8 exercises total per routine, with only one or two of them done in the cumulative-fatigue format. This should minimize the chance of overtraining.

d.  Persist with cumulative-fatigue training for any exercise for as long as you are gaining. So long as you can add a little weight every week or two, while holding consistently good form, keep at it.

e.  Use cumulative-fatigue training on exercises that are currently in your exercise program, to help reduce the severity of post-workout soreness. Even then you may still get very sore if you are used to performing no more than three work sets per exercise.

f.  If you do not want to drop your regular style of exercising which uses maximum weights, alternate both formats in the same cycle. On one day train with your maximum weight for 2–3 work sets, and on the next day you train that exercise, use the cumulative-fatigue method.

g.  As with any type of intensive training, religiously satisfy all the factors of recovery. [BB]

You will benefit from this book in direct proportion to how seriously you study it, how thoroughly you grasp the contents, how well you make the understanding one with you, and how resolutely you apply it.

Before thinking something important has been missed out of this book, please wait until you have read every page.

Without good exercise technique, even an excellent training program will fail. Not only that, but you can wreck your body in the process.

I know it may appear absurd, but gyms are usually terrible places for learning about good exercise technique. You must be sufficiently informed so that you can coach yourself and take responsibility for your own training. Put into action what this book teaches you!

Some popular and much-hyped bodybuilding exercises are abominable, even when done in the prescribed form. They have been responsible for hundreds of thousands if not millions of people getting injured and eventually giving up weight training. Stick to the safe exercises prescribed here and you can train safely for a lifetime.

# 10. Exercise Selection and Technique

10.1      Achieving your physique, strength or fitness goals hinges on the bedrock of correct exercise selection and technique. In order of priority, exercise technique comes *before* program design. Unless you *truly* know how to train with excellent exercise technique, and actually *practice it*, then no amount of advice on program design, training gear, diet, supplements, psychology or anything else really matters. *Technique comes first!* In fact, you can have a great training program, the best equipment, a perfect nutritional plan, an ideal rest and sleep schedule, and the most positive attitude in the world, but it will all be largely if not totally wasted if you do not use excellent exercise technique.

10.2      Exercise selection alone can make the difference between training success and failure. And even if you are using the best exercises, if you do not use perfect exercise technique you will get nowhere in your training but into the quagmire of injuries, frustration and failure.

10.3      Hundreds of thousands of people, if not millions, have been forced to give up weight training because of pain and injuries caused by using faulty exercise technique. The fact is, *improperly done*, weight training is one of the most dangerous activities around.

10.4      Excellent exercise technique is needed not just to avoid training injuries. The use of first-class exercise form is one of the essential requirements for stimulating the fastest rate of strength increase and muscular development.

10.5      The use of excellent exercise form is the exception in nearly all gyms, not the rule. Though it may seem unbelievable, gyms are usually terrible places for learning about good exercise form. You need to be knowledgeable enough so that *you* can take full responsibility for your own training.

10.6    Very few people practice truly good form because hardly anyone really knows what good form is, and this includes most gym instructors and personal trainers. In fact, much of the technique instruction given by gym instructors and personal trainers is so appalling that it is downright criminal.

10.7    Do not assume that anyone who claims to be a qualified personal trainer really knows what he is doing. Strings of letters that indicate certifications of various organizations, or degrees obtained, do not necessarily signify competence as a coach. Outrages are committed and stupidities are often babbled by holders of Ph.D. degrees, and by trainers who are "approved" by organizations. Be on your guard!

10.8    Exercise technique is taken too lightly by most people who lift weights. Form is wrongly thought to be simple, quickly learned, and a minor factor relative to program design and exercise intensity. With so much rampant ignorance it is no wonder that conventional weight-training instruction does so much harm.

10.9    Such is the paramount importance of exercise selection and technique that I devoted a whole book to it. There is not enough space in this book to incorporate the 214 pages and 244 photos of that other book. Please see THE INSIDER'S TELL-ALL HANDBOOK ON WEIGHT-TRAINING TECHNIQUE for the *full* step-by-step details on how to perfect your technique in the most productive and practical exercises, for injury-free maximum gains. Exercise technique needs to be covered in great detail if you are to grasp what good form is. A few bullet-headed points per exercise will not do. Exercise technique is too serious a matter to be treated skimpily.

## The bad luck myth

10.10    Weight training has dominated my life since 1973. I think bodybuilding and strength training are among the most thrilling and satisfying activities around. No one is keener to promote them than I am. But I do not just want to promote weight training per se. I want to promote *safe*, *productive* and *long-term* training.

10.11    Barring freak accidents, training injuries have nothing to do with bad luck. Injuries have everything to do with ignorance, following bad advice, and inattentiveness.

10.12    The exercise world has always played down the potential negative side of weight training. It has inadequately presented the specifics on safe exercise technique.

10.13    Done *incorrectly*, weight training is one of the most dangerous activities around. No matter how much you try to water it down, the danger aspect is always there. *Not* to explicitly state this betrays the training masses who need to know the truth, and perpetuates the harmful aspect of the Iron Game.

## Knowledge is power

10.14    In some circles, "injuries" and the term "safe exercise form" appear to be dirty words. Some people think that mentioning injuries produces fear and negativity. But you should be fearful of some lifting techniques, just like you should fear the effects of smoking or throwing yourself out of an airplane without a parachute. But a thorough understanding of training safety gives a positive feeling that you are not going to get hurt.

10.15    Here is what really produces negativity—getting hurt and frustrated by training. How is not alerting people of potential dangers in their best interest? And how is not letting them know of detailed technique instruction going to help?

10.16    Some people seem to think that little needs to be said about exercise technique. All they seem to think really matters is more and more on training intensity, program design, and the accomplishments of the big achievers. It is as if they think form is a simple thing that everyone can work out for themselves. But good technique is no simple matter! How are people going to find out about technique if they do not have it spelled out?

10.17    Few people have hands-on *well-qualified* coaching. Nearly everyone who lifts weights is at the mercy of the atrocious instruction most gyms offer, or the inadequate technique instruction that most publications offer.

## The macho fraternity

10.18    Some macho trainers promote the "no pain, no gain" mentality, bully students and inculcate in many people a life-long hatred of exercise (if they are school coaches, for example), consider anyone who does not battle through pain to be a wimp, and have a "you *must* do them" attitude to some exercises. These coaches are doing untold damage in the exercise world. Sure they have their training successes, but these coaches make the classic mistake of assuming that what their star charges succeeded on should be used by everyone. *Just because an exercise is demonstrably productive for some people does not mean that it is demonstrably productive for everyone.*

10.19    Over the years countless people have given up weight training due to having been hurt from following the prescriptions of the macho writers and coaches. But you do not hear from these people. You only hear the success stories of people who can break the rules and get away with it (at least over the short term). But even these people are usually forced to tidy up their acts eventually. If you live the macho "no pain, no gain" attitude now, you will regret it, and sooner rather than later.

10.20    Many people promote an "if it does not hurt, it is safe" school of thought, and do not count minor aches as pain. Minor aches are irrelevant, and must be ignored, they say. "Be a man! You have to suffer to succeed." So minor aches are tolerated, and eventually they turn into a serious injury. Even "men" get hurt.

10.21    Just because an exercise does not hurt you today, next week, or next month does not mean that it will not hurt you later on. Some weight-training exercises do not produce acute injury, but an accumulation of damage which, over time, will cause serious injury. So the theory of "if it does not hurt, it is safe" is no good. For example, I did squats for years with my heels raised, with no apparent damage at the time. The damage came later on.

10.22    Easy gainers do not suffer as much from exercise abuse as do hard gainers. But hardly anyone accepts that they are easy gainers. I am not talking about super easy gainers of the caliber of Reg Park, Bill Pearl, Sergio Oliva, Mike Mentzer, Lee Haney and Paul Dillett. I am talking about people who are able, *drug-free* but following years of dedication and hard training, to bench press 350+ pounds and squat 500+ pounds at under 200 pounds or so bodyweight. Anyone who can achieve these lifts has been blessed with a body *much* more responsive than the archetypal hard gainer's. I wish I had gotten a body like that.

10.23    Very high achievers need to appreciate that they were blessed with good genetics for building strength and muscle, and that blessing gave them a body more *robust* than the typical person's. *A minority of people do not get injured easily.* But it is that minority which has such a powerful influence in educating the exercise world. Because their bodies are so robust, many of them are largely unaware that certain practices may result in less robust individuals getting injured.

10.24    Easy gainers almost always fail to understand how it is on the other side of the gaining table, though some fail much more miserably than do others. A very few of these coaches, however, do know the real score because they have *sympathetically* worked with many archetypical hard gainers.

## Injuries arise from ignorance

10.25    There was nothing "unlucky" about the injuries I suffered. I got all my injuries because I used poor form in good exercises, and used some exercises that are bad almost no matter how you do them. *All the training injuries I have sustained were avoidable.*

10.26    I got hurt because I was so committed to training hard—I had the zeal that would make even the most macho coaches proud. I am all for training intensity; but first I am into proper and safe form, because full-bore intensity is ruinous when combined with poor form and/or bad exercises.

10.27    Good exercise technique and prudent exercise selection is so obviously the priority, when you really think about it. It should not be necessary to have to justify it.

## The conservative approach

10.28    I am more conservative in my exercise prescriptions and proscriptions than most trainers and writers. The exercise world, generally speaking, is not conservative. Consider all the exercise distortions that have been promoted over the years.

10.29    I am not the first person to criticize specific exercises. Dr. Ken Leistner has been criticizing the power clean for decades, and like me is no fan of the good morning, press behind neck, hack squat, or barbell and T-bar rows. Dr. Keith Hartman, Dick Conner, Dave Maurice and Rich Rydin have noted the dangers of squatting with your heels on a board. All this advice, and much more related to safety, has been published in HARDGAINER.

10.30    If there were only risky exercises, and it was either those or nothing, then there would be a case for using them. But the fact is that the risky exercises offer nothing positive that the intrinsically safer alternative exercises cannot provide. So why take a chance on the risky exercises?

10.31    I have been promoting the merits of the big basic exercises, in print, since 1981. I have been one of the staunchest champions of the squat and deadlift. But where I differ with most patrons of those exercises is that I do not give a blanket promotion. Done improperly, or done by people who are not structurally suited for training intensively on them, the squat and deadlift are among the most dangerous exercises around.

10.32    Such is my commitment to these exercises that I devoted 24 pages to deadlift variations in THE INSIDER'S TELL-ALL HANDBOOK ON WEIGHT-TRAINING TECHNIQUE. And I devoted 16 pages to the squat. My support of these exercises is not just rhetoric.

## Exercise selection

10.33    The 48 exercises explained in THE INSIDER'S TELL-ALL HANDBOOK ON WEIGHT-TRAINING TECHNIQUE can be divided into two categories: major compound movements, and important accessory exercises. It is from these 48 exercises that you should select the exercises for each training program you design. You must prudently select from the list while adhering to the tenets of abbreviated and basics-first training. If you cannot build an impressive physique by selecting from these exercises, you will not be able to build an impressive physique by selecting from any other pool of exercises. In such a case it would not be the exercises that would be limiting you, but what you are doing with the exercises, i.e., the program design, level of effort, and progression scheme you are using.

10.34    Stick to the safe forms of exercises as described in THE INSIDER'S TELL-ALL HANDBOOK ON WEIGHT-TRAINING TECHNIQUE, protect your joints, and then you will be able to train consistently over the long term. Being able to train consistently over the long term should be your priority, because without being able to do so you will never achieve your physique and strength potential.

10.35    But as critical as good exercise form is, for it to yield good results it must be combined with first-class training program design. If you overtrain, even while using good exercise technique, you can still hurt yourself. The main purpose of this book is to teach you how to design safe and productive training programs.

# Major compound exercises

10.36     In parentheses are the main muscles worked by each exercise.

1. squat
   *(quadriceps, thigh adductors, glutes, erectors)*
2. deadlift (i.e., bent-legged deadlift)
   *(erectors, glutes, front and rear thighs, lats, upper back, forearms)*
3. Trap Bar deadlift
   *(erectors, glutes, front and rear thighs, lats, upper back, forearms)*
4. partial deadlift
   *(erectors, lats, upper back, forearms)*
5. stiff-legged deadlift
   *(erectors, hams, thigh adductors, glutes, lats, upper back, forearms)*
6. sumo deadlift (hands in position *inside* the legs)
   *(erectors, glutes, front and rear thighs, lats, upper back, forearms)*
7. leg press
   *(quadriceps, glutes, thigh adductors, hamstrings)*
8. bench press
   *(pectorals, deltoids, triceps)*
9. dumbbell bench press
   *(pectorals, deltoids, triceps)*
10. parallel bar dip
    *(pectorals, triceps, deltoids, lats)*
11. pulldown
    *(lats, upper back, pectorals, biceps, brachialis, forearms)*
12. pullup (pronated grip)/chin (supinated grip)
    *(lats, biceps, brachialis, pecs, upper back, abdominal wall, forearms)*
13. machine pullover
    *(lats, pectorals, triceps, abdominal wall)*
14. prone row
    *(lats, upper back, biceps, brachialis, rear deltoid, forearms)*
15. press
    *(deltoids, triceps, traps)*
16. dumbbell press
    *(deltoids, triceps, traps)*
17. overhead lockout
    *(deltoids, triceps, traps)*
18. incline bench press/incline press
    *(pectorals, deltoids, triceps)*
19. incline shrug
    *(traps and entire upper back, deltoids, forearms)*

20. standing shrug
    *(traps, deltoids, forearms)*
21. calf machine shrug– *though recommended in the initial edition of this book, I now advise against it, due to the compression of the resistance on the working muscles, which can lead to muscle tears*
22. cable row
    *(lats, upper back, biceps, brachialis, rear deltoid)*
23. modified straddle/handle lift
    *(erectors, glutes, front and rear thighs, lats, upper back, forearms)*
24. decline bench press
    *(pectorals, deltoids, triceps)*
25. close-grip bench press
    *(triceps, deltoids, pectorals)*
26. dumbbell row
    *(lats, upper back, biceps, brachialis, rear deltoid, forearms)*
27. side bend
    *(erectors, quadratus lumborum, abdominal wall)*

## Accessory exercises

10.37      In parentheses are the main muscles worked by each exercise.
1. bench shrug
   *(pectorals, deltoids, traps)*
2. "breathing" pullover
   *(for rib cage enlargement)*
3. back extension
   *(glutes, lower back structure, hamstrings, thigh adductors)*
4. reverse back extension
   *(glutes, lower back structure, hamstrings, thigh adductors)*
5. crunch situp
   *(abdominal wall, especially the rectus abdominis)*
6. reverse crunch
   *(abdominal wall, especially the rectus abdominis)*
7. overhead pulley crunch
   *(abdominal wall, especially the rectus abdominis)*

---

**2004 revision**

I would now add the leg curl to this list of exercises, and include it in most training programs, one time each week. The leg curl is a valuable exercise that works the hamstrings differently than the compound exercises such as the stiff-legged deadlift, and deadlift. And, *prudent* use of the lateral raise is valuable, too.

---

8. calf raise variations
   (*gastrocnemius, soleus*)
9. barbell curl
   (*biceps, brachialis, forearms*)
10. dumbbell curls
    (*biceps, brachialis, forearms*)
11. supinating curl
    (*biceps, brachialis, forearms*)
12. finger extension
    (*finger extensors*)
13. grip machine training
    (*forearms, finger muscles*)
14. lever bar work
    (*forearms*)
15. L-fly
    (*shoulder external rotators, rear deltoid*)
16. neck work
    (*neck musculature*)
17. pinch-grip lifting
    (*forearms, finger muscles*)
18. thick-bar hold
    (*finger muscles—especially with a very thick bar, forearms*)
19. wrist roller training
    (*forearms*)
20. Rader chest pull
    (*for rib cage enlargement*)
21. pushdown/pressdown
    (*triceps*)

*The anatomy charts at the end of Chapter 1 show the main muscles of the body. The muscle groups are divided into their constituent parts.*

10.38    While most exercises are obviously "majors" or "minors," some (e.g., the side bend) could be placed in either, depending on individual value judgement. Do not get hung up on which group a particular "grey area" exercise has been placed.

10.39    With few exceptions, the exercises that are not included in the above lists are either dangerous, only of marginal value or no value to 99%+ of trainees (i.e., the myriad isolation exercises used for the detail training that is only relevant to the competitive bodybuilding elite), require machinery that is not commonly available, or are technically so demanding that expert hands-on coaching is needed. Grip training is an exception to this generalization.

## Machines and free weights

10.40    If you are unable to safely perform a recommended exercise
         with free weights, but you can safely perform a machine
         version of it, use the machine. But if you are able to safely and
         productively perform a free-weights exercise *and* the machine
         version of it, you are better off using the free weights version.
         Free weights involve more musculature than machine exercises,
         because the stabilizing muscles are involved to a much greater
         degree. In addition the free weights usually permit more
         freedom to adjust stance and/or grip in order to modify form to
         fit the individual. Machines are usually much more restrictive.
         Some are so restrictive that they hurt the users, over time. But a
         good machine used correctly can open new horizons for some
         people, e.g., the Tru-Squat can enable a person who cannot
         safely barbell squat to still squat intensively.

10.41    There are trade offs using machines, just as there are trade offs
         using free weights. Generally speaking, however, free weights
         are better tools than machines, along with being cheaper and
         more versatile. But the bottom line is safety. The decision on
         what type of equipment to use should be based on which
         allows *you* to push to your limits in the greatest safety.

## Fundamentals of excellent exercise form

10.42    Here are six basics of first-class exercise technique:

         a.  Before you can apply good exercise technique you first
             need to know what good exercise technique is. Please
             study THE INSIDER'S TELL-ALL HANDBOOK ON WEIGHT-TRAINING
             TECHNIQUE very carefully. This book covers all the major
             and accessory exercises just listed.

         b.  Before a set, review the correct exercise form you need to use.

         c.  Never charge into a set, grab the bar and then realize after
             the first rep that you took an imbalanced grip, the wrong
             stance, or are lopsided while on a bench. Get perfectly
             positioned for every set you do.

         d.  Be 100% focused and attentive while you train—always!
             Never be overconfident or casual.

         e.  For each work set, only use a poundage that lets you *just*
             squeeze out your target reps in good form. Most trainees

use more weight than they can handle correctly. This leads to cheating and a loss of control, and makes injury inevitable—and sooner rather than later.

f.   Lift the weight, do not throw it; and lower it, do not drop it. Use control at all times. Regularly perform the "pause test."

## The pause test

10.43   Most trainees lift and lower the resistance too fast. When doing the exercises listed in this book you should be able to stop each at any point, hold the weight briefly, and then continue. In an intensive set you will probably not be able to pause *and* get your target reps, depending on which rep you paused. The idea is that you *could* pause as a demonstration of control. Perform the pause test every few weeks, to check your control.

10.44   The more intensive any given set is, and the harder the reps become, the more critical it is that you pay attention to the negative (or lowering) portion of each rep. If you lower the bar slightly out of the groove you will be out of the groove on the positive (or lifting) portion, too, and risk missing the next rep and/or hurting yourself.

## The squat

10.45   The squat is *potentially* the most productive single exercise you can do *providing you can perform it safely and progressively.* The more efficiently you squat, the greater the potential benefits you can extract from it. How efficiently you squat is mostly a result of your relative torso and leg lengths, and relative femur and tibia lengths. While some people have much better mechanics for squatting than others, most people can squat well enough to obtain great benefits from the exercise, *if they have mastered the technique of squatting.* Whatever structural proportions you have inherited are all you are going to get. Never mind that some people can squat more efficiently than you, and obtain more benefits. What should matter most to you is learning how to fully exploit the squat in your own case.

10.46   The squat does not have a legendary reputation for nothing. So long as you are not prohibited from squatting by injury or serious structural limitations, you should squat hard and consistently. The sole addition of intensive squatting just once a week can turn an otherwise unproductive training program into a productive one. *The squat is that great an exercise.*

10.47    The squat has acquired its reputation for two main reasons. First, the squat is simply a super productive exercise. Second, it is possible to squat in almost every gym. The exercise is a universal one and many people have discovered its great benefits first hand.

10.48    One of the most important training-related projects you can set for yourself is the mastering of squatting. With improved understanding of squatting form, everyone can squat more efficiently. Even if you think you do not squat well, after truly mastering squatting form you may be able to squat much more efficiently and productively than you think you can. *Do not give up on the squat because of initial difficulties.* In THE INSIDER'S TELL-ALL HANDBOOK ON WEIGHT-TRAINING TECHNIQUE I devote sixteen pages to the squat, covering technique in extensive detail.

10.49    Mastering the squat, and then intensively and progressively squatting on a consistent basis is a linchpin of successful bodybuilding and strength training. Do not miss out on your chance to exploit this wonderful exercise. As tough as intensive squatting is, learn to love the exercise. It is because the exercise is so demanding that it is so productive. But be sure that you are experiencing the right type of discomfort. Pain and injury are not part of the package. Impeccable form is imperative.

10.50    Some people legitimately cannot squat well. This is usually due to injury limitations or structural restrictions. A tall person with, proportionately speaking, long legs and a short torso is always going to struggle in the squat, and perhaps to such a degree that he can never obtain any of the potential benefits from the exercise. For a minority of people the barbell squat is a high-risk exercise that should be avoided. Such people need to seek an alternative to the squat. Leg extensions will not cut it. A major multi-joint exercise is needed.

10.51    The Tru-Squat machine is an excellent substitute for the barbell squat, even for people who cannot squat safely and hard using a barbell. But Tru-Squat machines are few and far between. The Tru-Squat is a high-tech machine costing over $2,000, and can be found in only a very few gyms. If have access to one, or if you can afford to buy your own, exploit it to the full.

10.52    While the leg press can never be the equal of the squat, if you cannot squat, the comparison is irrelevant. But the leg press must be supplemented with a variation of the deadlift, because the leg press does not involve the lower back in the substantial way the squat does.

## The Trap Bar (or shrug bar) deadlift

10.53    If you cannot squat safely and productively using a barbell, and do not have access to a Tru-Squat or a good leg press machine, what are you going to do? Try the Trap Bar deadlift.

10.54    The Trap Bar deadlift is not just an alternative to the barbell squat. It is an outstanding exercise in its own right. Some form of deadlifting should be part of every program. But it need not be the Trap Bar (bent-legged) deadlift. It could be the stiff-legged deadlift with either a straight bar or Trap Bar, or it could be the sumo deadlift with a straight bar, the conventional deadlift with a straight bar, or the partial deadlift. (You may find the sumo deadlift a safer and more productive exercise than the straight-bar conventional deadlift, if no Trap Bar is available.) For bent-legged deadlifting, the Trap Bar deadlift is a superb option—it intensively works a great deal of musculature *and* reduces strain on the lower back. Because it so heavily involves the thighs, it could even be called a Trap Bar *squat*lift. If, however, you need to use a relatively wide stance (perhaps for knee comfort or care), you may not be able to use the regular Trap Bar safely, because the fixed gripping sites restrict stance width. A custom bar (trap bar or shrug bar) would be needed, with wider gripping sites.

10.55    While barbell squatting can be done in almost any gym, the Trap Bar deadlift requires a special rhombus-shaped bar, which few gyms have despite it costing no more than $200. The Trap Bar should be a required piece of equipment for all gyms. It is a wonderful training tool, and far more valuable and less expensive than many pieces of equipment that most gyms consider to be essential, but which in reality are either useless, downright harmful, or only marginally useful at best.

10.56    Very few people have experienced the tremendous benefits of the Trap Bar deadlift. This is purely because the exercise is a recent innovation and Trap Bars are so few and far between.

10.57    The Trap Bar deadlift is the equal of the squat for many hard gainers. And for some trainees it can be a more productive exercise. In fact, it has the potential to be the *number one* productive exercise for many hard gainers.

10.58    It is imperative that you know how to deadlift safely and correctly in all its important variations. Otherwise you will get hurt and never be able to profit from the deadlift. See THE INSIDER'S TELL-ALL HANDBOOK ON WEIGHT-TRAINING TECHNIQUE for how to perform all the important variations of the deadlift.

10.59    Easy gainers often have a "squatter's body"—a mesomorphic structure with legs and arms that are short relative to torso length. (This barrel-chested torso structure is also highly suited to bench pressing.) Hard gainers often have a "deadlifter's body"—legs and arms that are long relative to torso length. Hard gainers do not have the mesomorphic structure that is usually associated with a body that is very responsive to training, but some hard gainers have the structural proportions that are suited to efficient deadlifting.

10.60    In any type of bent-legged deadlift with a Trap Bar there are some big advantages relative to the squat:

   a.   The bar is held beneath the body rather than precariously near the top of the spine as in the squat, and thus there is no bar bearing down on you.

   b.   Good form is easier to maintain because the deadlift is technically less demanding than the squat.

   c.   Spotters are not needed.

   d.   No squat stands, power rack or safety bars are needed.

   e.   The exercise is easily done from a dead stop at the bottom.

---

The Trap Bar is not only terrific for many people who do not squat well with a bar over their traps. It can also be terrific for people who do squat well, but perhaps do not straight-bar deadlift well. However, depending on your leverages, the Trap Bar deadlift may not work your lower back adequately enough by itself. Stiff-legged or partial deadlifts may be needed too. And strength built by the Trap Bar may not necessarily carry over to the straight-bar deadlift, *depending on the individual.*

10.61    When comparing the same degree of descent of the hips you
         may even find that the Trap Bar deadlift works your thighs
         *more* than the squat. It is not necessary to descend in the Trap
         Bar deadlift until your thighs are parallel to the ground in order
         to mimic the effect on the thighs of the parallel squat. The effect
         on the thighs from the parallel squat can be produced from Trap
         Bar deadlifting from *above* the thighs-parallel-to-the-ground
         bottom position. (Some people, because of their body structure,
         do not get much thigh development from the parallel squat.)

10.62    I knew most of the benefits of the Trap Bar in theory, for years,
         but only when I actually used the rhombus-shaped gem did all
         those benefits become real. Designed by a man who was
         plagued with back problems (Al Gerard), it is tailor-made for
         hard gainers who do not squat as efficiently as they deadlift.

10.63    The Trap Bar will benefit *any* type of gainer. It reduces spine
         stress relative to that from a straight-bar deadlift, puts the arms
         into a more efficient position, and enables users to get the best
         from the deadlift while minimizing technique problems.

## Leg press

10.64    There are at least four main ways of looking at the leg press:

    a.  As one of the major multi-joint exercises in its own right,
        regardless of whether or not you squat well.

    b.  As an alternative to the squat when a break from squatting
        is felt to be needed.

    c.  As a squat substitute for people who have very poor
        leverages for the barbell squat that make the squat only a
        marginally productive if not dangerous movement. This
        group includes very tall people, and those of more
        average height but with proportionately long legs and a
        short torso. This group is also likely to be much more
        suited to the deadlift than the squat, thus making the
        deadlift and leg press an excellent pairing.

    d.  As a substitute for the squat when the latter can no longer
        be performed due to lower-back and/or knee limitations.

10.65    The critical condition in all these cases is that the leg press is
         performed safely and productively on a machine that suits you.

10.66    At least in some quarters, the leg press has acquired a stigma as being only for wimps—for those who lack the guts to squat. In part this comes from the "you must squat" camp. Any exercise selected as an alternative to the squat, in the view of this camp, is deemed as heresy and a cop out from the real work of squatting. I used to belong to this camp, and looked upon the leg press with scorn.

10.67    With maturity and experience I have come to see the leg press in a fair light. I am all for the squat *and* the leg press, *so long as both can be done safely and progressively.* If you can squat safely and progressively, then so you should—not necessarily in every training cycle, but certainly in most of them. Assuming that you can squat and leg press with equal safety, the squat is definitively the more productive of the two. But many people cannot squat and leg press with equal safety.

10.68    I should not have had a blind devotion to the squat that deflected me from serious pursuit of the leg press and variations of the deadlift. On hindsight, I should have focused on a different pair of exercises from cycle to cycle—e.g., squat and stiff-legged deadlift, leg press and Trap Bar deadlift, and squat and sumo deadlift. When recovery and training energy were very high I should even have trained the squat, leg press and stiff-legged deadlift in the same cycle. My aim should have been to exploit fully the great potential of the squat, deadlift, stiff-legged deadlift *and* leg press, not just one or two of them. I urge you to do the same, if possible.

10.69    The leg press is technically a much simpler exercise than the squat. Because of this it is easier to work yourself to the hilt on the leg press than on the squat. It is easier to maintain good form while leg pressing to failure than it is while squatting to failure. This is a big advantage.

10.70    By taking the lower back out of the exercise, *assuming you use good form,* the leg press enables you to work your thighs and glutes to the limit without having your lower back come into the picture other than as a stabilizer. This is great for people who have lower backs that fail before their legs do when squatting. With some machines, because of the control over pressing depth and foot placement, knee stress can be lessened substantially in the leg press relative to the squat, thus enabling people with knee limitations to get heavy work for their thighs and glutes.

10.71     Do not see the leg press as a cop out from squatting, or as a last resort exercise only for if you get injured and cannot squat. See it as a fine exercise in its own right. Do not wait until you get an injury that restricts or prevents squatting and deadlifting before exploiting the leg press. Pay your dues on it at any time and you will find it can pack muscle on your thighs. Not only that, but it may help increase your potential in the squat and deadlift because of its assistance value for those two great movements.

10.72     But to repeat a very important point, in a straight comparison, and assuming that you can perform both exercises safely and intensively, the squat *is* a superior exercise to the leg press— no question about it. The Trap Bar deadlift is also superior to the leg press. But if you truly cannot squat or Trap Bar deadlift well, despite having pursued all possible form modifications, the comparisons are irrelevant.

## The metabolic effect

10.73     Benefits from the squat and deadlift do not come merely from the localized muscular work, as important as that is. There is a metabolic effect that helps increase the body's overall growth potential. This effect is produced by only a very select few exercises, among which is the leg press, though its metabolic effect is less than that from the squat and Trap Bar deadlift *if* the latter two exercises can be done safely and intensively.

10.74     Here is how Jan Dellinger explained the metabolic effect in his article on the leg press in HARDGAINER issue #38:

> The effect on the cardiorespiratory system is an indicator of the value of an exercise. In my case, I noted that heavy, all-out sets of leg presses (especially those for reps of 8–20) got me significantly more breathless and rubber legged than squats under the same conditions. Of course, deadlifts for high reps was the ultimate self-torture with a barbell.
>
> Proponents of the squat rave on about its metabolic activation properties, and how this triggers growth. If I reach a higher state of stimulation with the leg press (or deadlift) doesn't this render the alternate exercises to squats better for me? The metabolic activation is what's supposed to trigger the body's gaining mechanism. The point is what gets the job done more efficiently. Due to unfavorable leverage (and, later on, injury) I could never

reach the poundage in the squat to match the higher level
of stimulation reached with the leg press or deadlift.
Which exercise, then, should I focus on most of the time?
What's wrong with propitious individualism?

## Leg press machines

10.75    The major problem with the leg press is the need for a safe
machine. This makes the leg press much more likely to be used
by those who train in commercial gyms as against home gyms.
Some leg press machines, at least for some body structures, are
destructive. *Great care* must be given to ensuring you use a
machine and style of leg pressing that do you no harm.

10.76    There are several types of leg press machines. Each can stress
the thighs and glutes slightly differently because of the
differing angles of body positioning. What is important is
finding a safe way of leg pressing over the long term.

10.77    The first basic type of leg press machine is the traditional
vertical one. This puts great stress on the knees and lower back,
and is not recommended. While this machine may not harm
young injury-free trainees, it can cause havoc for older people,
especially if they have had knee and back injuries.

10.78    Second are the $45^0$ or sled leg press machines. Some may
reduce some of the knee and lower back stress relative to the
vertical models, but can lead to excesses that cause damage.
Principally they lead to excessive poundage due to the
machine's design which permits very big weights to be used
relative to other models.

10.79    If used with caution and good form by a person with no injury
limitations to work around, the $45^0$ leg press models *may* yield
good results. But for most people, the leg press machine of
choice will be of the leverage-style, e.g., the models produced
by Hammer Strength and MedX.

10.80    A few leg press machines, e.g., one of the models produced by
Hammer Strength, can be used one leg at a time or alternately,
i.e., isolaterally/unilaterally. This contrasts with the usual
bilateral machines that have a single platform which is moved
by both legs pushing together. The unilateral leg press machine,
however, gives you the option of working both legs bilaterally,
too, though each leg will have its own resistance to overcome.

10.81    A unilateral leg press machine applies asymmetrical and
         rotational stress to your lower back because both legs are not
         pushing at the same time, *unless it is used bilaterally*. This may
         or may not pose a problem for you because technique and
         individual structural considerations are involved. To reduce the
         impact of asymmetrical stress, keep the non-working leg
         extended and braced against its resistance while the other leg
         works. But because the unilateral model can be used bilaterally,
         if unilateral use poses a problem for your lower back, then
         stick with using it in bilateral mode.

---

## Note of great importance

So long as you can squat at least reasonably well, you
will probably never find a more productive exercise
for growing bigger legs and putting your body in
anabolic mode. The benefits from the squat go well
beyond just developing the directly involved
musculature of the thighs, glutes and lower back.

If you do not squat, you must find an alternative that at
least approaches the quality of the squat. If you do not
squat (either with a barbell or Tru-Squat), you should
Trap Bar deadlift, or leg press, ball squat or modified
straddle lift/handle squat—see THE INSIDER'S TELL-ALL
HANDBOOK ON WEIGHT-TRAINING TECHNIQUE—*along with*
some form of deadlifting for the latter three. *If you do
not find a good alternative to the squat, you will greatly
reduce the potential value of your training.*

Many people have found that whenever they stop
squatting for a month or two they lose leg size *no
matter what exercise they substitute for the squat.* But
had they tried the Trap Bar deadlift they might not
have experienced that loss of leg size.

Intensive squatting once a week on a consistent basis
supplemented with a handful of multi-joint exercises,
supported with five or, even better, six nutritious
meals each day that supply a slight excess of calories,
along with lots of rest and sleep, can make anyone
gain lots of muscle. This combination really makes
things happen. *Do your utmost to master the squat!*

10.82   At least two potential advantages of using the unilateral leg
        press model will still apply even if it is used exclusively in a
        bilateral manner:

   a.   Each leg can work independently of the other, like
        pressing two dumbbells at the same time as against a
        barbell. While this may appear to be a disadvantage as far
        as control goes, at least to begin with, it permits limb
        strength differences to be allowed for. You could have
        your weaker leg loaded with a little less weight than the
        other side. Or you could load both sides with the same
        weight but control the set based on the performance of
        your weaker leg. In this case you would always keep your
        stronger leg working on a par with your weaker leg, and
        end the set for both legs when your weakest side has had
        enough. In either case this will help prevent the twisting
        (torsion) that can be a problem with a bilateral machine
        when both legs are not of the same strength.

   b.   The second potential advantage of using a unilateral
        machine, even in bilateral style, is if you have one leg
        shorter than the other. The unilateral machine, even used
        bilaterally, will naturally offset your leg length differences.
        This would help reduce the rotational stress that arises
        from using a regular bilateral leg press machine (and even
        squatting) with limbs of differing lengths.

10.83   The squat is used much more in the programs of this book than
        the leg press. The reasoning is twofold. First, not all trainees
        have access to a good leg press machine. Second, it is generally
        assumed that readers are *not* limited by injuries or *excessively*
        disadvantageous leverages for the squat. (And remember that
        the squat is potentially a much more productive exercise than
        the leg press.) But you do not have to have perfect leverages to
        get a lot of benefit from the squat. Even trainees with relatively
        poor squatting structures can get a great deal of benefit from the
        squat, and more benefit than they ever can from the leg press, *so
        long as they exercise good form and use a sensible progression scheme.*

10.84   If you can leg press safely and progressively, then for short
        periods you may substitute it for the squat. But keep in mind
        that the leg press, unlike the squat, does not heavily involve
        the very important lower-back musculature. Include a deadlift
        for your lower back, to complement the leg press.

10.85    See THE INSIDER'S TELL-ALL HANDBOOK ON WEIGHT-TRAINING
         TECHNIQUE for a comprehensive and illustrated description of
         safe and productive leg pressing technique.

# Shrugs

10.86    Few trainees are aware of any shrug exercises other than the
         conventional standing version done with either a straight bar
         or dumbbells. Dumbbells or a Trap Bar are best for this exercise
         because the straight bar drags against the legs. The standing
         shrug primarily works the upper traps.

10.87    Paul Kelso's evangelizing has been heavily responsible for
         publicizing shrug variations outside of the regular standing
         version, including the incline shrug which is strongly
         recommended in this book. His article in HARDGAINER issue #22
         is but one of many he has had published in the training world.

10.88    Shrugs done face-down on a bench set at about 45⁰ work the
         musculature of the upper back differently to the regular
         standing shrug. In the incline shrug the whole upper back is
         involved, especially the lower and middle areas of the traps,
         and the muscles around and between the shoulder blades.

10.89    There is even a shrug for the pectorals, together with the
         shoulders, called the bench shrug.

## Including shrugs in your program

10.90    To include an upper-back shrug *without* it adding much to the
         total load of your training, and to minimize if not eliminate any
         warming up, shrug after your final set of deadlifts. Perform
         one or two work set(s) of a shrug. But for your first few times
         out, use a light poundage and several sets, to learn how to do
         the movement properly. Once you have learned it, use a weight
         appropriate to your strength.

10.91    I rate the incline shrug as the most important shrug for regular
         inclusion in your training. You could substitute the regular
         standing shrug for an occasional spell. Use a rep target that
         you feel most comfortable with, e.g., 8, 12, 15 or 20, or vary the
         reps from cycle to cycle.

10.92    Build up your shrug poundage and you will build the strength
         needed for the top part of all variations of the deadlift (when
         you especially need to keep your shoulders pulled back). This

will help increase your deadlift poundages. Strength developed from incline shrugs will help you to keep the very important flat back while deadlifting and squatting. There are other important benefits, including strengthening the shoulder girdle, helping to keep your torso more solid, and putting muscle on your traps where you place a bar for squatting.

10.93    The incline shrug in particular will help improve posture for people who have rounded shoulders. In extreme cases where deadlifts cannot be done properly because of poor posture, incline shrugs need to be done until sufficient strength has been built to improve posture. Then, perhaps a few months later, the deadlift can be introduced and performed in good form.

## Bench press alternatives

10.94    The parallel bar dip works more muscle than does the bench press. Prior to bench pressing benches becoming standard fare in gyms, in the fifties, the parallel bar dip was a very popular exercise (as was the *strict* overhead press). Thereafter the bench press became a hugely popular exercise. The bench press is a very good exercise, but its degree of popularity today is excessive relative to the merits of the exercise. The parallel bar dip is potentially an excellent exercise, and one that does not require spotters or safety bars.

10.95    Though not working as much muscle as the parallel bar dip, the incline press (or incline bench press) should be considered as an alternative to the bench press, especially if only one pressing movement is included in a program.

10.96    The developmental effects of the bench press in your particular case should also be a consideration in exercise selection. If you find that you get overly heavy lower pecs from the bench press (or dip), the incline press should be a preferred choice.

## Bench press and overhead press relationship

10.97    A general rule is that the overhead press should be two-thirds of your bench press, comparing the same rep count and cadence. Increased overhead pressing ability can improve bench pressing ability, though some people can be good pressers but poor bench pressers.

10.98    One of the reasons why some trainees get stuck in the bench press is that their overhead pressing is weak. Compare your barbell bench pressing and barbell overhead pressing ability (for the same rep count and cadence). If the latter is less than two-thirds of the former, your overhead pressing is lagging behind your supine pressing. Spend a few months focusing on bringing your lagging overhead pressing up to par, and you may do more for your bench pressing potential than any extra attention given to actual supine pressing would.

## Essential isolation work: the support seven

10.99     There are seven small areas that should not be neglected during the focus on the core movements. This support seven can have a *big impact* for keeping you free of injuries. The support seven is made up of specific work for the calves, grip, shoulder external rotators, neck, midsection, lower back (isolation work from back extensions *additional* to that from deadlift variations), and finger *extensors* (to balance the strength of opposing muscles in your forearms).
*2004 revision: I would now add the leg curl to this support group.*

10.100    Midsection work is not just about the rectus abdominis (the "six-pack" muscle). It is about the whole of the midsection. It includes work for the internal and external obliques, and for the small muscles around and between the vertebrae.
*2004 revision: The side bend can provide this important strengthening work, but it is a risky exercise for many trainees. The* TWISTING *crunch situp is a safer alternative.*

10.101    Exercise for the obliques has received unfair press over the years, based on the mistaken view that it can add inches of muscle to the waist girth. The obliques have a *small* potential for hypertrophy. Regular, progressive exercise for the obliques will build *substantial* strength, and a little muscle. That strength and extra muscle should be welcomed for the stability and injury preventing potential it adds to your physique. And so long as you are lean enough for your waist musculature to be visible, development of your obliques will *add* to the impressiveness of your midsection.

10.102    Aim to have your neck about an inch larger in girth than your upper arm. To do this you will need to add some neck isolation work to your training schedule. Without isolation work, however, your neck will still be worked enough from deadlifts and shrugs to make it bigger and stronger than it was before you started lifting weights.

10.103     The support seven do their important work by maintaining strength balance in the body. (There is also aesthetic balance, especially in the cases of calf, grip and neck work). *Attention to the support seven is vital if you want to get big and strong.* By themselves they will not make you big and strong, but they play an important role in helping to keep you injury free in the exercises that *will* make you big and strong. Without being able to train long-term, hard and progressively on the key multi-joint exercises you will never be able to get big and strong.

10.104     The support seven do not need lots of work, and can even be dropped for short periods. But they must not be neglected over the medium and long term.

10.105     On the other hand, do not get so carried away with the support seven that you get distracted from the big basics. If you do three sets for each of the support seven, and do it all two or three times a week, you will never make progress on the big exercises.

10.106     Following a warmup set do one work set twice a week, or two work sets once a week, on each of these important small exercises. Do not do all of them twice a week because that would probably undermine your progress elsewhere. And do not perform all of them at the same workout unless you have a single session each week exclusively devoted to the support seven. Perhaps the best way to cover the support seven is to do two of them after your first workout each week, another two after your second workout, and the remaining three on an off day. Specific grip work can be done each workout. But you do not have to do specific work to train your grip. Deadlifts, shrugs and pulldowns (or chins) done without any support gear other than chalk will build a strong grip.

10.107     This is all the work you need to train the support seven well, so long as you slowly add resistance as the weeks and months go by. This can be done without getting distracted from the focus movements, and without making a significant demand on your systemic system except in the very final few weeks of a cycle. During the latter, when you are deep into new poundage territory in the major movements, temporarily either eliminate or severely cut back everything other than the major movements.

## Shoulder care

10.108   It is not surprising that shoulder injuries are almost universal among bodybuilders and lifters. There is a catalog of errors that almost all trainees are guilty of to some extent. Some of the errors have even been religiously promoted for decades by some trainers. The cost in terms of injuries is beyond measure. Be informed, apply what you learn, ignore those who promote destructive exercises, and save your shoulders.

10.109   While some people, over the short and medium term, may not appear to be suffering harm, watch out over the long term. Exercises notorious for causing shoulder harm include the press behind neck, upright row, lateral raise (especially with the little finger above the thumb), pulldown and pullup *behind the neck*, fly for the pecs, and pec deck work. There are very few experienced trainees who have not invested a lot of application in one or more of these exercises. Some of these movements are also very harmful for the rotator cuff.

10.110   The press behind neck is a traditional shoulder exercise, but one usually confined to trainees in their teens and twenties. Due to shoulder pain it is dropped from the routines of many people as they move into their thirties and beyond. The press behind neck is very severe on the shoulders, and is probably at the root of many shoulder and rotator-cuff problems. I do not recommend this exercise, not even for the very young. It is best not to start incubating shoulder problems in the first place, even though no apparent damage is felt to begin with.

10.111   Shoulder damage is also caused by potentially sound exercises which are ruined by distortions. These include the very wide grip bench press and overhead press, dip with the knuckles facing in, very wide grip dip, rock-bottom dip, bench press too high on the chest or to the neck, any press that uses an excessive range of motion (including the dumbbell bench press), and the pulldown or pullup to the front but with a very wide grip.

10.112   For lanky trainees the conventional range of motion on bench presses, especially with a close grip, is probably excessive and will cause shoulder problems.

10.113   Then there is very poor form in a good exercise that uses a safe grip. Such destroyers include not keeping tight at the arms-straight position in the pulldown, pullup or row, wrong bar path in the bench press, swinging and arching in the barbell curl, and slamming into the lockout of pressing moves.

10.114   Excessive training volume or frequency will damage your shoulders. Any shoulder, chest or back exercise heavily works your shoulders. Even on an abbreviated program—where, for example, you train each exercise once a week but while training three times a week altogether—you can overtrain your shoulders. Bench press on Monday, dumbbell row on Wednesday, and press on Friday, means three shoulder workouts per week. That will wear down even a superman's shoulders, eventually. Even two demanding shoulder workouts a week is too much for some people. Be careful how you structure your weekly training schedule. Give your shoulders plenty of recovery time.

10.115   Inadequately warming up your shoulders before performing any very demanding exercise for them will cause damage.

10.116   An excessive imbalance between the external (weaker) and internal (stronger) rotator muscles of the shoulders will produce shoulder problems. This, on top of the other sources of shoulder havoc just outlined, sets you up for rotator cuff problems. Train the L-fly once or twice a week, to strengthen your shoulder external rotators.

10.117   Rigorously analyze your exercise program, and discover where you are harming your shoulders. Rectify the problems, and you will hugely reduce the chances of shoulder problems ever impeding your training progress.

## Shoulder external rotators

10.118   The external rotators of the shoulder include two small muscles called the infraspinatus and teres minor. These are much weaker than the internal rotators, which include the pecs and lats. To distinguish between external and internal rotation of the shoulder, imagine you are standing and shaking hands with someone with your right hand. While in that position, if you move your hand to your right, you are externally rotating your shoulder. Move your hand to the left, and you are internally rotating your shoulder.

10.119   The infraspinatus and teres minor belong to a group of four muscles of the upper back that also include the supraspinatus and subscapularis. The tendons of these four muscles connect the scapula (shoulder blade) to the shoulder joint at the rotator cuff. Overuse and abuse of the rotator cuff and shoulders in general, together with weak external rotator muscles, make rotator-cuff injuries among the most common for weight trainees. (The book THE SEVEN-MINUTE ROTATOR CUFF SOLUTION by Dr. Joseph M. Horrigan and Jerry Robinson alerted me to the importance of specific exercise for the external rotator muscles.) Never try to work through pain in this area, or any other.

## Dumbbell work

10.120    Dumbbells are usually used for detail exercises which have very limited, if any application for the typical hard gainer whose priority is to build substantial size and strength. Barbells, generally speaking, have a tradition for being used for the big and most useful movements. If you have in mind doing the pec fly, lateral raise, concentration curl, triceps kickback and akin exercises with dumbbells, the 'bells will harm your training progress. But if, for example, you use them for one-arm rows instead of pulldowns, dumbbell presses instead of barbell presses, hammer or supinating curls instead of barbell curls, and one-legged calf raises instead of using a calf machine, then the dumbbells will be an asset.

10.121    While dumbbells provide variety relative to the straight bar, for some exercises, e.g., bench presses and overhead presses, they are very awkward to get into position. You may need two spotters for each dumbbell once you are using heavy weights. If the dumbbells fall out of the groove during a set the exercise can be very dangerous. Even if you escape injury, heavy dumbbells dropping to the floor risk damage to it and the equipment, and to anyone nearby at the time.

10.122    But most misuse of dumbbells comes from people who use 'bells that are too heavy for them. They are thus unable to

> **Depending on your leverages, the Trap Bar deadlift may not work your lower back adequately enough by itself. Stiff-legged or partial deadlifts may be needed too. For some people the Trap Bar deadlift is a great substitute for the squat but *not* for a deadlift variation. And strength built by the Trap Bar may not necessarily carry over to the straight bar deadlift, *depending on the individual.***

control the resistance properly, and thus put themselves and the dumbbells at risk. Use dumbbells properly, or not at all.

10.123   A barbell bench press can be easily set down on power-rack pins if you fail during a rep. Not so with a heavy dumbbell bench press where very alert, strong and competent spotters are needed at all times, and a power rack is unhelpful. But you could attach chains of the appropriate length to the dumbbells, and securely suspend them from overhead so that at rest the 'bells are at the bottom position of the exercise concerned.

10.124   Unless you have a full set of dumbbells available, the changing of the plates is a hassle and big disadvantage. But for some exercises—e.g., deadlifts, rows, curls and calf raises—there are fewer handling difficulties.

10.125   Keeping the potential negatives in mind, dumbbells offer some advantages relative to barbells. They demand greater control and coordination, and thus involve more musculature. They permit a greater range of motion in some exercises, e.g., the bench press and deadlift (but which may be harmful because too much range of motion may expose you to injury).

10.126   Dumbbells allow one-limbed work, which can be a terrific way of applying increased focus and effort on your body—train both sides of your body, but only one side at a time. At least in some exercises this permits you to use the disengaged side as the spotter for the engaged side, e.g., one-limbed curls and calf work. This can be very productive.

10.127   Very importantly, dumbbells enable the user to find the best rep groove for him. This may enable a given barbell movement that is not a success to be turned into a successful dumbbell version. The barbell forces the hands into a set position; but the dumbbells enable the hands to be held in whatever position is best for the user according to leverage or injury factors.

10.128   Many older trainees prefer dumbbells to barbells in many moves because the 'bells, with a slight change in wrist position, permit pain-free training relative to doing the same movements with a barbell. Of course you should avoid any training abuse that may cause damage to begin with; but if you are living with a legacy of mistakes from years gone by (not necessarily training related), then dumbbells may be particularly useful.

10.129   If you retain good control over the dumbbells, have their collars
         securely in place, do not expose yourself to undue injury risk,
         and are wise in your choice of exercises, the addition of
         dumbbells to your training can be invaluable.

10.130   The combined weight of two dumbbells is usually less than can
         be used in the same movement done with a barbell. The total
         used in bench pressing or overhead pressing with dumbbells
         will, typically, be about 80–85% of what can be moved in a
         barbell in those two exercises. This assumes familiarity with
         using the dumbbells. Until you are familiar with the tricky
         balance of using a pair of dumbbells, it is unlikely you will be
         able to handle 80% of your barbell weight. This dumbbells-
         versus-barbell comparison applies to exercises where two
         dumbbells are used simultaneously. It does not apply to
         exercises where one side is done at a time, e.g., dumbbell row.

## Thick-bar work

10.131   Using a thick bar (diameter of about 2 inches, or more) provides
         a challenging alternative to the regular-diameter barbell. You do
         not *need* to do thick-bar work to get big and strong, but
         including it can be a plus. Thick bars favor people with big
         hands, but all trainees can profit from them.

10.132   If you are a home gym user you can get yourself a thick bar in
         one of at least three ways. First, buy a ready-made thick bar;
         second, take a regular bar to a metal worker and have a metal
         tube of a diameter of your choice welded on between the inside
         collars; or third, get a metal worker to custom-make a thick bar
         from the materials he has available.

10.133   The ends of the bar need to be appropriate to the size of the
         holes in the plates you use. At a pinch, just a length of hollow
         heavy-duty pipe will suffice.

10.134   Similar comments can be made for getting your own thick-
         handled dumbbells. Get acquainted with a local and competent
         metal worker. You can then have other simple pieces of
         training gear produced conveniently, to your own design, and
         perhaps surprisingly economically.

10.135   Thick-handled dumbbells should be used with even more
         caution than thick barbells. For example, if your grip fails
         while performing thick-handled dumbbell curls, and you drop

the 'bells, you risk breaking a foot. But if while curling you drop a barbell loaded with anything other than only very small plates, your feet are not at risk. And if you properly use a power rack, then the barbell would never fall to the floor.

10.136    For pressing movements, a moderately thick bar (once you are used to it) will not greatly reduce the weights you use relative to those with a regular bar.

10.137    For curls, your poundage may suffer a little with the 2-inch bar, but a lot with a 3-inch bar. But for deadlifts and other pulling movements, and specific grip work, any thick bar will devastate the poundages you can use relative to a regular bar of 1–1.1 inch diameter. The thicker the bar, the greater your grip will limit you.

10.138    While you can use a thick bar for presses and curls, and still push all the involved musculature to the hilt, the same cannot be said for pulling movements. If you switch to using a thick bar for deadlifts and rows, your grip will severely limit the involvement from your back muscles and defeat the main purpose of those exercises, unless grip work is the focus.

10.139    Deadlifting using a thick barbell provides tremendous grip work. Add the thick-bar deadlift to your deadlift day's work, either on top of your regular work if you recuperate well, or *instead* of a little of your regular work, in order to keep the total volume of work constant.

10.140    While you will be able to get your fingers around or almost around a 2-inch diameter bar, you will not be able to encircle a 3-inch bar unless you have gigantic hands. For pulling exercises like the deadlift you will be faced with the alternative of holding the bar as if pinch gripping it, or by using your hands more like hooks (and be able to handle a bit more poundage), and in both cases have the choice of either the reverse grip (i.e., one hand facing forward, and the other facing to the rear) or a both-palms-facing-you (pronated) grip. Be consistent with the grip you use for record-keeping purposes, or use more than one grip and keep multiple sets of records.

10.141    The 3-inch bar is too thick for safe overhead pressing, but it *may* be satisfactory for bench pressing following a period of adapting to it, *if* your hands are larger than average.

10.142    If you were to get only one thick bar, the 2-inch diameter one (or one slightly less thick) would be the best choice.

10.143    Whatever thick bar you use for bench pressing or overhead pressing, do the work inside a power rack or an alternative apparatus that functions in a similar way. Position the pins/safety bars at the right height to catch the bar should you lose your grip or fail on a rep. There is less room for errors with a thick bar than a regular bar.

10.144    An unloaded, Olympic-length and solid 2-inch bar weighs about 75 pounds. A solid 3-inch bar of the same length weighs about 125 pounds, so a partially hollow one would be easier to handle. A regular Olympic bar onto which a 3-inch diameter tube has been welded between the inside collars weighs about 65 pounds. Hollow pipes are lighter *and* cheaper.

## Difficult-to-handle objects

10.145    You may want to follow the examples of Dr. Ken Leistner and Kim Wood and get yourself an odd-shaped and perhaps bulky object for some fun, challenging and potentially productive holding, lifting or carrying, to finish off a workout. A thick bar is just a starter. Logs, logs with handles attached, beams with handles attached, and sandbags can be used. *But be very careful not to over-extend yourself, use poor lifting form, get your toes caught under an object that crashes to the floor, or get injured in any other way. If in doubt, do not do it!*

10.146    Awkward-shaped objects are more difficult to handle than their weight may suggest. Be very careful! Wearing steel-capped boots is a necessity when lifting difficult-to-handle hard objects. And do not lift such objects on a surface that cannot stand having something dropped on it. To make it easier on the floor, and remove the chance of serious damage to your feet, use sandbags, with rope handles attached when necessary. Even if one should land on your foot while wearing shoes with soft uppers, it should not do any lasting damage. Play safe!

10.147    Something you could do with a thick-handled dumbbell is to fix up a "challenge" 'bell like some of the old-time strongmen did. Set it up just out of reach for your current strength at one-hand deadlifting (bracing your disengaged hand on your lower thigh), and work on it once a week until you can pull it. Then set up a new challenge dumbbell, and work on that.

10.148　　With dumbbells you can include the farmer's walk to end a
workout. Walk until the 'bells fall out of your hands. Only do
this on a surface that can withstand the dumbbells being
dropped on it—outside on a field, for example. And keep your
feet out of the way. Walk either for time or distance, and work
on increasing the time or distance. The field must have an
even surface—*you must not stumble and/or injure your ankle!*

10.149　　This type of training is an *optional* extra only. You can get very
big and strong without ever lifting any odd-shaped objects. Do
not let this type of training distract you from the priority
exercises. And do not injure yourself on the "icing on the cake"
extras. Always pay 100% attention to safety factors and good
form. Personally I would never do any heavy odd-object lifting
or carrying (but holding/supporting could be safe), and neither
should many others—because the risks far outweigh the
benefits. But for some people, when used carefully and
prudently, the odd-object lifting or carrying can be valuable.

10.150　　Never forget about the real ultimate weight-training challenges
such as 20-rep rest-pause squats. A period of *intensive* 20-rep
squatting will quickly get most other types of training into
perspective. Not only that, but a 20-rep squat program can build
a lot more muscle and might than can most other programs.

## Aesthetics and exercise selection

10.151　　Once you have built good overall development, aesthetics may
play a large role in the exercises or specific variations you employ.
If you are a function-first strength trainee, such as a powerlifter,
aesthetics may be of little importance but strength balance should
be very important. If you are primarily a bodybuilder, aesthetics
may heavily influence your exercise selection.

10.152　　As already noted in this chapter, training your neck, calves and
grip is an important part of overall aesthetics.

10.153　　You may choose exercises for specific purposes, or you may
*avoid* certain exercises. If your pecs respond well to the supine
bench press, and are large, do not hammer away at the same
movement and overdevelop your pecs. Move to the incline
variation instead, or perhaps the parallel bar dip. If you get little
or no lat development from dumbbell rows, find a core exercise
that does develop your lats. If you get little or no biceps
development from lat work, include direct work for your biceps.

10.154   Once you are already well developed and know how specific exercise variations work for you, you may select or modify your exercises accordingly.

10.155   Regardless of whether or not you put aesthetics high on your priority list, you will probably find an exercise or two that you can, relatively speaking, do much better at than the other exercises. You will then have the option of making a natural strength more outstanding. This will let you achieve something exceptional (both in poundage and development) in that limited area. Alternatively you could back off in your natural bias(es), to try to get balance throughout your body. My advice is to make the most of any natural strength(s) you have. But the final choice is yours.

10.156   As explained in Chapter 4, there is the matter of how lean you are and how visible your development is. For an appearance-first bodybuilder this is a major factor.

10.157   Finally, remember to pay attention to your posture and gait. How you hold your body, and walk, has a big bearing on how you present your muscular development. [BB]

---

Exercise selection alone can make the difference between training success and failure. And even if you are using the best exercises, if you do not use perfect exercise technique you will get nowhere but into the quagmire of injuries, frustration and failure.

---

The understanding of good exercise technique is one thing, and vital in its own right. But being able to practice it yourself is another matter. Intelligent use of a video camera will help you to develop good exercise form. See THE INSIDER'S TELL-ALL HANDBOOK ON WEIGHT-TRAINING TECHNIQUE for detailed instructions on how to use a video camera to increase training productivity.

*Many people get themselves so concerned with what is the "best" rep cadence (and rep range, pace of training, and many other matters) that they forget that of first importance is good and safe form, hard work, and progressive poundages. Even if you had the "perfect" combination of rep cadence, rep range and pace of training, if you use sloppy form, do not train hard, and use stagnant training poundages, you will never build a big and strong physique.*

# 11. How to Perform Your Reps

11.1 Most bodybuilders and strength trainees perform their reps too quickly. Many take only about one second to raise the weight, and another one second to return the resistance to its starting position. A 1/1 cadence is not controlled lifting and lowering, but throwing and dropping. Changing to a slower rep cadence is, for those trainees, probably the single most dramatic improvement in training safety that can be made.

11.2 I am talking exclusively about traditional bodybuilding exercises, i.e., bench press, squat, deadlift, pulldown, chin, row, curl, etc., not skill-first, highly technical and explosive Olympic-style weightlifting exercises such as power cleans, cleans, snatches, and jerks. The latter are not necessary for bodybuilding and strength training because there are plenty of alternative exercises that are super productive but technically much simpler. *Mastering* the Olympic-style lifts is *far* more difficult than mastering the traditional bodybuilding exercises.

11.3 Olympic lifting can be a fine way to train *if* the coaching is hands-on and expert, and the subject is injury-free and physically well-suited to this type of training. But unless you have access to expert hands-on Olympic lifting coaching, and are physically well-suited to this type of lifting, leave it alone. There are safer ways to train which are technically much less demanding—i.e., those which are promoted in this book.

11.4 Very importantly, even a well-controlled rep cadence will injure you if your biomechanics are all wrong. *Good form is not merely about rep cadence.*

11.5 Focus on getting each rep right, one at a time. Do not concern yourself with the whole set, but with each individual rep. Getting each rep right involves a number of factors: form, rep cadence, and between-rep pauses.

# Form and cadence

11.6    Rep form is related to rep cadence and between-rep pauses, but
        slow cadence does not necessarily mean good form, and fast
        performance does not necessarily mean the use of poor
        technique. Slow does not always mean strict, just like fast does
        not always mean cheating. And heavy low-rep work does not
        necessarily mean fast reps.

11.7    A slow rep can still involve terrible exercise form, and some
        exercises—e.g., snatch, clean and jerk, clean, and other
        explosive movements—must be done quickly.

11.8    Any exercise can be performed in an explosive way, but
        explosiveness is not promoted in this book or in THE INSIDER'S
        TELL-ALL HANDBOOK ON WEIGHT-TRAINING TECHNIQUE. These
        books are concerned with minimizing the risk of injury while
        maximizing the potential for muscular size and strength.
        There is no need to increase the demands on technical
        expertise, or to expose yourself to exaggerated muscle and
        connective tissue stresses in order to gain size and strength.
        Stick to the exercises promoted in this book and you can
        realize your potential for muscle and might while minimizing
        your risk of injury.

11.9    More important than rep speed per se, is rep *smoothness*. If your
        reps are smooth, you are using the control that is necessary for
        safety *and* applying great stress on the involved musculature.

11.10   Smoothness and a moderate or slow tempo of rep cadence are
        not necessarily the same thing. It is possible, for example, to
        perform a three-second bench press ascent that involves an
        explosive start. The first few inches might take a split second,
        but the rest of the rep could take almost three seconds. That
        very explosive initial thrust greatly exaggerates the stress on
        the involved musculature and connective tissue, and is an
        unnecessary risk. But you probably could have performed a
        smooth two-second ascent with the same weight. In this case,
        the two-second rep would be safer than the three-second one.

11.11   Recall the pause test given in the previous chapter:

        When doing the exercises listed in this book [in Chapter
        10] you should be able to stop each at any point, hold the
        weight briefly, and then continue. In an intensive set you

will probably not be able to pause *and* get your target reps, depending on which rep you paused. The idea is that you *could* pause as a demonstration of control.

11.12    If you can pass the pause test, you have control over the bar, and can focus your attention on intensity of effort and poundage progression. But if you do not have control over the bar, you need to fix that before you focus on intensity and poundage progression. Sloppy reps done with intensity will hurt you, and sooner rather than later.

11.13    Let rep smoothness and the pause test be your guides for rep performance. It is not necessary to count seconds, or to lock yourself into a specific cadence for each exercise. In practice, however, smooth reps that pass the pause test will take about three seconds for the positive (or longer for the final rep or two of a set) and at least three seconds for the negative.

11.14    At the beginning of each set of multiple reps you are stronger than you need to be to perform the reps. You will not need to use your full degree of effort until the final reps of each set. But even using the maximum power output possible over the final rep(s) of a set will move the resistance only relatively slowly.

## Rep pauses

11.15    Reps can be done in a continuous cadence or with a pause after each rep. The continuous-cadence style restricts the size of the poundages that can be used, but shortens the duration of the sets and heightens the aching in the muscles. Using a short pause between reps enables greater poundages to be used. Taken to an extreme of 30–60 seconds between reps, a single set almost becomes a series of single-rep sets. This exaggerated rest-pause training usually necessitates putting the bar down (or racking it) between reps.

11.16    Some exercises are more suited to one style than the other. Calf raises are suited to the continuous style, but are more effective with a brief pause at the top. Squats and bent-legged deadlifts provide an almost overwhelming urge to take a brief pause between reps, at least towards the end of a set. *Generally speaking*, continuous reps are not as productive as those done with a pause before each. Continuous reps produce quicker muscular fatigue, and the perception of intense stimulation, but that can be deceptive as far as growth stimulation is concerned.

# General recommendation

11.17    Take about three seconds for the positive stroke and at least
         another three for the negative stroke, performing every stroke
         of each rep *smoothly*. If you move faster than at about 3/3 you
         will be unable to exercise the necessary control. For the positive
         phase of the very final rep of a set, when you almost grind to a
         halt, you may need over five seconds. For a few workouts have
         an assistant count the seconds as you perform each rep, and
         give feedback while doing so, to ensure you do not move faster
         than at about a 3/3 cadence. Once you get the feel for a smooth
         cadence you will be able to exercise it without needing to have
         the seconds counted. If in doubt, go slower rather than faster.
         Some exercises have a longer stroke than others, e.g., the
         pulldown and overhead press need more time per rep than do
         the calf raise and bench press, to show comparable control.

11.18    Do not try to count seconds *and* reps. You can successfully
         count one or the other, but not both simultaneously. If you
         want to count both cadence and rep number, get a helper to
         count one of them, and you count the other. While a 3/3 or so
         cadence is the general recommendation, *do not* get so locked
         into a precise number of seconds that you become a slave to
         time. *The focus should be on control, form and progression.*

11.19    Perform each rep as an individual unit that ends with a brief
         pause prior to performing the next rep. Take the time you need
         to set yourself to perform the next rep perfectly. As a set
         progresses, your pauses will tend to become longer. But overdo
         the pause and you will fail the set prematurely. Experience will
         teach you what is an excessive pause for you in each exercise.

11.20    In exercises that can involve a sustained contraction in the
         flexed position, e.g., calf raise, curl, pulldown and supported
         row, hold the resistance for a second or two in the position of
         full contraction. This will tighten your form and intensify the
         contraction. In effect, briefly squeeze in the contracted position.

11.21    While you can do this "squeezing" in single-joint exercises, you
         cannot do it in all multi-joint exercises. For example, in the calf
         raise—a single-joint exercise—there is no easing of stress on the
         muscle when you are in the extended position. But in the
         squat—a multi-joint exercise—the stress is taken off the
         muscles in the extended position (where the legs are straight).

*Please read the box on page 353 for "More on rep speed."*

## Double-pause reps

11.22    Some exercises naturally lend themselves to a pause at both the bottom *and* top of each rep, e.g., curl, pulldown, and prone row. But only one of the pauses is actually a resting pause. The other is a contraction squeeze, which is very demanding. It would be accurate to call these "single-pause" reps. (At the bottom of the pulldown, chin, shrug and any row, do not relax or allow your shoulders to slump. Stay tight or else otherwise you may injure your shoulders.)

11.23    Many exercises do not permit a pause at the top *and* bottom of the exercise, at least not when done in the conventional down-and-then-straight-up manner of performance, e.g., squat, bench press and overhead press.

11.24    But with modification these exercises can easily be performed in a pause style—actually a "double-pause" style. Set the pins of a power rack at the appropriate height for the bottom position of the chosen exercise, and briefly rest the barbell on the pins at the bottom of each rep. A pause for just one second is enough to ensure that you start each rep from a dead stop in the bottom position. This is sometimes called "from the bottom" bench pressing, squatting, etc. This is a rigorous and highly productive way to train. It is strongly recommended— not necessarily for year-round training, but at least for some cycles. You could even mix double-pause and single-pause reps in the same workout for a given exercise, but in different sets.

11.25    You can rest longer than just a second or two at the bottom of the press and bench press, but not in the squat. You must keep very tight at the bottom when doing from-the-bottom squats. If you pause for more than a second or so you risk losing the necessary tightness. If you need to take longer pauses at the bottom of the squat, stand between reps with the bar resting at the bottom position (across the pins). Keep your feet and hands in position, descend on a deep breath, hold that breath and quickly get under the bar, and then immediately drive the bar up, and exhale. (If you exhale before you drive the bar up, you will lose the tight torso that is essential for safe squatting.) Pause at the top position, and then carefully descend and set the bar down on the pins ready for the next rep.

11.26    Especially for long-limbed and narrow-chested trainees, an extended pause at the bottom of the bench press and overhead press may not be safe, due to the extreme range of motion and shoulder extension. Better to keep the pause to the minimum, and perhaps reduce the range of motion a little.

11.27    The deadlift can be done with a pause at both the top and bottom (double-pause style), but fatigue can quickly lead to form deterioration. For control and safety, reduce the range of motion for double-pause deadlifting—take the bar from off pins set in a rack at knee height or a little lower. Release your grip on the bar while it is set on the pins, to let your hands and forearms recover adequately to be able to hold the bar securely for the next rep. Such a partial deadlift is actually a partial *stiff-legged* deadlift because knee flexion is taken out of the exercise.

## Priority of practical application

11.28    It is practical application that determines whether or not a certain training modality works for the individual concerned. When properly supervised on someone who is not restrained by injuries or structural limitations, and who is not at the limit of his muscular potential, all the interpretations of training described in this book have the potential to deliver substantial muscular development. But each interpretation must be done well and on a sustained basis. It has to be done for a whole cycle of a few months, or longer, to deliver noticeable results.

11.29    No matter how good something may be in theory, or in practice for *some* people, if *you* cannot put it into practice for long enough to see results, it is not productive for you. You must find an approach that *you* enjoy, that *you* can do consistently, and that delivers results for *you*.

11.30    I want you to train long-term—for life. You need to maintain your enthusiasm for training, and not exhaust your enthusiasm and end up skipping the gym for a while. *You cannot keep whatever gains you have made unless you keep on training.*

> **When experimenting with a particular change in your training, it is not necessary to implement it in all your exercises. Try the change on just one exercise; but be sure you really try it! Then if you like what it does in one exercise, extend it to other exercises. No need to put all your eggs in one basket, so to speak.**

## Range of motion

11.31    While making an exercise harder usually makes it better, there
         are many exceptions. Increasing the depth of squatting and
         deadlifting, for example, makes those exercises harder, but for
         some people that "harder" means harmful, if not ruinous.
         Generally speaking, you should use as full a range of motion as
         possible *so long as it does not hurt you.*

11.32    There are some exercises, however, where the range of motion
         is intentionally reduced *even when a greater range of motion can be
         performed safely.* For example, in THE INSIDER'S TELL-ALL
         HANDBOOK ON WEIGHT-TRAINING TECHNIQUE the partial deadlift
         and the overhead lockout are described and recommended.

11.33    Using a four-post power rack, or the smaller half rack or open
         rack, it is easy to break exercises into their component parts—
         the start, the finish (i.e., the lockout), and the part in between.
         The start would go from the very beginning of the rep—e.g., at
         the chest in the bench press—until *only* about the sticking
         point, before pausing, and lowering the resistance to the
         beginning. The lockout would be just the last few inches of the
         rep, usually starting from above the sticking point. But the
         "part in between" could go from about a third of the way up
         till about two thirds of the way up—i.e., the middle phase only,
         just through the sticking point—*or* it could go from at about the
         sticking point right to the finish.

11.34    Doing lockouts often enables weights to be used well in excess
         of what can be handled for the full rep. On the one hand this
         can be useful for overloading, but simultaneously it provides
         the most dangerous aspect of partial-rep training—excessive
         demands upon the skeletal structure of the body. Never mind
         that some people can use colossal weights in many partial lifts
         without apparent harm. Those people are *not* role models for
         you or any other typical person because most of those strength
         phenomena are genetically blessed with unusually robust joints
         and connective tissue. But even some of these gifted people
         suffer damage over the long-term. It is much safer to stick to
         working a component of a rep other than the lockout part, if
         you want to try partial-rep training.

11.35    This does not, however, exclude *careful* and intelligent use of
         lockouts in the occasional cycle, at least in some movements,
         but *not* in movements where you have a structural weak link.

Start relatively light, and take a couple of months of progressively building up before you start to use your limit weights for lockouts.

11.36      For lockouts, your form must be *absolutely impeccable*. If you get out of the groove with the very heavy weights that lockouts in some exercises permit, you will expose your body to potentially very dangerous levels of stress. Be careful! Generally speaking, non-exaggerated full-range training is a much safer way to train.

11.37      Using a restricted range of motion *other* than the lockout part can be a safe and very productive way to train even on a regular basis. Training the bench press from two inches above chest height, and the squat from two inches above the point where the thighs are parallel to the ground, are examples of reduced-range-of-motion training that do not necessitate the big (and potentially risky) loads that lockouts do.

## One-and-a-half reps

11.38      Full reps and partial reps can be blended in the same set. This is a very demanding way to train, and a potentially productive addition to your arsenal of training tools. But do not apply it to too many exercises at any one time, or else you will risk overtraining. Be conservative and use it on no more than two exercises in any given routine. Over time, vary the exercises to which you apply one-and-a-half reps training.

11.39      There are two ways to perform one-and-a-half reps:

a.   Using the bench press as the example, imagine the bar at arm's length. Lower the bar under control, gently touch your chest a little below your lower pec line, and press the bar back to arm's length. Pause for a second or two and then lower the bar approximately half way down, stop, and then press the bar back to arm's length. Alternatively the half rep could be done *before* the full rep. In both cases this is one-and-a-half-rep work going *down*.

b.   Again imagine the bar at arm's length. Following a short pause, lower the bar all the way to your chest. Then press the bar only half way up, and return the bar to your chest. Then press the bar all the way up. This is one-and-a-half-rep work going *up*. The half rep is done before the full rep.

11.40    Both ways can be productive. You may find one is better suited
         to some exercises than the other—experiment to find out. You
         may, however, prefer to use *both* ways in a systematic way for
         the same exercise—for example, alternate the two approaches
         from set to set, or workout to workout.

11.41    A full rep and a half rep counts as a single one-and-a-half rep.
         Naturally you will have to reduce your poundages relative to
         what you would use for sets of the same rep count but of
         exclusively full reps. And, of course, you would focus on
         progressive poundages in good form for this training approach,
         just as you should for any format. When you return to sets of
         full reps after a period of using one-and-a-half reps for that
         exercise, you should be able to work into new personal best
         poundages—perhaps, though, only after a short period of
         readaptation to using purely full reps.

## The pilgrimage

11.42    No matter what style of training you use, each set needs to be a
         pilgrimage. There is no room for anything other than 100%
         application if you want to make good progress. Pay homage to
         focus, perfect form, and effort. And make each set perfect by
         making each rep perfect! BB

> Elite bodybuilders, lifters and athletes can tolerate and
> even prosper on explosive training because they have
> the required robustness of joints and connective
> tissue. But even they often pay a heavy price in terms
> of injuries, *eventually*. There is absolutely no need to
> take any risk with explosive training. A slower and
> controlled rep tempo—as promoted in this book—is so
> much safer, and by far the best option for typical
> trainees. Why seriously risk pushing your body
> beyond its structural limits, and possibly suffering
> *permanent* injuries, when there are safer ways to train
> that are super productive?

Had all hard-gaining trainees followed programs akin to those promoted in this book, there would be tons more muscle in the world. There would also be much less drug use because it would no longer be necessary to take steroids to make training programs work. And there would also be a lot less use of the label "hard gainer" because so many people would consider themselves relatively easy gainers.

To maximize your gains in muscular size and strength you must organize your training, nutrition, rest and sleep in order to ensure progressive training poundages. Everything you do must be built around providing the optimum environment for the production of progressive training poundages while using consistently good exercise form. To ensure that the strength gain yields growth, you may, however, need to avoid very low reps, partial reps, low-rep rest-pause work, and overly infrequent training.

# 12. How to Design Your Own Training Programs

12.1     A general framework of training that delivers results for everyone does exist, but each trainee must individualize it in order to maximize gains. Here are six of the most critical lessons you can learn concerning program design:

       a.   Focus on no more than a handful of big basic exercises each workout.

       b.   Do not neglect important accessory movements.

       c.   Train hard but within the context of intensity cycling.

       d.   Get more rest days than weight-training days.

       e.   If in doubt always do less training rather than more.

       f.   Stress progressive poundages in good form.

## Exceptions

12.2     All six of these key lessons are broken by some successful trainees. These exceptions are, however, *not* the typical trainees I am aiming my writing at. Of course teenagers and those in their early twenties who have low-stress and well-rested lives (relative to those of us who are over thirty years old with demanding careers and families) can train differently, at least to a degree, or train on similar routines but with greater volume and frequency. And genetically gifted or drug-assisted people can break all the "rules" and still gain very well.

12.3     The instruction in this book is geared primarily for people who neither have near-ideal training conditions nor near-ideal recuperation capabilities. But should you be fortunate to have circumstances more suited to quicker gains, make the most of it while it lasts. Follow the training methods promoted in this book and you will gain in abundance—far more than you would on conventional programs.

# Six Frameworks for Productive Training Programs

*This section is a revised and expanded version of the section of the same name in* THE MUSCLE & MIGHT TRAINING TRACKER.

12.4    As far as training programs go, here are six frameworks to be used as *starting points*. Each should be personalized by each individual according to the advice given in this book. In keeping with the spirit of abbreviated training, the routines are short and simple, and dominated by major exercises.

12.5    Abbreviated training is the most productive type of training for typical drug-free trainees. The potential huge productivity of abbreviated training rests on the brevity of its routines and its infrequent workout frequency relative to conventional training methods. If you complicate the routines by adding exercises and/or training days, you will dilute the effort given to each set, increase the demands on your recovery ability, seriously risk overtraining, water down your enthusiasm for working out, and undermine if not destroy the potential value of the routines. Then you will be back at square one—with a conventional routine that yields little or no growth for everyone except the genetically gifted and drug-assisted.

## FRAMEWORK 1
### Full-body-routine program

12.6    This involves a single full-body routine that is performed only as often as can be coped with, e.g., twice a week, or once every fourth, fifth, sixth or seventh day. Because each workout is identical, the same exercises get trained each workout. Here is an example of a full-body-routine program:

*General warmup*
   a.  Squat
   b.  Parallel bar dip
   c.  Stiff-legged deadlift
   d.  Dumbbell press
   e.  Pulldown or pullup
   f.  Barbell curl

    g.  Calf work

    h.  Crunch situp

*Cool down*

12.7    Assuming you really are training intensively, to train twice a week on the same full-body routine is too much for many if not most drug-free typical people.

12.8    Particularly in the pre-steroids era, working out three times a week on a full-body routine was a common way to train. But the factor often responsible for making this type of training productive was that only one of the three weekly workouts was intensive. The other two weekly workouts were performed in a relatively leisurely fashion, with reduced weights—i.e., "light" and "medium" workouts.

12.9    To train hard and productively on the same set of exercises every workout, most people need to reduce their training frequency to no more than once every four or five days, or three times every two weeks. Many people would be better off training just once a week when using a single high-intensity full-body routine. This can be a super-efficient way to train, especially for people with busy lives.

12.10    You may be able to train some exercises productively with full-bore intensity more often than others. Perhaps you can train your accessory exercises (e.g., calf, neck and waist work) productively twice a week, but only be able to train your major core exercises really hard once a week. Few drug-free trainees can train with 100% effort in the squat, deadlift, stiff-legged deadlift or bench press twice a week every week. You could, however, still train your big core exercises twice a week, but make one of those workouts only moderate-intensity for those specific exercises, e.g., train them using your usual rep count but with only about 80% of your usual weights. However you train, though, you must stimulate growth without overtraining.

> **If, for example, you overhead press following the bench press, your performance in the press will suffer. And if you perform the L-fly immediately after the curl, your performance in the L-fly will suffer. Arrange your exercises so that none suffer in this way.**

## Possible shortcomings

12.11     Serious trainees love to train, and train hard. To train just once a week is not enough. But training must not be done so often that overtraining is the outcome. Satisfaction from weight training comes from good results, not just hours spent in the gym. But the greatest return arises from great results plus the satisfaction that comes from being able to weight train productively two or three times a week.

12.12     To weight train productively twice a week, see Frameworks 2, 4, 5 and 6. To possibly train productively three times a week, see especially Framework 3.

12.13     A single full-body schedule has only one routine. This limits the number of exercises you can productively include in your program. With divided programs you have two or three different routines, and scope to include, productively, more exercises. With the potential for productive inclusion of more exercises, assuming they are the right exercises, a more balanced exercise program can be designed. A balanced weights program produces balanced musculature throughout the body.

12.14     Having a one-routine weight-training program can become monotonous, because every time you train you perform the same routine. (But a raw beginner is usually best off following a one-routine program so that each exercise is trained often enough for lifting skills to be learned quickly.) Having two or three different routines—which are alternated, or rotated— provides built-in variety on a steady number of exercises. This provides the training variety—for non-beginners—that produces increased motivation and enthusiasm for many trainees, and delivers best results.

# FRAMEWORK 2

## Twice-a-week divided program

12.15     This program involves twice-a-week training, alternating two different workouts and training each exercise once a week. Here is an example, mixing major and accessory exercises at each workout:

### Monday

*General warmup*
   a.  Squat
   b.  Bench press or parallel bar dip

    c.  Pulldown or prone row
    d.  Calf work
    e.  Back extension
    f.  Crunch situp
    g.  Grip work (including finger extension)
*Cool down*

### Thursday
*General warmup*
    a.  Sumo deadlift or stiff-legged deadlift
    b.  Overhead press
    c.  Curl
    d.  Side bend
    e.  Neck work
    f.  L-fly
*Cool down*

## Dangers

12.16    If you have excessive overlap between the two workouts you will produce two different but nevertheless full-body workouts. This would mean that you would be training all your major musculature twice a week. This is excessive for many typical drug-free trainees if the training is done with real effort each session. To produce routines with minimal overlap—but some overlap is inevitable—put exercises that involve a lot of common musculature into the same workout, or only use one of the involved exercises in the whole weekly program.

12.17    The above program is an example of two routines that have considerable overlap. Day one includes the squat and bench press as its major exercises, and day two could include the sumo deadlift and overhead press as its majors. The squat and sumo deadlift involve the same thigh, glute and lower back musculature. So that means you would be blasting your lower back at both training days each week. On such a course overtraining is likely for many trainees, and sooner rather than later. Bench pressing on one day, and overhead pressing on another, means two major sessions per week for your upper-body pushing structure. This may cause overtraining of the shoulders for many trainees.

12.18    In these cases the problem lies in there being only three or four days of rest between training the same major structures, which may not be enough recovery time for many trainees. Instead, arrange the same exercises so that you get a full week of rest between major strikes on the same musculature. For example, day one's major exercises could become the squat and stiff-legged deadlift or sumo deadlift, and day two's major exercises could become the bench press, overhead press, and pulldown. Then you would have all major thigh, glute and lower back work on day one, and all the upper-body pushing on day two.

12.19 To see the impact of this type of rearrangement of exercises while using the same training frequency and volume, experiment in the course of a training cycle. Start the cycle with an interpretation that has a lot of overlap across the two routines. Stick with it until poundage progression grinds to a halt in all your major exercises. Then rearrange the program, using the exact same exercises, so that there is no serious overlap across the workouts. Then you should see a new lease of life and many weeks of small but regular poundage gains across all your exercises.

12.20 To make faster progress you may need more recovery time between workouts. Try alternating the two workouts on a Monday-Thursday-Wednesday-Monday basis. If your gains improve, or even stay at the same rate, stick with the less frequent training schedule. If progress slows or regresses, return to the twice-weekly schedule.

## FRAMEWORK 3
### Three-days-a-week divided program
12.21 This program is similar to Framework 2 but puts all accessory exercises into a single routine, and increases the training days to three each week. Three intensive weight-training days each week is a risky strategy for most

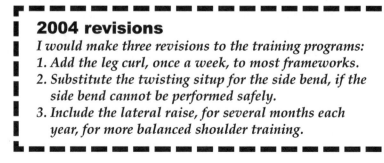

**2004 revisions**
*I would make three revisions to the training programs:*
*1. Add the leg curl, once a week, to most frameworks.*
*2. Substitute the twisting situp for the side bend, if the side bend cannot be performed safely.*
*3. Include the lateral raise, for several months each year, for more balanced shoulder training.*

trainees—because of the big chance of overtraining—but it may work if the middle day has accessory exercises only, and if there is no serious overlap between workouts. But to have major exercises at each of the three different workouts is training suicide for most drug-free trainees, especially if there is serious overlap between the workouts.

12.22    Here is an example of a three-days-a-week divided program that might be productive because it minimizes the overlap between workouts:

### Monday
*General warmup*
   a.  Squat
   b.  Stiff-legged deadlift
   c.  Pulldown or prone row
*Cool down*

### Wednesday (accessory day)
*General warmup*
   a.  Calf work
   b.  Crunch situp
   c.  Grip work (including finger extension)
   d.  Side bend
   e.  Curl
   f.  Neck work
   g.  L-fly
*Cool down*

### Friday
*General warmup*
   a.  Bench press or parallel bar dip
   b.  Overhead press
*Cool down*

# FRAMEWORK 4
## Twice-a-week three-day-divided program
12.23    This program is similar to Framework 2 but spreads the same number of exercises, or a slightly increased number of exercises, over three workouts (mixing major and accessory exercises) but while training only twice a week. This increases the rest period between workouts for a given exercise relative to Framework 2, and gives the chance to include more exercises without overtraining.

12.24   Here is an example of a twice-a-week three-day-divided program:

### Monday (of week 1)
*General warmup*
  a.  Squat
  b.  Bench press or parallel bar dip
  c.  Pulldown or one-arm dumbbell row
  d.  Standing calf work
  e.  Crunch situp
  f.  Grip work
*Cool down*

### Thursday (of week 1)
*General warmup*
  a.  Stiff-legged deadlift
  b.  Overhead lockout
  c.  Dumbbell curl
  d.  Side bend
  e.  Neck work
  f.  L-fly
  g.  Finger extension
*Cool down*

### Monday (of week 2)
*General warmup*
  a.  Leg press
  b.  Machine pullover or incline shrug
  c.  Back extension (conventional or reverse)
  d.  Barbell curl
  e.  Reverse crunch
  f.  Grip work
  g.  Seated calf work
*Cool down*

### Thursday (of week 2)
Same as Monday of week 1

## Dangers
12.25   Similar danger points apply to this schedule as they do to
        Framework 2. You should not have full-body workouts. If you
        do, you will probably be unable to recuperate properly. Avoid
        excessive overlap between workouts. For example, to squat at
        the first workout, bent-legged deadlift at the second, and then
        stiff-legged deadlift at the third would give your lower back a

very stressful workout every session, and overtraining would be likely. Divide your chosen exercises over the three days so that no musculature other than your abs and forearms is heavily involved in more than two of the three workouts.

## Two important additions for frameworks 1–4
### a. Rib cage work

12.26    Add the "breathing" pullover or the Rader chest pull to each workout. (See THE INSIDER'S TELL-ALL HANDBOOK ON WEIGHT-TRAINING TECHNIQUE for how to perform these valuable but too-rarely performed exercises.) Perform a couple of sets with the focus on maximum chest expansion. Neither exercise is systemically demanding, so the inclusion of one of them should not mar your recovery ability.

12.27    Some trainers are vigorously opposed to the possibility of increasing chest size through rib cage enlargement, and claim that chest girth can *only* be increased by muscle growth. But the fact is that many people *have* increased their rib cages. I am one of them.

12.28    While even middle-aged trainees have modestly increased the size of their rib cages through the breathing pullover and the Rader chest pull, some young trainees have greatly increased the girth of their rib cages. Rib cage enlargement will produce a deeper and broader chest, wider back and shoulders, and, as a bonus, perhaps help improve posture.

12.29    The breathing pullover and the Rader chest pull are usually performed immediately after an exercise that gets you heavily winded, e.g., high-rep squats, deadlifts or leg presses. But you can do the rib cage work whenever you want to, and without having done any exercise before it. You may even find that if you are heavily winded you will not be able to do either of the rib cage expansion exercises properly. You may even do a set or few of rib cage work every day for a few months if you want to specialize on enlarging your rib cage.

12.30    Go easy at the beginning, especially if you are not performing the rib cage stretching when winded from a heavy exercise. The forced and exaggerated breathing may make you feel dizzy unless you work into it over a period of a few weeks. Your chest may get very sore, too, if you do not work into the rib cage stretching exercise gradually.

### b. Shrugs

12.31    As explained in Chapter 10, upper-back shrugs have sufficient value to warrant their inclusion in your regular training. To include an upper-back shrug *without* it adding much to the total load of your training, and to minimize if not eliminate any warming up, shrug after your final set of deadlifts. Just one or two work set(s) of the shrug will do the job. The incline shrug is the best all-purpose upper-back shrug.

## FRAMEWORK 5
### Super-abbreviated program

12.32    The first four frameworks are already abbreviated relative to conventional training. But even these abbreviated programs can themselves be abbreviated. This is done primarily by dropping all the accessory exercises. And even the major exercises can be pruned back. Pruning back in this way does not mean you must neglect big areas of musculature. It is possible to work all the body's major musculature with just a few exercises, so long as only the very best exercises are selected. A single routine of just three exercises—e.g., Trap Bar deadlift, parallel bar dip, and pullup—covers all the major musculature of the body. Rid yourself of the notion that a lot of exercises are needed to build a big and strong body.

12.33    But why use super-abbreviated programs? Because they can be even more productive than "regular" abbreviated programs for producing gains in muscular mass.

12.34    Note that a super-abbreviated routine is at the core of every abbreviated training program. All other abbreviated routines are in essence super-abbreviated routines together with a few additional exercises.

12.35    There are several powerful applications for ultra-abbreviated routines, including:

         a.    For extending the gaining lifetime of a routine. Once a routine has run dry of gains, drop everything but the absolute essentials, perhaps add more rest days, and then you may get additional weeks of gains from an otherwise finished routine.

         b.    For extreme hard gainers, an ultra-abbreviated routine may be the only way to go, right from day one. Later programs may use more rounded abbreviated routines, once a substantial foundation has been built.

   c.   For people with very little time in which to train, ultra-abbreviated routines are perfect. With little training time so much strength and growth can be stimulated.

   d.   For people who want to try the epitome of abbreviated training for the pure sake of it. Do this at least once in your training career, even if you are never forced to by circumstances. Choose three of your favorite major exercises and devote at least a few months to gaining as much as you can in them. Then you may find the gains so startling that you regularly repeat such a tight focus, but not necessarily using the same exercises each time.

12.36    In all four applications, exercise focus is taken to an extreme, and the demands on the recuperative abilities pared back to a minimum. The time commitment for training is also greatly reduced relative to regular abbreviated training (which is already much briefer, more practical, and more effective than conventional routines). While ultra-abbreviated routines can be used for maintaining overall strength when training time is very short, they are wonderful for making terrific gains when time is at a premium. A very busy life should never preclude good gains in size and strength, so long as you know what you are doing.

12.37    The gains that can be made from specializing on only two or three exercises does not just benefit those exercises. Get yourself bigger and stronger in two or three big exercises and you will increase your ability in other exercises. There is a crossover effect from one set of exercises to another, though it may not manifest itself until after a short period of getting to grips with the grooves of the other exercises.

12.38    Here is one example of a super-abbreviated program:

**Day one**
*General warmup*
  a.  Squat
  b.  Bench press or parallel bar dip
  c.  Overhead press
*Cool down*

### Day two
*General warmup*
  a.  Stiff-legged deadlift
  b.  Pulldown or pullup (or chin)
*Cool down*

12.39    The training frequency could for example, be Monday-Friday
         of each week. If more recovery time is needed, use a Monday-
         Friday-Wednesday (three times every two weeks) schedule.

12.40    The above is a divided program with different musculature
         focused upon each day. Below is an example of very abbreviated
         *full-body* routines to be alternated every five days or so:

### Routine one
*General warmup*
  a.  Squat
  b.  Parallel bar dip
  c.  Prone row
*Cool down*

### Routine two
*General warmup*
  a.  Trap Bar deadlift
  b.  Bench press or incline press
  c.  Pullup (or chin)
*Cool down*

12.41    The program can be even simpler. It is possible to make very
         good overall gains by training just once per week on a single
         very abbreviated full-body program of just three exercises, e.g.,
         the squat or Trap Bar deadlift, parallel bar dip, and pulldown or
         pullup. If you had only 45 minutes to weight train each week,
         perhaps due to extreme demands from work and family, this
         program could be perfect. Rid yourself of the notion that you
         must do a lot of exercise in order to get bigger and stronger.

12.42    A super-abbreviated program is, out of necessity, imbalanced to
         a degree. Though it can cover all the major musculature of the
         body, some of the smaller areas are neglected. While an
         occasional imbalanced program will not cause long-term
         problems, the consistent use of the *same* imbalanced program
         will set you up for possible postural problems and an
         unacceptable imbalance in muscular development.

12.43    Do not make a single super-abbreviated program a year-round schedule. Vary the exercises over successive cycles. And if you alternate a cycle of regular abbreviated training (e.g., Frameworks 2–4) with a cycle of super-abbreviated training, you are not going to produce any serious imbalances.

# FRAMEWORK 6
## Specialization program

12.44    Frameworks 1–5 are designed to produce strength gains and muscular growth throughout the body. In a specialization program, focus is given to a single body part or specific exercise. Progress is only targeted in the focus body part or exercise. Good progress means a substantial increase in strength relative to your recent personal bests in the exercises concerned—not necessarily relative to the cycle's starting poundages because they will likely be less than your personal bests, especially if you have not done the exercises concerned for a while.

12.45    The existing strength and development of the rest of your physique should be maintained with the minimum of exercise and effort. Any effort to progress in the rest of your physique must be temporarily suspended. Then the effort and recovery ability that is "saved" from easing back on the rest of your physique can be channeled into the focus body part or exercise.

12.46    Specialization is not needed by beginners and intermediates. At those stages you need overall growth and strength. Trying to produce a big increase in size in a single body part, or poundage gain in a single exercise, without first having the main structures of the body in impressive condition by the standards of non-competitive bodybuilding and lifting, is to have made a mockery of weight training.

12.47    To get big and strong you have to consider the body as a whole, not as a collection of parts. The hard gainer can only tolerate and respond to a small-to-moderate amount of training. Exceed this and you will get nowhere, or perhaps even regress. Concentrate on your thighs, hips, back and upper-body pushing structure. Hard gainers *cannot* be concerned with keeping everything in perfect balance while building themselves up. Of course you do not want to end up with a body way out of proportion, but if you concern yourself with "perfect" balance right from early on in your training, you will have to use so many exercises and train so much that you will lose your focus upon the best exercises, and make overtraining and stagnation inevitable.

12.48      If instead of being concerned about biceps, delts, triceps, pecs and lats specialization all hard gainers were concerned with getting stronger and stronger, and then stronger still in the squat, deadlift, bench press, overhead press and a row, with the addition of no more than a few single-joint exercises, there would be tons more muscle in the world within a few months. And all without any specialization programs, leg extensions, lateral raises, pec-deck work, cable cross-overs, etc.

12.49      Here are three of the benefits of a specialization program for those qualified to use it:

      a.   Enables you to bring up a lagging body part or exercise.

      b.   Introduces variety and heightens training enjoyment and satisfaction due to different challenges and targets.

      c.   Exploits an existing strength and enables you to make it outstanding. This breaks the concept of a balanced physique, but if you have a natural strength, whether it is a body part and/or a particular exercise, and want to see how far you can take it, you need to specialize on it and make it into an even greater strength. This greater strength should, however, have some beneficial carry-over effect to the rest of your physique.

12.50      While balanced development has its merits, exploiting a natural advantage to make it into something exceptional may satisfy you more. Consider the stellar example of Bob Peoples, who, in 1949, deadlifted in competition (with an overhand hook grip) a gigantic 725.75 pounds at a bodyweight of just 189 pounds. Had Peoples kept his deadlift and back development in proportion with his other exercises and body parts, he would never have become a colossus of Iron Game history.

12.51      The basic hard-gainer specialization formula, following the development of the necessary foundation, is less work for the rest of the body than usual, and not pushing yourself to your limit in those exercises—keep yourself a little below your absolute best there. When the specialization area is the grip, calves or neck, intensity in other areas does not have to be kept in check, but I believe that it does when you specialize on other areas.

12.52    Successful hard-gainer training is about riveting attention on abbreviated routines, the best exercises, and progressive poundages. Specialization focuses this basic approach onto a small area of the body, or a single exercise. It is *not* about adding lots of additional work (especially a lot of detail exercises) to an already extensive and excessive training program, as it is in the conventional approach to specialization.

12.53    Here is an example of a body part specialization program, for the upper arms:

### Monday
*General warmup*
   a.   Seated barbell curl (in effect a partial curl)
   b.   Shoulder-width bench press
   c.   Seated supinating dumbbell curl (one arm at a time)
   d.   Parallel bar dip
*Cool down*

### Thursday
*General warmup*
   a.   Squat
   b.   Stiff-legged deadlift
   c.   Calf work
   d.   Ab work
*Cool down*

12.54    Here is an example of a single-exercise (deadlift) specialization program:

### Monday
*General warmup*
   a.   Trap Bar deadlift: warmups plus 1 x 6–8
   b.   Trap Bar deadlift: 3 singles
   c.   Partial deadlift from knee-cap height, in a rack: 2 x 10
*Cool down*

### Thursday
*General warmup*
   a.   Leg press

    b.  Parallel bar dip

    c.  Curl

    d.  Calf work

    e.  Ab work

*Cool down*

12.55    For the specialization body part or exercise you need to select one or more specific formats from those explained in Chapter 9, i.e., different training intensities, and cumulative-fatigue work. You also need to select rep and set performance styles from those explained in Chapter 11, i.e., rep cadence, single- or double-pause reps, one-and-a-half reps, and possible use of partial reps. And you need to choose an appropriate rep count, exercise selection, training volume, and between-set rest periods, as detailed elsewhere in this book. Do not try to combine many formats in a single specialization program. Be prudent in your selection, then stick with your choice for at least 6–8 weeks to give it a fair trial. Later on you can try another program with different formats, and compare results.

12.56    During a specialization program, experiment with training the focus body part or exercise twice a week (or three times every two weeks), rather than just once a week. For just a few weeks, or even a couple of months, an increased training frequency during a specialization program may be productive, but only if...

    a.  you severely cut back on training for the rest of your body,

    b.  you are making no effort to progress in those areas,

    c.  you are fully meeting your nutritional requirements, and

    d.  you are getting lots of rest and sleep.

12.57    If you try this increased training frequency for the focus exercise or body part, you can either use the same specialization workout more frequently, or use two different specialization workouts (for the *same* focus exercise or body part) and alternate them. If or when the specialization work falls on the same day as the maintenance work for the rest of your body, perform the specialization work first, rest ten minutes, and then do the exercises for the rest of your body. The focus body part or exercise must get priority.

## Eclectic training programs

12.58    A single training program does not have to use the same
         format of cadence, rep count, sets, intensity, rep pauses, rest
         periods, etc., for all exercises. You may even use a different
         specific format for each exercise in the program. There are
         many potentially productive ways to interpret the same
         framework of abbreviated training. Different exercise choices
         and varying numbers of exercises make up only part of the
         rational variety you can use.

12.59    Following on from the different interpretations of hard work
         explained in Chapter 9, and the different ways of performing
         reps explained in Chapter 11, here is an example of an eclectic
         program based on Framework 2. Only work sets are listed.
         Warmup sets would be additional.

### Monday
*General warmup*
  a. Squat: *1 x 20 rest pause reps, very hard training*
  b. Parallel bar dip: *3 x 6 one-and-a-half reps, four minutes rest
     between sets, very hard training*
  c. Pulldown: *6 x 6 cumulative-fatigue with a contraction squeeze
     on each rep*
  d. Calf work: *6 x 10 cumulative-fatigue with a contraction
     squeeze on each rep*
  e. Back extension: *1 x maximum reps, 5/5 cadence*
  f. Crunch situp: *2 x 10–12, 3/3 cadence with a contraction
     squeeze on each rep*
  g. Thick-bar holds, inside a power rack: *hold for 60 seconds,
     one minute rest, hold the same resistance for 30 seconds*
*Cool down*

### Thursday
*General warmup*
  a. Stiff-legged deadlift: *2 x 8, 3/3 cadence, four minutes rest
     between sets, hard training*
  b. Partial deadlift from knee height, alternate weeks only:
     *1 x 10, 3/3 cadence, double-pause reps, very hard training*
  c. Overhead press: *2 x 6–8 double-pause reps in a power rack,
     starting each rep from the bottom, four minutes rest between
     sets, very hard training*
  d. Dumbbell curl: *one arm at a time (unilateral), 2 x 6–8, three
     minutes rest between sets, brutally hard training*
  e. Side bend: *6 x 8 cumulative fatigue, 3/3 cadence*

   f.   Neck work: *2 x 10–12, 5/5 cadence, hard training*
   g.   L-fly: *2 x 6–8 per arm, 5/5 cadence, hard training*
   *Cool down*

## Critical reminders for all training programs

12.60    Though you may be making some gains on your current
         training program—even an abbreviated program—you may
         make better gains if you trained each exercise and/or body
         part less often. The additional rest and/or reduced demands
         on your recovery system may be what your body needs to
         make a full recovery from each workout—and thus be able to
         progress faster.

12.61    Put this recovery-priority thinking to the test. But this assumes
         that you are training hard. If you are loafing in the gym, then
         increasing recovery time will not help your gains. You must
         trigger the growth mechanism through hard work.

12.62    Before you ever jack up your training intensity you must first
         ensure that you are not training with excessive volume and/or
         frequency. Some people who are told they must train harder
         are already training hard enough to make progress—it is not
         necessary to train until you collapse in order to stimulate gains.
         The explanation for their poor or non-existent gains is that they
         are not resting enough between workouts to permit their
         bodies to grow. And because they are overtraining on their
         current training volume and intensity, to train even harder will
         only make matters worse.

## The barometer of success

12.63    Never get caught up, like so many people do, in the near
         religion of gym visits, as if gym attendance is the barometer of
         success. If your training poundages are moving up steadily,
         and your form is consistently good, then you are bang on
         course. To be able to gain like this you may not need to train

> This book teaches enough variations of abbreviated
> training to last you a training lifetime. These include
> different set and rep schemes, rep styles, intensity
> formats, cycling methods, ranges of motion, choice of
> exercises, equipment selection, rest periods between
> sets, and use of specialization programs.

any exercise more often than once every seven days. And there are some people who are better off training some of their exercises and body parts less often than once a week.

12.64    Most trainees would greatly improve their rate of gaining if they would halve their training volume per workout, double the rest days between workouts, get serious about delivering real effort in the reduced training time, and pay more attention to ensuring that enough calories and nutrients are consumed daily.

12.65    To maximize your gains in muscular size and strength you must organize your training, nutrition, rest and sleep in order to ensure progressive training poundages. *Everything you do must be built around providing the optimum environment for the production of progressive training poundages while using consistently good exercise form.* To ensure that the strength gain yields growth, you may, however, need to avoid very low reps, partial reps, low-rep rest-pause work, and overly infrequent training.

12.66    If at the end of a training cycle you are the same bodyweight as you were at the start of that cycle, and you are only capable of handling poundages that are the same or just marginally more than they were at the start, then you cannot expect to have bigger muscles.

## Training diversity

12.67    The need for training diversity varies among trainees. Training diversity for its own sake is a mistake. As-the-mood-takes-you training is a recipe for ruin because there is insufficient structure and consistency to it. There are so many productive ways to train that there is no reason why anyone should ever get bored with weight training—even within the constraints of abbreviated training. But results are what will satisfy you most of all. Training diversity is only valuable *if* it helps your overall progress. So use diversity and variety intelligently, and judge the changes you experiment with by the results they produce.

## Caution!

12.68    Many people only turn to recovery-dominated abbreviated training as the final resort. They seem to insist on first wasting years of their lives on other methods before finally finding the courage to swim against the training tide. But once they put recovery-dominated abbreviated training into determined practice they start making great progress. Then they become annoyed with themselves for having used as the last resort what should have been the first resort.

12.69    But even within the philosophy of abbreviated training there is a "more is better" mentality. Because the difference between conventional training methods and abbreviated training is so great, many people think that they cannot possibly overtrain on abbreviated routines of just 6–8 exercises at any single workout. *But the reality is that many people will still overtrain on such routines* (which are at the upper end of abbreviated training programs). In fact, many hard gainers need to use super-abbreviated programs in order to make decent gains. *You may need to use ultra-abbreviated training programs in order to experience your fastest possible rate of gain.*

12.70    Frameworks 1–4 and 6 may be excessive *for you*. You may need to prune them back in order to make them productive for you, or perhaps move straight to Framework 5. Results are what count, not gym attendance hours! So if your training is not delivering the goods—and assuming that you are satisfying all the out-of-the-gym components of bodybuilding and strength-training success, and you have no serious physiological problems—then you need to change your training. *Remember, more of what did not help you over the last few months is not going to help you over the next few months.* **BB**

> **Generally speaking, the routine illustrations in this chapter have the big exercises listed to be performed before the small ones. This is a good general guideline, as is performing any specific arm work last in a workout. But a more important guideline is to train progressively *all* exercises in a routine. If scheduling your exercises in a different way suits *you* better, so be it. If, for example, to squat or deadlift first in a workout wipes you out so that you cannot do justice to any other exercise, you would be better off to squat or deadlift at the end (and shorten your routine too).**

> Chapter 21 has important additional information on program design, including another Framework, as part of the changes for the revised edition of this book.

## How to train hard but with discipline

Some people find visualizations helpful; others find them a distraction. Try some and see if they help. Either way, the essence of training well is to work hard, without rushing, and while holding good form. Good form means perfect technique *plus* a controlled rep tempo. Executing this demands great discipline. It is not about just banging out reps to failure.

With the bar loaded for a work set, switch onto training mode. Switch off from your life. "Become" your training. *Nothing else matters now.* Visualize huge muscles and power to spare to complete your set.

Perform the set one rep at a time. Look no further than the current rep. Do not rush. *Use perfect exercise form.*

When the discomfort intensifies, dissociate yourself from it. Imagine you are watching yourself on film. Push on. Do not rush. *Use perfect exercise form.*

Regroup your thoughts during the brief pause between reps. Remind yourself of how much you want a stronger and better physique. Keep the reps coming. Do not rush. *Use perfect exercise form.*

To be able to train hard is a privilege. Remind yourself of this during the between-rep pauses. Think of people less privileged than you—those in nursing homes, and those in graves. Resolve not to quit before you are spent. Forge on. *Use perfect exercise form.*

As the set nears completion, and you are at your hilt, visualize a vivid life-or-death situation where if you fail to make the rep, you die. Then squeeze out a rep or few more. *But use perfect exercise form.*

Training intensively is no excuse for getting sloppy with exercise form. *In fact, the harder you train the more important that good form is.* Remember, intensity *together* with disciplined good form is what successful training is about, not just banging out reps to failure.

*The instruction in this book is geared primarily for trainees who do not have optimal responsiveness to training, ideal recuperation capabilities, or perfect conditions for working out. But should you be fortunate to have conditions more suited to quicker gains, make the most of the situation while it lasts. Follow the training methods promoted here and you will gain in abundance—far more than you would on conventional programs.*

*The more progressive workouts you put in, the faster your overall progress will be. But if you train too frequently you will not be able to produce many if any progressive workouts.*

# 13. How to Personalize Your Training Programs

13.1    A single package of prescriptions does not exist that will deliver equally good results for everyone. Even "standard" hard-gainer-style routines with a proven track record for many people do not always fit the bill. Even sensible training programs built around the basic frameworks outlined in the previous chapter need to be personalized by each individual trainee.

## Individual variation

13.2    A training program consists of many components, including exercises, set and rep schemes, intensity level, training frequency, and cycling procedure. There are many potentially productive ways to employ these variables. But as so many people discover the hard way, there are far more useless and even destructive applications.

13.3    It is impossible to give a list of training measures and assume that the package will work equally well for all users. Here are three of the reasons why:

    a.  No two people can interpret and implement a set of measures identically.

    b.  Identical brothers or sisters aside, no two people are identical physically and thus do not have the same "response package."

    c.  No two people endure the same out-of-the-gym stresses, which can greatly influence how well you respond to a set of training measures.

13.4    There are many out-of-the-gym variables that can hugely affect response to training. Individuals vary in many ways including age, genetic ability to grow muscle, physical weak links, tolerance of exercise-induced discomfort, motivation and training zeal, training supervision, demands of family and work, sleep and rest habits, nutritional practices, discretionary income, time available for training, training knowledge, and equipment availability. Because of these variables, a program that works very well for one trainee can fail to deliver the goods for another similar individual.

13.5    And what worked well for you when you were 25, unmarried, well rested, well nourished and relatively stress free will probably fail to work now that, for example, you are 35, married with children, cutting corners with your diet, overworked, and highly stressed from many directions. As your circumstances change, so must your training.

# Personalizing Your Training Programs

13.6    There are many factors you can manipulate to personalize any training program you use. Intensity cycling has been covered in Chapter 7. Here are other ways in which you can personalize a training program, to help maximize your progress.

## Training volume

13.7    Your individual level of "hardgainingness" determines the volume of training you use. Generally speaking, the harder you find gaining to be, the less training you should do.

13.8    My general recommendation for the average hard gainer is to use about 6–8 exercises per workout early on in a cycle (e.g., four major movements and two accessory ones), while training twice a week but using a different set of exercises each session. Then, *and only if necessary*, reduce the number of exercises during the very final stage of the cycle. But if you can keep gaining on all the exercises without having to cut back on any of them, do so.

13.9    The cutting back on volume of weekly training can be done in at least three ways:

   a.  Reduce the number of exercises in your training program.

   b.  Do the same number of exercises and training days, but spread the exercises out more, e.g., train some exercises alternate weeks instead of each week.

      c.  Do the same number of exercises and training days, but do fewer sets per exercise.

13.10     For most hard gainers for most of the time, training twice a week is probably more productive than three times, *even* if different exercises are done on each of the three workouts. Working out with weights *more* than three times a week is training suicide for most people, and even "just" three weight training days is too much for many hard gainers. But as noted in Chapter 12 you may want to experiment with weight training three times a week but make the middle session an accessory day only. Then focus on just the major movements on your other weight training days. In Chapter 21 are other possible suggestions for weight training three days per week.

13.11     Many hard gainers are not average in their "hardgainingness," but are genetically disadvantaged and may, at least temporarily, need no more than six exercises spread over two workouts each week to *start* a cycle with.

13.12     Some people have consistently trained long enough on abbreviated routines that they have become very big and strong. They have become so big and strong that no one would ever believe these trainees could possibly have been hard gainers. And some better-than-average gainers have trained like genuine hard gainers should, and have achieved awesome levels of muscle and might. Learn the great lesson: abbreviate and grow.

## Training frequency

13.13     Most people weight train too frequently and do not provide enough time for their bodies to grow stronger and bigger. Thus they fail to progress; and in addition they accumulate wear-and-tear injuries because their bodies are being worn down.

13.14     The relatively low frequency of training recommended in this book refers only to weight training. If you do cardiorespiratory work on non-weights days, you would have a total of four or five training days each week, but only the weight-training days would be the tough ones.

13.15     Intensive weight training is very demanding—*much more demanding than most people realize.* The publicity of the astonishing gains that the super-responsive elite have achieved from their high-volume and very frequent training has blinded people to just how very severe the demands of intensive weight training are upon drug-free and genetically typical trainees.

13.16     The more progressive workouts you put in, the faster your overall progress will be. *But if you train too frequently you will not be able to produce many if any progressive workouts.* Not training as often as conventional training recommends is in no way a measure of lack of dedication to training. *It is a dedication to results that counts most, not a dedication to mere gym attendance.* If I thought that weight training four, five or six days a week would help you to progress, I would advocate it.

13.17     Once you get the full measure of your body's real need for recovery time, you can keep gaining for season after season without a break or even any cycling of training intensity. You can even keep a cycle going for over a year without needing to change your program. That is over fifty consecutive weeks of poundage gains from the same program. They will not be big weekly gains, but you can do it safely and without having to kill yourself every workout.

13.18     You need to find the right training regularity but without working out on such a rigid schedule that you train when you are not fully recovered. If you normally weight train on Mondays and Thursdays, and your Monday workout in a given week went very well and you really delivered some effort, you would naturally feel fatigued on Tuesday and Wednesday. If you had an unusually heavy work schedule on those two days, or if there was a family crisis that devastated your sleep on those two nights, you would not be fully rested for Thursday's workout. So postpone that workout a day or two, until you are fully rested. Do not weight train if you are still dragging your feet from the previous workout.

13.19     Do not confuse this sort of rational rescheduling of weight-training workouts with laziness and lack of dedication. You should be dedicated to getting optimum results from your training. Results from your weight training come from using progressive poundages. To achieve progressive training poundages you must rest between workouts long enough to recover from the impact of each workout, and then rest *a bit longer* so that your body can build a bit of extra strength and muscle (i.e., overcompensate).

13.20    *Rescheduling of exercise sessions should be the exception, not the rule.* If you find you often need to reschedule an exercise session due to fatigue, you need to redesign your program so that you are not overtraining and/or under-recovering.

13.21    Successful weight training is about stringing together as many progressive workouts as possible. Twenty progressive workouts over ten weeks will produce far better results than thirty workouts over the same period but with only a handful of them being progressive. Weight-training success is about results, not just about how many hours you clock up at a gym.

## The bottom line on training frequency

13.22    Experiment with training frequency to see what delivers steady and consistent exercise poundage gains *for you.* This will be relative to your individual recovery ability and the type of training program you use.

13.23    The training frequency that best suits you for your current program may not be what is best for you for your next program. The type of training approach used, the way you organize the exercises over the workouts, specific exercises selected, the degree of exercise overlap and duplication over the course of the training week, the intensity and volume you are using, and rest and nutrition habits, can all influence the optimum training frequency of each of your exercises.

13.24    What one person may gain quickest on can be very different from what another person gains fastest on. If you can squat

> The recommendation to delay training if you are not recovered from your previous workout is not license to be lackadaisical with your training. Training consistency is absolutely essential. But only consistent dedication to something that works is going to do you any good. You could be the world's most dedicated trainee, but if your training is not working, then all that dedication and training consistency will not produce bigger and stronger muscles. Find a training volume and frequency that work well for you, and then become a super-consistent trainee, only delaying or skipping a workout under exceptional conditions.

twice a week and add a pound each workout to your top work set, you will make much faster progress than someone who can only add a pound a workout if he squats once every 7–10 days. But if the latter fellow squats hard twice a week, he will stagnate, get overtrained, and *lose* strength. The faster gainer is better off than the slower gainer, but there is nothing (drug-free) that the slower gainer can do to improve matters *assuming* that he is truly *fully* attending to all the components of recovery, and is training well on an abbreviated program. The slower gainer should not copy the faster gainer, and the faster gainer may not want to train less frequently if he is gaining well on his current schedule. But, the faster gainer should experiment with once-a-week squatting for a couple of months—he may find that on that training frequency he can gain in strength, per week, at a faster rate than he was while squatting twice a week. There may not, however, be an increase in muscle gain at the reduced training frequency to accompany the strength gain.

13.25    I am not promoting a radical training frequency for the sake of it. I am promoting it because it is a *necessity* for many trainees. What matters most is what works best *for you*. If training on one frequency does not work well for you, but a lesser frequency does, then train on the lesser frequency. Despite this being so obvious, many people continue to imprison themselves in a training frequency that is excessive *for them*.

13.26    Coaches and trainers need to be very careful when prescribing training frequency for their charges. Training frequency should be personalized for the individual concerned, not dictated based on the success of star pupils and/or the coach or trainer himself. Considerable input from each charge must be provided, and some experimentation through rational trial and error needs to be carried out. Some coaches and trainers have such rigid training principles, including training frequency (both gross weekly frequency, and of how often each exercise should be hit) that they take any suggestion of a different frequency being better for some people, as an affront. Rather than having a sympathetic understanding of different needs among their charges, and a flexible training methodology, the coaches and trainers often vent their frustration by slamming as "wimps" anyone who cannot gain on their prescriptions.

13.27    Volume and intensity of training are reflected in frequency of training. Hard training can be productively done with slightly greater volume and frequency than can very hard training, which in turn can be done with slightly greater volume and frequency than can brutally hard work. (See Chapter 9 for definitions of effort levels.)

13.28    The more intensive and demanding the training, the greater the recovery time needed. Smaller doses of growth stimulation, but a greater number of them, may produce the same end result as that from larger but fewer doses of stimulation, but then again they might not. For the sake of variety, and to make the most of each interpretation, you could alternate the approaches over successive training cycles.

13.29    Do not misinterpret this advice and think you can periodically get into *any* sort of training volume and frequency. The range I am discussing contrasts, for example, one very hard set of 20 squats once a week, and squatting three hard work sets of 5–8 reps three times every two weeks. There is a big difference between these two options, but no connection with the instruction that wreaks havoc in gyms today.

**Example experiment**

13.30    You may find that some exercises and body parts respond best if trained twice a week, others more like three times every two weeks, and others once a week. Training some exercises less often than once a week, especially the squat and deadlift, may be best in order to keep poundage gains coming, at least for some people. On such a schedule a light session for the exercise(s) concerned could be tucked in midway between the heavy workouts. You need to experiment, but within reason. Do not try training six days a week with 20 sets per muscle group.

13.31    For the experiment, make it specific. Getting the frequency right is especially important during the hard-work stage of a cycle, not during the very early not-so-hard stage. During the hard stage, keep the volume and intensity of your workouts as consistent as possible (and other variables including rest, sleep and nutrition), and just vary the workout frequency. Work each exercise twice weekly for a few weeks, except for any deadlift variation which should be trained only once a week at most.

13.32    As this experiment progresses, find the exercises you are not able to add weight to. Drop their training frequency to three times every two weeks and see how you go for a few weeks. If the poundages move up nicely, and you are recovering well, stick with that. But if you are still dragging your feet a bit on some exercises, then drop those to once a week and see if your training energy and poundage increments pick up. If so, then you are better off with the less frequent schedule.

13.33    Follow how *you* respond to your training, rather than get locked into a calendar-dictated schedule. This complicates training somewhat, and you will need to juggle your schedule to accommodate the likely different training frequency needs of at least some exercises and body parts, but you will be learn about how best to train yourself. Training regularity is still imperative, but only if you are recovering fully from each workout.

13.34    Especially if you are an advanced trainee, experiment with a training frequency for some exercises of less often than once a week. When training full-bore and with personal best poundages, try deadlifting heavily only once every two weeks. Try heavy squatting once every ten days, as another example. Be intelligently radical in your experiments—keep what helps, drop what hinders. But as noted earlier in this section, it may be a good idea to perform a light workout midway between the infrequent intensive sessions for the biggest exercises.

13.35    As you do any fine-tuning that may be necessary, do not disturb a formula that is working well. Always remember that the aim is to find the *optimum* intensity, volume and frequency of training for a given exercise that enables *you* to consistently add poundage to it in good form, *and* which produces growth.

13.36    Some people who have a history of injury in a particular location may find that a little very light but regular work for that area is helpful. Done several times a week it keeps them in good shape for their infrequent heavy workouts.

## Fixed-day vs. variable-day training

13.37    Most people probably find fixed-day training more practical and successful than variable-day training. Being locked into the seven-days-per-week life program also locks training into that program. Training every fourth day would mean, for example, Monday, Friday, Tuesday, Saturday, Wednesday, Sunday, etc. That is six different training days over the course of three consecutive weeks. This is impractical for many people. A fixed Monday-Friday, Tuesday-Saturday, or Monday-Friday-

Wednesday-Monday schedule is likely to be more practical. But with fixed training days you can approximate ideal rest intervals. The Monday-Friday-Wednesday-Monday schedule comes close to training every fourth day. The big advantage of having fixed gym days is that you know your training days and non-training days, and can organize your weeks accordingly.

13.38    But a fixed schedule of training days should not be written in stone. You must be constantly alert to the signs of impending overtraining, and be ready to adjust your training days, routine design, and volume of training accordingly (not just weight training, but aerobic work too).

## Adapting to trying circumstances

13.39    "Listen" to your body, be aware of changes in your lifestyle, and tailor your training accordingly. The more demanding your life is out of the gym, and the less rested and well fed you are, the more you need to cut back in the gym. You only have a limited recovery ability to begin with, and if you have had that shrunk by out-of-the-gym factors, then you will not have much to play with in the gym. This forces you to cut your training to the bone if you are to have a chance of progressing.

13.40    While you probably cannot control all the out-of-the-gym factors, you can at least shore up some of them. If you cannot get time to prepare decent meals when you are out of the house, prepare a nutritious easily digested blender concoction, put it in a thermos, and take it with you and use it for liquid feeds every three hours. This will keep you steadily supplied with nourishment. *Skipping feeds will kill your gains.*

---

A good training program that does not yield good results can often be made productive by supplying more rest, sleep and nutrition. When you are experimenting with training frequency you must keep other variables constant. Use a good abbreviated training program suited to you, train hard, rest and sleep well, and fully satisfy your nutritional needs— only then should you experiment with training frequency to discover what works best for you. "Best" is defined as what consistently produces poundage gain on all your exercises.

13.41   Try to arrange your life so that you are well rested during the 24 hours before you train. While you can occasionally psyche yourself up to train when you are very tired, or depend on a stimulant such as coffee to do the job, you cannot do this indefinitely. (Do not become dependent on taking a stimulant in order to be able to get in an intensive workout. You need to be able to train hard under your own control.) A good night's sleep prior to a training day can transform you. Select your gym days so that you train when at your least tired.

## Rep selection

13.42   Productive routines can draw on many rep formats. The rep number is not the most important factor—effort, form and progression are. You can gain muscle *and* strength from low, medium and high reps. Some people are more suited and responsive to one range than another, and this can vary from exercise to exercise in the same person.

13.43   *All* rep ranges are dangerous if form is poor on a consistent basis, or is usually good but just occasionally breaks down in a serious way, especially at the end of a set. Increasing reps as a response to hurting yourself with lower reps is not addressing the root of the problem if your exercise technique is flawed.

13.44   Here is the critical qualification to the "all rep counts should be safe *if* you use very good technique" statement: Your body must be accustomed to the rep count you are using *before* you start to push yourself very hard at it. This especially applies to singles (one-rep sets) and very low rep work (sets of 2–4 reps).

13.45   Singles and very low reps have more potential for causing injuries than higher reps. This is because the per-rep stress on joints, muscles and connective tissues is much greater from singles and very low rep work. Comparing the *same* degree of form error, if you get out of the ideal groove during a maximum single you are more likely to hurt yourself than if you get out of the groove during a hard set of medium or high reps. *But this does not mean that high reps with reduced weights are guaranteed to be safe.*

13.46   Even with high reps and reduced weights, if you use poor technique and/or a jerky rep cadence, and train intensively, you will hurt yourself. During the severe fatigue from intensive high-rep work you must be *especially* vigilant not to let your form break down. An advantage of single-rep work is that there is no accumulation of fatigue to contend with during the set. There is just one rep to do, and one rep to get right. But many people simply cannot train on singles because their bodies are unable to tolerate the heavy weights that are necessary, *no matter how carefully they build up over several months.*

13.47    I make no apology for harping on about the need for good exercise form. It cannot be stressed enough. You must learn what good technique is, and *put it into practice.*

13.48    Even some people who, when training others, generally stick to certain rep ranges, apply something else in their personal training. Experience has shown them that, at least for some exercises, they have very specific rep needs if they are to gain in their own training. For example, Dr. Ken Leistner in HARDGAINER issue #33 stated this:

> What I have found in both my own case and those of so many others, despite what is written in the books, is that the effective number of reps will vary from exercise to exercise, and to body part within any individual trainee. Forget the comparison of individuals to each other. Some do really well if their rep range is 10–12 for direct biceps or triceps work, 6 or so in the bench, and 15 for the low back; or vice versa.
>     In my own case, all of my pressing movements make no progress whatsoever if I work over 3–5 reps. Except for the skill work necessary for contest preparation, I never recommend reps that low, but for me, it is a necessity in the overhead press, push press, and bench press.

13.49    Through the experience of sensibly trying different reps for different exercises you may find for a given exercise the rep number you can increase your poundages most easily on. This will not be the same for all exercises you do. While some people gain well on reps over 10, others find reps of 5 or fewer to be more productive. Some people try low reps and cannot gain much from them, but gain well on reps over 10. In some exercises, perhaps especially the squat and deadlift, you may gain well from high and low reps, done in different cycles.

## The "ideal" rep count
13.50    With experience you may get to know—for a given exercise—the rep number over which it is almost impossible for you to

go even if you stick with the same weight for a few weeks. But at that ceiling you can probably get it again next time *with a pound or two more on the bar*, and then again the next week with another small increment on the bar, and again the next week. When you get to know what that rep number is for a given exercise, do not try to exceed it. Keep to it, or better still choose a rep target under it, and then focus on adding poundage.

13.51    Some people prefer a fixed rep number for a given exercise, while others prefer the double-progression method. In practice, and over the long term, most people use a mixture of both approaches.

13.52    Do not lock yourself into traditional rep ranges for specific body parts. For example, calf and abdominal work are traditionally done with reps of about 20, or more. Experiment here with lower reps—10 or perhaps even as few as 5 or 6— using heavier weights, and you may find that you make better progress. But make a careful transition between the high reps and low reps. Do not, for example, add 100 pounds to your usual calf machine 20-rep poundage and immediately start performing full-bore 6-rep sets. Instead, move to 6-rep sets but increase your poundage by 10 pounds maximum a week, and later on increase by no more than 5 pounds weekly, and then later on by smaller increments.

13.53    Knowledge of your personal rep preferences will influence the type of program you choose. It may also lead to modifications of any training program you consider appropriate for you.

**Twenty-rep work**

13.54    Though not popular today, in the pre-steroids era the 20-rep squat was very influential. It was hugely productive back then, when used as the cornerstone of an *abbreviated* training program, and it can be hugely productive today. Anyone who

> **Find what you can do well and with substantial effort (within the context of intensity cycling), actually recover from, really enjoy doing, and then you will obtain what you are supposed to from weight training—bigger and stronger muscles. Never blindly follow a given program. Tailor it to fit *you*, always.**

thinks that high reps do not build muscle and strength is totally out of touch with Iron Game history. This special 20-rep rest-pause work does not have to be limited to the squat. It is very well suited to the bent-legged deadlift, *especially when using a Trap Bar*. In fact, for deadlifting, the Trap Bar is far superior to the straight bar.

13.55    There is nothing magical, however, about the number 20. If 21, or 18 had been chosen and initially championed, the muscle-building results would have been the same. But 20 is a round number, and what was initially championed.

13.56    Twenty-rep rest-pause squatting and deadlifting are extremely demanding, which is why they can be extremely productive, but only when combined with a very abbreviated training program, lots of recovery time, and plenty of quality nourishment. Never go through the rigors of 20-rep squatting or deadlifting unless you know you can fully satisfy the rest, sleep and nutritional components of recovery. Otherwise you will knock yourself out in the gym for nothing.

13.57    The rest-pause 20-rep style means performing one rep at a time—absolutely no continuous reps. This permits the heaviest poundage. In the squat you keep the bar over your shoulders, stand upright between reps, and take as many deep breaths as you need—increasingly more as the set progresses.

13.58    For 20-rep deadlifting you can set the bar on the floor and stand between reps. If you pause between reps as you stand while holding the bar, your grip will fail before you have adequately worked your legs, glutes and back.

13.59    Between reps in the squat you must hold your body safely and securely, without rounding your back, without losing or exaggerating the natural arch in your lower back, and without any swaying at your hips.

13.60    Intensive 20-rep squatting and deadlifting need to be experienced before they can be fully appreciated. A single set is a workout in itself—a test of both the body and spirit. You must take your time to adapt to the rigors involved. Do not jump in at the deep end. While a few people survive on that approach, the great majority fail. You must condition your body to withstand the rigors of 20-rep work. The demands are not just muscular. The heart and lungs need to adapt, as does your entire supporting structure including your shoulder girdle, vertebral column, and even the arches of your feet.

13.61    For 20-rep work to be productive it needs to be implemented in a prudent way. There is a macho and foolish tradition attached to 20-rep squatting that wants to exaggerate the severity of the exercise, i.e., "Take a weight you can only squat 10 reps with, and then force yourself to get 20 reps!" While unnecessarily exaggerating the severity of the exercise, this foolishness also increases the chances of failure and injury.

13.62    Adopt a sensible, progressive approach. Start using a weight with which you could do about 40 reps if you were to go to your limit, but stop at 20. Add 5 pounds a week until you get to the point where you could only get 25 reps if you went all the way, though you still stop at 20. Then drop to a 2 pounds or 1 kilo a week increment. Keep that slow rate of progression up for six months and you will add 50 pounds to your 20-rep squat. Though this 20-rep squatting will be very hard it will never totally crush you so that you become fearful of your training. Training enthusiasm must be sustained.

13.63    If you had to almost die in the effort, and yet still failed to get all 20 reps, you will probably fail to get the same "failed" rep count next time, let alone the full 20. Train hard, for sure, but do not go over the edge and kill your gaining momentum. Take the extra months to progress slowly and steadily, rather than try to pack all the gains in 6–8 weeks and burn out after four.

13.64    Consider the following two scenarios, and see which one is best. The first scenario is the macho one. The starting weight is absolutely at the hilt of the trainee's capabilities, e.g., 260 x 20. Despite being totally crushed, with sore arches in his feet, a strained lower back, and a fear of ever doing anything like that again, he gets psyched up the following week and makes all 20 reps with 265 pounds. Then after a week of 20-rep squatting nightmares, and with all aches and pains apparently gone, 270 is tried, but only 18 reps are completed. Disastrous! And the final 2 reps of that failed set were done with loose form. A week later, with a few aches still resident, and despite all the cajoling of a supportive audience, again 18 reps cannot be beaten. Then with a crushed spirit, and a crushed body, the 20-rep squat is discontinued. The fallout includes injuries and a hatred of a potentially super-productive way of training.

13.65    Here is the second scenario, the conservative one. Start with 225 x 20. All 20 reps are made with lots of room to spare. Over the next five weeks, squatting once a week, 5 pounds is added to the bar each week. Your mind and body adapt, your supporting structure toughens, your cardiorespiratory system adjusts, and good form is maintained. After five weeks you will be at 250 x 20. Though it will be demanding it will not push you to your limit. You will mentally and physically adapt to the rigors, and enjoy the challenge. Then you get out your little discs and start adding 2 pounds per week. Five weeks later you will be using 260 for 20. Though it took you ten weeks to get where you could have been if you had started off with 260 x 20, you have laid the ground for much further progress, and you are mentally and physically challenged to push on. Five weeks later you make 270 x 20, with room to spare. A further five weeks you make 280 x 20, again with room to spare. Though the work is darn hard, you always have a little room to spare each session. Then after ten more weeks of further slow and steady but safe and sure progress, you hit the "magic" 300 x 20, which is an outstanding achievement for any hard gainer. And you still have the gaining momentum going, so further progress is possible if you feel inclined to continue with 20-rep squatting.

13.66    Which is the best way to approach 20-rep squatting or deadlifting, macho or conservative?

13.67    But the macho approach described here is mild compared to what some people urge. I described intensive squatting just once a week, but some people have promoted full-bore 20-rep squatting *three times* a week. And they want you to add 5 pounds to the bar each week if not each workout. Such instruction is a road to ruin for most trainees.

13.68    As far as where in your routine to position the 20-rep squatting or deadlifting, there are two common alternatives. One is to open your routine with it (following warmup work), when your energy is supposed to be at its highest. The other extreme is to do the 20-rep work at the end of the workout, because after going full-bore on the 20 reps you may not have enough energy left to do justice to much else. You could do the 20-rep work first, take a break for 20 minutes, and then resume your workout and do justice to the exercises that remain.

## Singles

13.69    Single-rep work is exaggerated rest-pause training where the pause between reps is extended to several minutes, making the individual reps into sets of one rep each. Single-rep training *does not* use true maximum singles, but about 90–95% of your limit weights (once you have first acclimatized to the program using lighter weights). Single-rep training is dangerous if not done properly, or if used by people who have no business performing such high-force training. But single-rep work can be safe and productive for some trainees. It is not the rep count per se that determines safety, but how the reps are performed.

13.70    The ability to benefit from singles and very low reps is at least in part related to one's physical structure. Most advocates of singles, and most success stories from using singles, are mesomorphs not ectomorphs. Mesomorphs, who are usually easy gainers, are blessed with thicker joints and connective tissue than are ectomorphs, who are usually hard gainers. Mesomorphs can usually safely respond to intelligently applied singles and very low reps. Hard gainers *can* greatly increase the robustness of their joints and connective tissue, but their ultimate potential for robustness is much less than it is for mesomorphs. *Generally speaking, medium and high reps are much safer and more productive for hard gainers than are singles and very low reps.* And also generally, singles and very low reps favor pure strength development, while higher reps favor strength *and* size development.

13.71    If you want to try singles, and feel that your body is robust enough, gradually convert your current program into one in which the core exercises are done as singles. Stay with your regular reps and sets for waist, calf, neck and direct arm work.

13.72    A key to safety and success with singles—in addition to using excellent form—is that you start with weights well under your true 90–95% maximums, performing 3–5 singles. Take just enough rest between singles so that you comfortably make each one. Until you are working your singles at the 90–95% level, perform one or two demanding sets of five reps in the respective exercises, to maintain your strength. Once you are at the 90–95% level you can drop the five-rep sets and focus on the singles.

13.73    Take about six weeks or so to build to the 90–95% level, reducing the number of singles to three if need be. Then increase the poundage *slowly*, to avoid jumping to your absolute limit, and take enough time between singles so that you can make each one relatively comfortably. By adding poundage at a rate your body can build strength you will be consistently working at the 90–95% level for many weeks if not a few months, but with ever-increasing poundages. This will translate to a much bigger true maximum single.

13.74    For example, say your current maximum one-rep bench press is 300 pounds. You would take about six weeks to build to 95% of 300 for 3–5 singles, which is 285. Then by adding 2 pounds a week for ten weeks you would get to 305 pounds for three singles. This new 95% of maximum translates to 320 pounds or more for a true maximum single. This is a terrific gain for a drug-free advanced man, taking approximately four months for the entire cycle.

13.75    If after you have followed these guidelines you still get a negative reaction in your joints when you start handling weights that are 90–95% of your current maximums, do not persist with single-rep training. *Remember, many if not most people simply do not have the robustness of joints and connective tissue needed to prosper on singles.*

13.76    When establishing your current maximum single for an exercise, in order to calculate your singles progression scheme, you do not have to actually lift a maximum weight and risk injuring yourself. Use the conversion charts given in Chapter 4. Then no matter what rep count you normally use you can compute the equivalent single-rep maximum.

## Exercise selection

13.77    Choose exercises you can safely perform over the long term. With experience you will find the exercises that best suit your body structure and personal preferences. Once you have found your preferred major core exercises, then you can stick with them over the long term. It is a fallacy that you must regularly change your exercises in order to keep progressing. Changing your exercises around *excessively* is even counterproductive because it stops you from applying yourself to a given group of exercises for long enough to really milk them dry.

13.78    One person's selection of a safe, enjoyable and productive core group of exercises may be very different from another's. This is why many exercises and variations are described in THE INSIDER'S TELL-ALL HANDBOOK ON WEIGHT-TRAINING TECHNIQUE.

13.79    In my youth, the squat and bench press were core exercises that I did with almost religious consistency, and later on the barbell deadlift became a core exercise. But due to abusive exercise technique, and downright foolishness, I damaged my back and knees. I was not using good exercise technique, and I paid a heavy price. As a result I now cannot safely perform the barbell squat and conventional deadlift. I also cannot safely perform the Trap Bar bent-legged deadlift. So my core leg and back exercises have had to change—to the leg press and Trap Bar stiff-legged deadlift for a period, superceded by the Tru-Squat and stiff-legged deadlift from just below knee height. (The Tru-Squat is a unique patented machine manufactured by Southern Xercise—see page 481.) And purely out of personal preference I no longer bench press. I prefer the parallel bar dip.

## Exercise overlap

13.80    When constructing an abbreviated and basics-first program of exercises, there are two basic structures:

   a.    Put movements that overlap (i.e., those that exercise similar muscle groups) into the same workout, e.g., bench press and overhead press at the same session, and squat and bent-legged deadlift at the same workout.

> Once you have designed a good program along the lines promoted by this book, and have fine-tuned it according to the guidelines of this chapter, stop looking for another way to train. Instead, get set for a long training period steadily accumulating gains. Rather than look for a better way to train, look for ways to recover better between workouts, and to focus better during your workouts so that you can train harder and with better form. These two strategies will improve your gains, for sure. But looking for another way to train, when you have already found a good one, is almost certainly not going to improve your gains.

b.  Divide the overlapping movements (i.e., those that exercise similar muscle groups) over two days per week. For example, do the bench press on Monday and the overhead press on Thursday, and squat on Monday but deadlift on Thursday.

13.81   When putting overlapping exercises into the same workout, the involved musculature is trained as often as you use that routine. But when the overlapping exercises are divided over the week's training, the same basic structure is trained perhaps every time you get in the gym. Training each exercise just once a week does not necessarily mean training each body part only once a week.

13.82   Squatting and deadlifting on separate days each week, for example, means your lower back in particular gets two poundings a week. Put both exercises on the same day—with plenty of rest in between them so that the second does not suffer from the first—and the lower back gets trained hard only at that workout. You will then have as much rest for your lower back as you have between sessions of the squat and deadlift workout.

13.83   Squats and deadlift variations are not the only exercises to stress the lower back heavily. Overhead presses, and bench pressing with an exaggerated arch, put a great deal of stress on the lower back. This can raise your potential for injury from the squat or deadlift. Reduce this source of lower-back stress to a minimum—avoid exaggerated arching—and be sure that your back is adequately rested before squatting and/or deadlifting.

13.84   In the same cycle, you cannot productively use many exercises that heavily work your lower back. But the degree to which any exercise affects the lower back varies among individuals. Technique and leverage differences can greatly influence the degree of impact the same exercises have among different people. Experiment rationally to find what works best for you.

13.85   Putting the overlapping exercises into the same workout gives you greater control over the recovery period between working the same body part. But it delivers a greater pounding at a single session to that body part, thus requiring you to rest more between workouts relative to the other approach. Some trainees prefer to do the smaller amount of work for a given body part twice a week, whereas others prefer the bigger amount of work (from two or three exercises that overlap) once a week.

13.86    During the early stage of a cycle when it is exercise form and getting a gaining momentum going that are the priorities, it probably does not matter which way you handle overlapping exercises. But later on in the cycle when the training is intensive, how you handle overlapping exercises may affect your rate of progress.

13.87    If you find squatting and deadlifting with your top poundages on different days each week means that your lower back is overtrained and ripe for injury, put both exercises into the same workout. Alternatively you could train the deadlift less often. As another option you could work both exercises in the same cycle, but stop the non-focus lift at a maximum of 90% of your previous same-rep best, so as to concentrate on getting the focus lift to well over your previous best. Next cycle, reverse the focus.

## Another aspect of overlapping exercises

13.88    This concerns the timing of a minor exercise relative to a major exercise. For example, if you perform arm work before chest and back work in the same workout, the latter will suffer. This would only be acceptable during an arm specialization program.

13.89    If you do accessory exercises on say Wednesday, including work for your shoulder external rotators, and then bench press on Friday, you could risk injuring your rotator muscles. This is because the rotator muscles are heavily stressed during the bench press, especially during the final rep. If the rotator cuff muscles are still fatigued from Wednesday they would be much more likely to let you down on Friday than on the following Monday. Better to do your shoulder rotator work after your benches rather than shortly before.

13.90    While there is much in common between the bent-legged and stiff-legged versions of the deadlift, because of the overlap, there are considerable differences. Because you are used to one of them does not mean you can train the other heavily without easing into it over at least several weeks. If you do not get adjusted like this you could be in for debilitating soreness and possibly injury. Similar comments can be made for other groups of overlapping exercises.

13.91    Another aspect of exercise overlap concerns safety. Suppose you perform the stiff-legged deadlift quite soon after the squat or leg press in the same routine. As you deadlift, your legs may tremble to such a degree that you cannot control them adequately. This can lead to back injury.

13.92    A similar comment can be made for other pairings, e.g., side bend and stiff-legged deadlift, shrug and deadlift, shrug and pulldown, pulldown and parallel bar dip. But avoid intensive stiff-legged deadlifting immediately *before* the squat. That is not recommended because fatigue in your glutes and lower back could expose you to an increased risk of injury from the squat.

13.93    Whenever you find that safety is compromised in one exercise because of it following closely behind a specific other exercise, rearrange your exercises.

## Avoid excessive duplication

13.94    While some overlap between exercises is fine and even desirable, getting carried away can be destructive. If you are bent-leg deadlifting in a cycle, do not stiff-leg deadlift heavily as well. You could perform some light stiff-legged deadlifts to maintain flexibility, but do not push the exercise hard as well as the regular deadlift. An exception to this may be during deadlift specialization.

13.95    If you are bench pressing on a regular horizontal bench, do not go adding decline *and* incline benches. If you do not overdo the volume and frequency of each, you may be able to gain on two chest-shoulder-triceps exercises—e.g., the bench press and the parallel bar dip—but add a third one and you are likely to halt progress in them all. The exception to this generalization is during *advanced* specialization work, when multiple exercises for the same body part in the same program can be productive.

## Physique imbalance

13.96    Many people have a natural body structure that is imbalanced, possibly exaggerated by a lifetime of activity. This needs to be considered when fine-tuning a program. A not uncommon imbalance is a lower-body structure and development that is considerably heavier than the upper-body. In such a case, if you give the same focus to the squat and deadlift as you do to your major upper-body exercises, you will make the situation even more pronounced. Instead, do some maintenance squats and perhaps make it challenging by performing very high reps once a week, adding a few pounds to the bar once you hit 100 reps, dropping the reps and building up again. Focus on your upper-body structure and substitute stiff-legged deadlifts for bent-legged ones. Give it time, as in a year or two, and you will even out the imbalances considerably, though your lower body will probably always easily get ahead.

13.97     Keep in mind that if you want to exploit a natural strength or bias, especially in a particular exercise, you need to live with imbalances, and even intentionally exaggerate them.

## Opinion bias

13.98     If you align yourself rigidly with one strand of training opinion you can get so locked into it that you never apply yourself with zeal to any other line of opinion. Therefore the other opinions are never going to work for you. On the other hand, you can argue that once you have found something that works very well for you, why try anything else?

13.99     Some people rave over how well they do on a 5 x 5 program— two or three progressive warmup sets followed by three or two work sets with a fixed poundage. Others do not get much out of a 5 x 5 program, but sets of 10–12 work well. Some people like the cumulative-fatigue approach, which involves holding back on the first few sets, but other people prefer to go full-bore on all their work sets, and thus do fewer sets. And many people prosper on advanced work in the power rack, whereas some advanced trainees do not.

13.100    Some people only like to squat for 20-rep sets. Others hate high-rep squats and never get into them hard enough and long enough to get much out of them, though they can reap lots of benefit from performing sets of five reps.

13.101    Some people rave over very slow reps, whereas most trainees find them so boring that they cannot deliver consistent effort over long enough to make the very slow reps deliver growth.

13.102    Some people are terrific natural squatters; others have poor leverages for squatting, but can become terrific deadlifters.

13.103   Some people respond well on a "blood and guts" single-set-to-failure-per-exercise type of routine—if it is well cycled, with plenty of rest between sessions, and if supervised by a like-minded training partner or trainer. But left to their own devices there is no way they can deliver the intensity needed, though they can do very well on a 5-x-whatever format.

13.104   You have to be very keen on a program to commit yourself 100% to it. If you apply anything less than 100% commitment, the results will be way under what you could get on the program if you really applied yourself to it.

13.105   You must not only find something that is practical for you, but something you like doing, and can do well for long enough to earn good results.

## Between-set rests

13.106   At one extreme there is the take-as-much-time-as-you-want philosophy. At the other there is the take-as-little-as-possible approach. The former does not want to sacrifice the weights by hurrying through the workout, and is a physically less uncomfortable way to train. The latter philosophy is heavily concerned not only with the intensity of each individual exercise, but the overall intensity of the short-duration workout. This style of training usually consists of a single work set per exercise, taken to failure. The poundages suffer when exercises are done almost back to back, but this is supposed to be offset by the overall metabolic stimulation for muscular growth that the body may get if you can deliver the necessary intensity.

13.107   Both approaches can build big and strong bodies, as can different twists in between the two extremes. What matters most is finding an interpretation *you* can do consistently and with progressive poundages. You may be able to benefit from more than one approach.

13.108   Not hurrying between sets is the most practical way for most people to train—about two minutes between work sets of the smaller exercises, and more like four minutes between work sets of the biggest exercises. Shorter breaks can be taken between warmup sets. Make ninety minutes the *upper limit* for a workout, with an hour being a better ceiling, excluding the general warming up work, and cooling down. Organize your workout design, number of sets, and rest periods accordingly.

13.109    For many people the most practical between-sets rest period is the time it takes for a training partner to perform his set, and for weights to be changed. If there is no partner, then the time to change weights and catch one's breath is what many people apply. The more demanding a given exercise is, the more time that is needed to catch one's breath between sets. So naturally more time is taken between sets of squats than calf raises.

## One-minute rest periods

13.110    Taking one-minute rests between sets is a quite fast pace of training, but not a back-to-back pace. When taking only a minute of rest between sets you cannot maintain the same poundage for all your work sets in a given exercise unless you let your reps drop with each set, or unless you hold back on the first set(s).

13.111    Take an example of being able to do three sets of six reps with 300 pounds in the squat if you rest five minutes between sets. But if you take only one minute between sets, your three sets will be something like 300 x 6, 300 x 3 and 300 x 1. To keep the reps up, reduce the poundage each set and be rigorous about only taking one minute between sets—use a clock.

13.112    Experiment to see what reduction you need in order to keep the reps up. Using the same squat example, to keep the reps up to six in each set, you may need to use weights of 300, 260 and 235. You may prefer to use a percentage method, or a fixed poundage drop per set for a given exercise. The percentages or fixed poundage drops will not be the same for all exercises because the big movements suffer more from short rests between sets than do smaller exercises. Once you have found what suits you for a given exercise, be consistent. Keep records of your poundages, and concentrate on progressive poundages across all the sets.

13.113    Intensity of effort in each individual set is more important than rushing between exercises. Do not compromise on the quality of a set by rushing from one to another quicker than you can manage. Getting each set right is much more important than getting all the sets over as quickly as possible. If you need several minutes between sets to get each one done well, fine.

13.114    You have to enjoy the challenge of training. If you step it up so much, including rushing between sets, that you make training something you no longer enjoy, then that is no good *for you*.

The individual set and *your* training performance are most important, so never let anything mar them for you.

### Adaptation to faster training

13.115    If you want to try faster-paced training, move to it over a period of a couple of months or so, to give your body a chance to adapt. If you pick up the pace too quickly you will become light-headed and perhaps even nauseous. Start with at least two minutes rest between sets, and take at least two months to gradually cut back the rest period until you are working at the pace you want. But do not rush it too much or else you will end up not working the muscles properly, and your training will deteriorate into a mere race against the clock.

### Another interpretation of faster-paced training

13.116    Another way of training quicker is to sequence groups of exercises. For example, do a set of bench presses and then after no more than a minute of rest perform a set of pulldowns or cable rows. You could even sequence three different exercises. After the two- or three-exercise sequence, take your regular between-sets rest period before repeating the sequence.

13.117    This can work well so long as you train at a quiet time at a gym where it is practical to work out like this. It will probably be best if you are using reps on the medium to low side and thus are not getting heavily out of breath. If you are in a hurry to finish your workout, and do not want to reduce the volume of work you do, this is a good strategy to use.

### Limited back-to-back training

13.118    Back-to-back training does not have to be for all exercises in a routine, or none of them. It can be for specific pairings of exercises. Three particular pairings come to mind for those who want to test their mettle and boost their training intensity.

> Though not popular today, in the pre-steroids era the 20-rep squat was very influential. It was hugely productive back then, when used as the cornerstone of an *abbreviated* training program, and it can be hugely productive today. Anyone who thinks that high reps do not build muscle and strength is totally out of touch with Iron Game history.

These pairings are the squat and stiff-legged deadlift, the leg press and stiff-legged deadlift, and the bent-legged deadlift and leg press, but, for safety, *not* the leg press followed by the bent-legged deadlift, or any type of deadlift followed by the squat.

13.119    In order for the two exercises of each pairing to be done back to back, the equipment and weights for both movements must be set up in advance.

13.120    The second exercise in each pairing will suffer as a result of the effects of the first exercise. You must reduce the poundage of the second movement accordingly.

13.121    Done intensively, especially for high reps, each of these pairings will crush you, but the growth stimulation can be huge. But do not drop into it without a progressive preparatory period. Stick with it, rest adequately between sessions, build up the weights in both exercises of each pairing, and you will get bigger and stronger as a result.

13.122    Safety must be uppermost in your mind if you use any of these pairings. Because you will be crushed after the first exercise, you need 100% attention to using perfect form on the second exercise. Consider the leg press and stiff-legged deadlift combination. As you do the stiff-legged deadlift your legs will tremble and you could lose control over them. This could be very dangerous. If you cannot exercise perfect control in the second exercise, then *do not* do the exercises back to back.

13.123    Even following waiting several minutes after performing the leg press, your legs may still shake when you stiff-legged deadlift. If this happens to a degree that your form is

> **If you rest too long between training a given exercise or body part you will stagnate or even get weaker, and lose muscular size. More rest is only good up to a certain point. But what that "certain point" is varies from person to person, exercise to exercise, and according to the volume and intensity of training used. *Find the training frequency that is best for you and each exercise or body part.* To do this, experiment sensibly with the guidelines given in this book.**

compromised, then reorganize your program. Arrange it so you have sufficient rest between the two exercises that the second of them can be done in perfect form.

## The back-down set

13.124    The back-down set is done with a weight less than that of the last work set you did on an exercise. Strip off enough weight so you can do about twice as many reps as you normally do in that exercise. This is sometimes called a "pump set," but if you use it, it should be for a lot more than a mere pump. The pump is a good indication of where an exercise stresses your musculature, but it is not necessarily an indicator of growth stimulation.

13.125    If you reduce an exercise's poundage by about 30% and rep out to the maximum, not only will you get lots of pump but you will stimulate growth—unless this extra set causes you to overtrain. But if you reduce the weight by 60% and rep out to the maximum, you will get lots of pump but no growth stimulation.

13.126    Piling back-down sets on top of your regular work sets is likely to overtrain you. To counter this, do not do a back-down set in each exercise every workout. Alternatively you could substitute each back-down set for one of your regular work sets.

13.127    The principle of progressive poundages applies in back-down sets just like it does in regular work sets.

13.128    The back-down set may be a productive addition to your training. Once beyond the beginner stage, consider including a *single* back-down set to finish off an exercise. But you need to be very alert to the danger of overtraining, and take precautions to ensure you train within the limits of your recovery abilities. If in doubt, do not do back-down sets. BB

---

**This book is devoted to helping *you* to further *your* progress to achieving *your* potential. It is not concerned with the achievements of others. What matters most to you (training wise, that is) is *your* physique, strength, health and fitness, *not* the exploits of others. The physique that concerns you the most is the one you see, use and think about the most—*your own*. This book is dedicated to YOU and YOUR physique.**

*Too many sets, exercises and workouts are the factors usually thought of as being the villains behind overtraining. There is much more to overtraining than this gross oversimplification.*

*If you are alert to the symptoms of overtraining, and become aware as soon as you start to overdo your training, you can take action and nip overtraining in the bud.*

*Do not be macho and battle on to see how many of the symptoms of overtraining you can withstand, and yet continue to at least maintain your strength.*

# 14. How to Avoid the Plague of Overtraining

14.1    The inability of most trainees to recognize the symptoms of overtraining is at the root of their training problems. But recognizing the symptoms is only the start. You need to know how to respond to the early symptoms—*immediately*—if you are to escape the frustration and misery that accompanies chronic overtraining. *This is a very serious issue.*

14.2    Serious hard-gaining trainees have the grit and character to soldier on even when the going gets tough. This is usually a desirable trait, but when it comes to dealing with the warning signs of overtraining, this grit can be destructive. Watch out for your emotions getting the better of your reason. You *must* train within *your* body's ability to recuperate. Never mind what someone else can recuperate from. Someone else is not you.

14.3    Overtraining arises when the body is exposed to more stress than it can deal with. It may be that you are training too frequently for the exercise load you are under, or that you are training too much each workout for the frequency you are using. But overtraining is usually much more complex than that.

14.4    Overtraining does not occur overnight unless you greatly increase your training load and/or have some drastic reduction in the quality of your rest, sleep and nutrition, and/or have some calamity in your personal/family life that wipes you out. Overtraining is usually an accumulative process of weeks and months of demanding too much from your body, and ignoring the warning signs of impending chronic overtraining.

14.5    When on the edge of overtraining you may still creep forward in the gym; but things will fall apart as you reach the exhaustion point of your recovery abilities. Then, unless you back off in a big way, your body will crumble.

14.6     Growing bigger and stronger is your body's response to the stress you impose on it by lifting progressively heavier weights in good form. The stress you impose is essential. Getting unusually strong and big demands an unusual degree and type of stress, but there is a fine line between doing enough and doing too much.

14.7     Even when you think you can cope with a very heavy stress level, such as at the end of a training cycle when you are pushing full-bore, your body is taking such a battering that your immune system is suppressed to a degree. This increases your chance of infection. When you are riding the crest of a wave of effort and progression in the gym, do not think you are indestructible. At such a time, take an extra day or two of rest between workouts, reduce your training volume a little, sleep more, eat better, and be super attentive to recovering fully between workouts. Do all this so that you do not go from being "indestructible" one day, to being laid low with a viral infection the next.

14.8     Stress itself is not bad, but an excess of stress relative to what you can deal with *is* bad. An over-stressed body regresses. This is Nature's way of forcing you to cycle your training intensity. Whether you like it or not, you will end up cycling your training intensity to some degree, whether you do it intentionally (by deliberately backing off at times) or have it forced upon you by injury or illness.

## Symptoms of overtraining

14.9     Before you can take action in response to warning signs of overtraining, you need to know what signs to look for. While the following symptoms are accurate for the typical non-competitive trainee, including those who are advanced, the *very* advanced *and* competitive elite may exhibit different symptoms of overtraining. This list is not presented as an exhaustive study.

         a.  Stagnated training poundages, perhaps even before you have reached your most recent best training weights. One or two bad workouts do not necessarily mean you are overtrained. All people have the occasional bad workout that should be written off. But when you have three or four consecutive bad workouts, then you are almost certainly overtrained.

b.  Reduced enthusiasm for training, i.e., not looking forward to training as much as usual, and having trouble getting a workout finished without cutting corners. (This could be caused by out-of-the-gym distractions, not necessarily overtraining.)

c.  A body that is more tired and sore than it usually is in the days following training. You will not bounce back from the healthy feeling of fatigue that follows a great workout. And despite perhaps sleeping more than usual you still feel drained.

d.  Even though you feel very tired you may have trouble getting to sleep and/or have trouble getting back to sleep when awoken during the night.

e.  An increasing number of minor aches and pains, and ones that do not heal.

f.  Reduced appetite and food intake.

g.  Reduced level of concentration during each set.

h.  Being more irritable and less patient in your life in general.

i.  Being anxious about your training not going well.

j.  Feeling under the weather.

k.  Getting frequent colds.

l.  Diminished endurance—formerly moderate-intensity aerobic work starts feeling quite demanding. The perceived exertion from the aerobic exercise increases.

m. Legs feel heavy, in and out of the gym, and all activities seem to involve more effort than previously.

n.  Increased resting heart rate.

o.  Increased diastolic blood pressure.

p.  An inclination for corner cutting in any training-related issue, including your nutrition.

q.  Losing interest in reading training magazines and books.

14.10   *Many of the above can be the result of out-of-the-gym factors. Even in those cases it is still wise to back off to a reduced training intensity until your life and recovery machinery are back to normal.*

14.11   Be totally honest with yourself. Discover if you have any of the symptoms of overtraining. You probably suffer from at least several of the symptoms. If so, face the fact that you are overtrained and need to adjust your training so the symptoms of overtraining do not persist. Do not be guilty of denial. *You will not increase your muscle and might through overtraining!*

14.12   Local soreness and systemic fatigue are part and parcel of training. There is, however, a huge difference between post-workout systemic fatigue that is a high from training, and the fatigue that is almost debilitating. To train hard, and have a shower followed by a good meal, leaves a sense of achievement and worked feeling that is a joy. To beat yourself into the ground once you are already tired and dragging yourself around, as in the overtrained state, produces no post-workout high.

## Causes of the overtrained condition

14.13   Too many sets, exercises and workouts are the factors usually thought of as being the villains behind overtraining. In addition, a few people train too hard especially through the excessive use of forced reps, drop sets and other intensifiers. But there is much more to overtraining than this.

### a. Factors outside of the gym

14.14   While a major if not *the* major source of physical stress in your life is your training, stress from all aspects of life can wear you down. Depending on your circumstances, the non-training contribution to stress may exceed that from your training. If your recovery machinery goes out of order due to employment, personal or domestic factors, do not expect to continue with your usual training program and still make progress.

14.15   Here are real-life situations that can destroy your body's ability to cope with what was previously a productive training schedule: going through a major relationship problem or serious financial difficulty, working at two jobs, caring for a sick child, travelling a lot, not sleeping well, skipping meals, moving home, changing jobs, preparing for examinations.

14.16    When you are feeling well and your life is running smoothly, and thus your recovery machinery is in good order, your body has a much greater capacity for coping with and responding to training than it has when you are run ragged from your life out of the gym. This is why you should always modify your training to reflect how your life is going outside of the gym. It also explains why what worked for you last year when your life was running well will fail this year if your life is in a mess.

14.17    The conventional approach for dealing with overtraining neglects to consider seriously enough the impact of the circumstances of life outside of the gym. *Training cannot be seen in a vacuum.*

## b. The contribution of exercise technique to overtraining

14.18    Training too much, too often and with poor exercise style— e.g., heaving instead of pushing, dropping instead of lowering, going too deep when squatting or dipping, squirming when benching, yanking when deadlifting and rowing—not only fails to deliver size and strength gains, but wreaks havoc on your body. Such abuse delivers aches, pains and even serious injury, and all of this in amongst the frustration that results when no gains in muscle and might are being produced.

14.19    Exercise technique is not about excellent form or terrible form. No one can use terrible form for long without being forced to stop training through injury. But very few people use really good exercise technique. The nearer you are to using perfect exercise technique, the less of a negative effect exercise form is going to have your body. The poorer your form, the more of a negative effect the *same amount* of training will have on your body. Poor form wears your joints and connective structures down, and takes more out of your overall recovery abilities.

14.20    Good exercise form is important for many reasons, one of them being to deliver the most positive effect from your training, but with minimum negative effect. Always keep your form tight. Never loosen it in order to get more weight on the bar.

14.21    Poor form is not only about obviously dreadful technique, but about perversions of exercises that in the short term appear to do no damage, but over the long term are destructive for many people, e.g., squats with heels raised excessively, bench presses with a grip too wide or too narrow, pulldowns with a very wide grip, pulldowns to the rear of the head, overhead presses with an excessively wide grip, behind-neck pressing, and excessive arching of the back while bench pressing.

### c. Gross overtraining

14.22    Gross overtraining, *even if you are using good exercise style*, will wear you down, deliver injuries, and make you prone to infections. This is not just a product of excessive training volume in each workout. It is also a product of how often you train and how your exercises are spread over the week. Even a good abbreviated program of a low volume of exercise can fail if you divide the exercises up inappropriately *for you*.

14.23    Shoulder and lower back injuries are among the most common in the gym. To discover why, look at how the shoulders and lower back are battered, either directly or indirectly, on conventional training routines. Even when using abbreviated workouts, design your routines so that your shoulders and lower back are not pounded each time you work out.

### d. The contribution of other forms of exercise

14.24    You may be performing other types of exercise on top of your weight training. Moderate aerobic work should not impede your gains in the gym, so long as you set about it properly, and assuming your weight-training program is sound. In fact, moderate aerobic work will improve your overall physical conditioning. This will increase your ability to train well with the weights and recover from workouts. But overdo the aerobic work, and you will kill your progress in the gym.

14.25    If you are seriously into other athletic activities you will make gains in the gym much harder if not impossible to produce. While your body's ability to recuperate from exercise and make progress can be improved, there are limits. The source of your overtrained state with the weights may rest with the other exercise you do, and thus you need to make changes there if you want to progress with your resistance training.

> **Do not wait until you get buried in full-blown overtraining before you appreciate the devastating impact it has, and how, on an accumulative basis, it can cost you years of your training life.**

# How to react to signs of overtraining

14.26    If you are alert to the symptoms of overtraining, and become aware as soon as you are starting to overdo your training, you have the opportunity to nip overtraining in the bud. Stay out of the gym an *extra* couple of days before your next workout, rest and sleep a bit more, pay more attention to nutrition, and then reduce your work sets when back in the gym.

14.27    If you need to plug in an extra day or two of rest between workouts on a regular basis, revise your whole training program so that the required rest days are actually scheduled. Or maybe the training frequency that you are currently overtraining on will be fine if you do fewer sets and/or exercises at each workout.

14.28    If you *still* feel stagnated in the gym after taking an extra day or two of rest, take another *extra* few days of rest and good nutrition before your next workout, to total at least a full week off. Then when back in the gym, back pedal a little. Cut back all your poundages by 10% and take a month to build back to your best of four weeks earlier. This one-month down period can restore you, avoid full-blown overtraining, and set you up for a period of gains.

## Two areas for action

14.29    There are two areas for action when responding to warning signs of overtraining—in the gym, and out of the gym. Cut back in the gym—do less work each session and/or train less often. If you are being run ragged by your life in general out of the gym, then do something about that area.

14.30    Cutting back in the gym and mere fiddling with out-of-the-gym factors are not enough. You need major overhauling to ensure that you *consistently* rest and sleep enough, attend to meeting nutritional needs, and work to solve whatever sources of distraction and anxiety are ruining your training.

14.31    Never mind that easy gainers can, apparently, at least over the short term, break many of the rules of proper rest and nutrition, and yet still make progress in muscle and might. Hard gainers have *far less* room for corner cutting than do easy gainers. And keep in mind that the most successful easy gainers usually do not cut corners when meeting their rest and nutritional needs.

## Laying off, and coming back

14.32    If you are overtrained to a frazzle and suffering from most if
not all of the symptoms listed earlier, you need to have a
layoff for a couple of weeks. A layoff means not only doing
*nothing* in the gym, but not even going to the gym. Stay out of
it. You need a complete rest. Even a bit of aerobic work, or
just a few sets of curls, will delay your recovery. Stop
exercising other than doing some stretching and leisurely
walking. Sleep early and get up late whenever possible, eat
well but not excessively, and get thoroughly rested. As you
restore yourself, your training zeal will start to return.

14.33    Let this feeling of anticipation and vigor build up. *Do not* get
back in the gym as soon as possible and risk having the
fledgling zest extinguished. Let your enthusiasm build up until
you are almost rabidly keen to train.

14.34    Now get back in the gym on a new program—one that is more
abbreviated than your former one, and with reduced
poundages. Take it easy, use *immaculate* exercise technique,
and build back to your best working poundages *over six weeks*.
Gradually let your body adapt to the reintroduction of
increasing training poundages, *without* experiencing severe
systemic fatigue and local soreness, or any of the warning
signs of overtraining. While avoiding overtraining you will
build up the conditioning needed to forge into new poundage
territory in the final stage of the cycle. If you rush back you
will return to the overtrained state.

14.35    And be sure to rest, sleep and eat better than you did when
you got overtrained in your previous program. So long as
your training program is reasonable, the major factor
determining whether or not you gain from it is how well you
satisfy the recovery component—rest, sleep and nutrition.

14.36    Taking a couple of weeks layoff as a response to chronic
overtraining, and then returning to the *same* training
program that got you overtrained in the first place, is *not* the
way to go. You have to take action to ensure that you do not
repeat the scenario that got you into a mess of overtraining
in the first place. And even if you thought that what you
were doing in the gym prior to the layoff was modest relative
to what some people can grow on, if it overtrained you, then
*you must still cut back.*

14.37    Forget about what others can gain on. What matters most to *you* and *your* training is what *you* can gain on. Always remember that reducing training volume and frequency nearly always produces more gains, both for hard gainers *and* for not-so-hard gainers.

14.38    Never continue with a training program that produces symptoms of overtraining, no matter how little you may be training relative to elite bodybuilders. What matters in your personal training is what works *for you*. Overtraining will not make your muscles grow!

## Training variety

14.39    Some people stress the importance of training variety as a means to prevent overtraining. If they mean rational training variety within the confines of what works for the drug-free typical trainee, fine. But if they mean, as they usually do, to change the routine every so often despite the training volume, frequency and/or intensity being beyond the recovery abilities of the trainee, that is no good. And if they mean chopping and changing exercises every week or few, that is training suicide to a hard gainer.

14.40    Hard gainers need to stick to a pool of safe major exercises, and a fixed sensible training format for a sustained period of months before making any changes. Only in that way can they get full value from each exercise. How can you get the most from an exercise, or a rep or set format, if you do it for only a few weeks? You will forever be getting used to exercise changes—i.e., learning or revising the grooves, finding the right working poundages, and familiarizing yourself with changes. You will never have sufficient time to dedicate to consistent workouts to build up your poundages into new personal bests.

14.41    The most important factor behind sustained training motivation is sustained progress, and *excessive* variety will kill your gains.

## Combining the training variables

14.42    Find the minimum volume, intensity and frequency of training that will deliver consistent gains. Then you will have a margin for error so that you can stay below the threshold of overtraining. In this way you will minimize the chances of being so near the edge that just a little more work will push you over it. Most people design their routines with the attitude of doing as much as they can get away with. Some just manage to keep it a tad under overtraining, but most do not, which is why most non-beginners stagnate for years on end.

14.43   Be on the lookout for warning signs of overtraining, and act on them *immediately* if or when they appear—to nip overtraining in the bud. Do this to get control over your bodybuilding and strength training. Never surrender control to another person.

## What if you train while severely overtrained?

14.44   Your body's immune system works to prevent invading organisms—bacteria and viruses—causing illness. A healthy person can deal relatively easily with everyday bacteria and viruses. When you repeatedly push your body to the limit there is heavy disruption of your immune system. Though an individual weight-training workout is very unlikely to devastate you like a marathon run would, for example, if you persist in consistently training beyond your ability to recover, the effect will be similar.

14.45   The harder you train, the more careful you have to be to look after yourself well, because now is the time when your defenses are lowered. The effect of short-term overtraining is one thing, but if you overtrain over the medium and long term you will get so worn down that almost any bacterium or virus could strike you down. You may consider yourself big and strong, and everyone else in your family is weak in comparison. But when it comes to being able to resist infection, you may find *you* are the weak one if you are overtrained.

14.46   Some former elite track athletes have had their sporting careers wrecked because they persisted in training hard despite already being severely overtrained. After being supremely fit these athletes suffered from severe immune system suppression, and long-term illness/injury.

## Sleep

14.47   Sleeping well on a regular basis is of critical importance. *You need to take concrete action to correct any sleeping inadequacies you may have.* Otherwise your inability to sleep adequately will continue, your recovery will be compromised, and your rate of gain in muscle and might impaired.

14.48    The advice to get enough sleep is good, but not enough.
          Developing the discipline to go to sleep earlier is the only
          action most people need to take to ensure that sufficient sleep
          is had each night. But for some people other action is needed
          because there are legitimate sleeping difficulties.

14.49    If you do not sleep well, and/or if you know you need more
          sleep but your body will not currently cooperate to let you
          sleep well, you must investigate the problems and find
          solutions. Your sleeping difficulties may be easily fixed. Visit
          a library or bookshop and select a book or two on sleeping
          disorders and solutions. There are a number of simple
          practical measures you can take to improve the quality and
          quantity of your sleep. If these measures do not help, there
          may be a medical problem, in which case you should consult
          your doctor or a sleep clinic.

**The acid test**
14.50    Unless you wake *every* morning feeling *fully* rested, and
          *without* having to be awoken, you are not getting enough
          sleep. And even if you are making gains in the gym, more rest
          and sleep could substantially increase your gains. While the
          realities of life will at least occasionally disrupt the full
          satisfying of your sleep requirements, if you have the
          necessary determination you can ensure that you get your full
          sleep quota at least *almost* every night. Dedicate yourself to
          doing your absolute best to make the exceptions to the rule
          only *very rare* occurrences.

14.51    To get more sleep you will have to have fewer hours awake.
          There are only twenty-four hours in a day. You cannot burn
          the candle at both ends and expect to make decent
          bodybuilding and strength training progress. When you know
          that it is time to get to sleep, but you are tempted to watch an
          extra video or TV program, stay out an extra hour or two, or

> If you are undereating you will seriously impair your
> recovery ability, which will lead to overtraining. But
> overeating cannot compensate for overtraining. Eat
> very well every day and never cut corners with your
> nutrition; but get your workouts in really good order
> and train *within* your recovery means.

chit chat for a while longer, etc., remind yourself that your training and physique are more important than entertainment. Then get to sleep on time.

14.52    If you are a hard gainer, then eight hours of sleep each night should be your *minimum* if you are serious about making decent progress. Do not try to get extra sleep. Focus on getting what your body naturally needs. Go to bed immediately when you start to feel sleepy.

14.53    Here are ten tips to help improve your sleeping ability:

a.  Do not weight train late in the day. Train in the morning or afternoon if possible, or early evening at the latest. Intensive training gets your body charged up. The body needs a number of hours to calm down before being ready to sleep.

b.  Low-intensity cardiorespiratory work late in the day may help you to fall asleep.

c.  Do not drink coffee, tea or any other stimulant before sleeping. It is best to avoid stimulants completely.

d.  Sleep in a dark room. Take action to eliminate light sources, e.g., use curtains that do not allow light to pass through.

e.  Eliminate as much as possible all sources of noise, and sound proof your bedroom as well as you can.

f.  A warm shower or bath before going to bed should help prepare your body for sleeping.

g.  Stretching immediately before going to bed helps some people to relax.

h.  Before closing your eyes and trying to go to sleep, read something that relaxes you.

i.  Shortly before bedtime, do not watch anything on TV or at a cinema that stirs up your emotions in a major way.

j.  Establish regular sleeping habits. Going to sleep at 11PM one night and then 1AM the next is not regularity. Make it

10.30PM till 7AM on a regular basis, for example. And much better than catching up on lost sleep is not losing any sleep in the first place.

14.54    When you have an unusually good night's sleep, determine the conditions that brought it about. Then try to create the same conditions in future. Conversely, when you have an unusually bad night's sleep, determine the conditions that brought it about. Then avoid setting up those conditions in future. [BB]

## Note on the Trap Bar and shrug bar

Where the Trap Bar® is referred to in this book, you may also read "shrug bar." The shrug bar came on the market after BEYOND BRAWN was first published. The two bars are produced by different manufacturers. Both are excellent training tools. The shrug bar provides more knee room because it has a hexagonal shape as against the rhombus shape of the Trap Bar. Please see page 481 for how to find more information on the shrug bar. You may, however, find the *standard* shrug (or Trap) bar too restricting for safe bent-legged deadlifting, and require a custom-made bar with gripping sites placed wider apart.

Because I am only interested in drug-free training, and primarily concerned with satisfying the needs of the hard-gaining masses, some of the methods and values promoted in this book are heretical relative to much of what is customary in gyms today. There is no other approach to take if training methods that are practical and helpful for drug-free typical people are to be promoted.

You will benefit from BEYOND BRAWN in direct proportion to how seriously you study the book, how thoroughly you grasp the contents, how well you make the understanding one with you, and how resolutely you apply what you learn.

*The harder you train, the less of it you can do, and the less of it you can stand. If you have not cut back your sets and/or training frequency, and have not boosted your diet, rest and sleep, a hike in intensity will wipe you out, overtrain you, and cause you to lose strength.*

*While most trainees are guilty of not training hard enough, some are training too hard. They train at an intensity beyond what they can respond to.*

*To make the most of the final leg of each cycle you have to be dedicated to your training and training-related matters to the point of almost being obsessed. As soon as you start compromising on one thing or another, you will start compromising on your gains.*

# 15. How to Milk Your Training Cycles Dry of Gains

15.1    Implement the following thirteen-point strategy—some of which connects information given earlier in this book, especially related to avoiding overtraining—and you can extend the growth stage of a training cycle considerably. Then you can notch up more muscular gains before finally starting a new training cycle.

## RULE #1
### You must be a model of dedication and commitment

15.2    To make the most of the final leg of each cycle you must be *101%* dedicated to training and training-related matters. Compromise on anything and you will compromise on your gains.

15.3    But maintain an extraordinary level of dedication *without* neglecting the rest of your life. Remember that what is very important to you is unlikely to be as important for your family, friends and fellow workers. Just get on with applying your dedication in your own private way.

## RULE #2
### You must train hard

15.4    All the talk, study and whatever else about training counts for nothing when you have to give your all to squeezing out another good-form rep, and then another, and then another. Here is when you discover how much you want bigger and stronger muscles. Here is when your mettle is tested. Here is where the buck stops with you. If you do not deliver the effort, then forget about gains no matter how conscientiously you may satisfy all the other requirements of productive training.

15.5    Relish the hard work. Savor the final and most taxing reps of a set—the domain of the growth zone. Revel in the opportunity to stimulate further growth; and then give your pound of flesh.

# RULE #3
## Get your training well supervised

15.6    Good supervision, whether from a training partner or
        someone else, is a first-class way of getting you to deliver
        more than you would by yourself. Do your utmost to get
        supervised over at least the final leg of cycle—when you need
        all the encouraging and even bullying you can get to push
        yourself to new heights of effort. Quit on the effort, and you
        will quit on the gains.

# RULE #4
## At the end of a cycle, reduce your training for each
## exercise to warmups plus one intensive work set

15.7    The harder you train, the less of it you can do, and the less of it
        you can stand. The greater the volume of your training, the
        more you will need to dilute your effort to survive each
        workout. Reduce your training to the absolute minimum—i.e.,
        warmups plus a single work set, per exercise—and focus all
        your usual efforts on the reduced training volume. Then you
        should see an increase in your training intensity. That can make
        the difference between growth stimulation and muscle
        maintenance. You will also demand less from your
        recuperative powers and better enable your body to respond to
        the growth stimulus.

15.8    To ensure sustained progression on the biggest and most
        important exercises during the final leg of a cycle, severely
        reduce, or temporarily eliminate, all other exercises. You may
        even need to drop one or two of the biggest exercises in order
        to keep progressing on the others. For example, your progress
        may grind to a halt in the squat and deadlift, each trained
        once a week. But drop one of them and then progress in the
        other may keep moving forward and the cycle can continue
        for a while yet.

# RULE #5
## Train each body part less often

15.9    Following on the heels of training volume is training frequency.
        At the end of a cycle you may need less of both (depending on
        what you were doing earlier on). Arrange exercises so that
        overlapping ones—e.g., bench press and overhead press, squat
        and bent-legged deadlift—are done the same day, so you have
        sufficient rest days in between "hits." If in doubt, take an extra
        day or two of rest. Experiment with less frequent hard training

for the biggest exercises. For example, squat and deadlift
intensively only once every ten days. See if that helps you to
keep adding weight each session.

# RULE #6
## Use small poundage increments

15.10    The closer you get to the limits of a given cycle, the more
         important it is to add only a very small increment when you
         increase the poundage of a top set. The typical minimum jump
         of 5 pounds is out. An exception here is if you are performing
         some big-poundage, extremely short range exercise, where you
         can keep going with relatively large increments.

15.11    Add 1 pound next workout and you should still get your
         target reps, especially in the big exercises. You may even be
         able to keep 2 pounds a week coming for quite a while
         towards the end of a cycle in the very big exercises such as
         the squat and deadlift. In smaller exercises like the curl, add
         half a pound a week, or two 100-gram discs.

# RULE #7
## Boost your diet

15.12    It is at the end of a cycle—when you are pushing yourself to
         the hilt, and wanting to do it again and again—that you must
         be absolutely certain you are not compromising on your diet.
         Boost your diet. Hike up your intake of animal protein—
         make it specific, like the addition of two cans of water-
         packed tuna a day, or two protein shakes you can easily
         digest. Such a protein boost will also give you a calorie boost.
         But all trainees do not need a boost in their caloric intake in
         order to keep gains coming.

15.13    If you cannot afford to gain any bodyfat, then compensate for
         the protein boost by clipping calories from your fat and
         carbohydrate intake so that you end up with a diet having the
         same calories as before but with about 100 grams of
         additional protein. And make sure every scrap of food you
         eat is high quality.

15.14    If you are not already doing so, take a broad-spectrum
         vitamin and mineral supplement. Your micronutrient needs
         may increase at the end of a training cycle. But taking a multi
         vitamin-mineral supplement may not be enough. There are
         micronutrients that are not available in supplement form. Be

sure, in particular, that you consume more green leafy
vegetables, yellow/orange vegetables, and seeds (e.g.,
pumpkin and sunflower).

## RULE #8
### Go overboard with rest and sleep

15.15    The harder you train, and the deeper you go into new poundage
         territory, the more you demand from your powers of recovery.
         Therefore you need to deliver more rest and sleep than usual.
         Not only do you have to provide the rest and sleep needed to
         recover from the immediate effects of training, but you have to
         provide *additional* rest and sleep so your body can grow.

15.16    Getting adequate sleep is pivotal for enabling your body to
         recover optimally from training. Most trainees shortchange
         themselves in the sleep department, and as a result restrict
         their rate of progress in the gym.

15.17    As noted in Chapter 14, if you are a hard gainer in intensive
         training, eight hours of sleep each night should be your rock-
         bottom *minimum* if you are serious about making good progress.

15.18    A full quota of sleep means getting to sleep as soon as you feel
         drowsy in the evening, and sleeping until you wake naturally.
         If you are awoken by some other means, then you cannot have
         had your full quota of sleep.

15.19    To milk a cycle dry, cut back aerobic work to the minimum
         intensity and duration, or temporarily eliminate it.

## RULE #9 (OPTIONAL)
### Further increase training intensity

15.20    Once you are consistently applying rules 1–8, you could try to
         increase growth stimulation by raising training intensity a
         notch. This option, however, is not for everyone. Many of you
         may be better off moving to rule #10 and skipping #9.

15.21    If you are up to it, and want to see if it helps you to keep
         adding a little poundage every week or two, do not end a set
         after the very final full rep you can squeeze out. Go to the next
         rep and do as much of it as you can. Do not cheat it up. Keep
         your form tight and do as much of the rep as you can. Put your
         heart into it. Do not relax the effort once you have got the bar

as high as you can. Now you have reached concentric failure. Give your all to holding the resistance at the highest point you can get to, which will not be far into the rep if you have gone to the limit in the complete reps. Maintain the static hold for as long as you can, and then fight like hell to stop gravity pulling the bar down. You will then have reached isometric failure. Then resist the eccentric as if your life depended on it.

15.22    If you have strong and competent spotters, and are really up to the absolute limit of intensity, then have your spotters lift the resistance for you so that you can resist another eccentric. Continue this procedure for another eccentric or two or three, until you cannot control the descent. (Control means that you can take *at least* four seconds to lower the resistance.) Your spotters must be super vigilant and ready to take the resistance from you as soon as you can no longer control its descent. This final stint of "paralytic" training will take you to eccentric failure.

15.23    Do this properly and you will have trained to utter failure. Supply the necessary factors for recuperation, and this to-utter-failure training of just one set for an exercise at the end of a cycle *may* help you to get more growth mileage out of the cycle. But if you have not cut back your sets and/or training frequency, and have not boosted your diet, rest and sleep, the intensity hike will wipe you out, overtrain you, and cause you to lose strength.

15.24    For this intensity hike do not go to eccentric failure on all the exercises in a given workout. Isometric failure is enough for most exercises, and perhaps more than enough. Only go to eccentric failure for one or at most two exercises per workout, varying which exercises you select from week to week. Do not go to eccentric failure for any given exercise more than once every four weeks. Use a less severe training intensity the other times you train the exercise.

# RULE #10
## Cut back a little, get some momentum going again, have some coasting weeks as well, and then forge on

15.25    When you have applied rules 1–8 (and perhaps #9 too), and you cannot add a single pound to any exercise, you could try back cycling to get some gaining momentum going again. Take a few days extra rest and then cut back 5–10% in all your top sets.

Drop the to-absolute-failure training if you were implementing rule #9. Take 3–4 weeks to inch back to where you were, and then forge on to a few weeks of new poundage territory. Then, to drag it out a little more, have some coasting weeks where you intentionally repeat the poundages and reps from the previous week or two, and make *no attempt* to increase poundages or reps. This lull will enable you to garner your mental and physical resources for another spell of gaining.

## RULE #11
### As an alternative to Rule #9, increase pauses between reps in order to permit more poundage increments

15.26   While increasing the rest period between sets and exercises will help you to keep up your reps as the poundages increase, especially if you are performing multiple work sets per exercise, increasing the between-reps pauses may make a bigger contribution. As an alternative to *Rule #9*, take a few more seconds rest before each rep.

15.27   Only increase the length of the between-reps pauses once you have exhausted the first eight rules for sustaining progress. As you keep notching up the poundages, you can take a bit more rest between reps. This should be enough to get an extra few weeks of poundage progression out of your current program. This can gradually move you from a regular-style of rep performance to a rest-pause one. You can even let it take you all the way into a full-blown rest-pause program where you rest up to a minute between reps, actually setting the resistance down during the pauses.

15.28   Do not take each between-reps pause in a way that you increase fatigue, e.g., do not hang from the overhead bar when taking a pause while chinning; stand on a bench instead.

## RULE #12
### If you know you are already training very hard, but have stagnated, try reducing your training intensity

15.29   While most trainees are guilty of not training hard enough, some train too hard. (Please review Chapter 9 for details.) This appears to contradict some of the points of this chapter, but I want to cover more possibilities.

15.30   If you know you are already training darn hard, and have *everything else* in good order but are still not gaining, try *reducing* your intensity a little. Drop your poundages by 5–10%, and stop taking your sets to failure. Train hard, but not all out. Stop your work sets 1 or 2 reps short of what would be your actual limit. Increase the poundages by a little each week or two, so long as you get your target reps *without* having to go absolutely all out on the final rep or two. With time you may build back to your previous limit poundages, for the same reps, but without having to go 100% all out. Then work into new poundage territory.

# RULE #13
## Get rid of negativity

15.31    A mind occupied with negative thoughts will limit your progress. Be aware of your thoughts, both while training and not training. Do not allow negative thoughts to dwell in your mind. Set them aside as soon as they appear. A period of practice will be needed before you can control your thoughts and get rid of negativity. [BB]

---

If you are gaining in some body parts or exercises, but not in others, there are at least two explanations. First, you may have more potential in some areas than others. Second, and perhaps more likely, you are overtraining the stagnated areas. Discover what you are doing in the successful areas that you are not doing in the others, and apply the successful strategies elsewhere. For example, perhaps you are making good progress deadlifting just once a week, for 3 sets of 6–8 reps, but are getting nowhere with your biceps by barbell curling three times a week for 3 sets of 8 reps followed by 2 sets of 6 reps of alternate dumbbell curls. There are lessons there.

*This chapter provides important practical instruction that applies to every training program you use. Draw on it as you plan your next training cycle, AND when you put the training into practice.*

*Learn from the costly experiences of those who have been through the mill of desperate frustration with conventional training advice. This book is not based on only one man's journey, but is a distillation of the experiences and acquired wisdom of generations of people.*

# 16. Twenty-Three Extras for Maximizing Your Training Productivity

16.1 Successful training depends on *much* more than exercises, goals, effort level, form, and rep, set and cycling schemes. Here are twenty-three other factors to apply to your training.

## 1. Timing of training

16.2 Train during a time of the day that suits you. Some people can train first thing in the morning, but probably most people do not feel right for training so early. Some people like training in the evening. Others have trouble sleeping if they train late. Find the time of day that is practical and agreeable to you, both physically and mentally. By scheduling one training day at the weekend, most people should have at least one workout a week at the optimum time of the day for them.

16.3 If practical, schedule your training so you have enough time after each workout for more than one meal before you go to sleep. If you train at 6PM you may have time for only one meal before you sleep (unless you go to bed very late, which is not recommended). If you train at 4PM you will have time for a post-workout liquid meal followed about two hours later by a solid-food meal. The few hours after training are especially important nutritionally, so providing two or more high-quality meals after training (and before you go to sleep) should be your target. This will get your recovery off to a fine start.

16.4 To perform your best at a workout, try to avoid doing anything very unusual in the twenty-four hours or so before the session. If you usually sleep eight hours a night, then if you got just five the night before a workout, your training may suffer. If you had an *extraordinarily* tiring day yesterday, that could mar your workout today. Better to train tomorrow instead.

16.5      If there is a major event that follows shortly after a scheduled
          workout, and you cannot get it out of your head, e.g., a very
          important meeting or examination, postpone the workout.
          Better to wait a day and get in a perfect and progressive
          workout rather than stick rigidly to a schedule that results in a
          poor workout because you could not focus properly.

## 2. Pre-workout feeding

16.6      Neither wait too long after a feed before training, nor train too
          soon. Have a simple meal that you can digest easily, and train
          about two hours afterward. Some people can train well on an
          empty stomach, others cannot. Discover how much time you
          need for a meal to be processed enough so that you can train
          hard without any digestive tract discomfort or nausea.

16.7      The meal should be carbohydrate-rich, but the carbohydrates
          should not just be simple ones. Complex carbs are needed to
          sustain your energy at a high level throughout your workout.
          Through trial and error discover the food types, balance and
          quantities that will carry you through an intensive workout
          without any waning of energy. It may, for example, be a bowl
          of wholegrain pasta topped with grated cheese, a couple of
          baked potatoes and two scoops of cottage cheese, or a liquid
          meal perhaps based on a meal replacement product. Find what
          works best for you, and then stick with it.

16.8      If you have something shortly before you work out, even if it is
          an "energy drink," you may set yourself up for vomiting if you
          train very intensively. If you ever barf during a workout, or get
          very close to barfing, then in the future consume less food
          before training, select easier-to-digest items, *and* wait 30–60
          minutes longer before training.

16.9      Surprising yourself with very intensive training, especially
          squats or back-to-back leg and back work, when you usually
          train at a lesser intensity, is often at the root of nausea *regardless
          of pre-workout food considerations.* If you want to try very
          intensive squatting or deadlifting, or any back-to-back sets of
          big exercises, gradually increase the training intensity over
          several weeks, to give yourself a chance to adapt.

## 3. Before each workout

16.10     Check that planned poundages, pin settings in the power
          rack, set and rep targets, etc., are correctly written in your

training diary. Look back at the records of previous workouts, and check that you have entered the correct weights and other targets for today's workout. As you look back, recall lessons learned that you can apply to make your training better, and be sure to act on them.

16.11    Immediately before you train with weights, spend 5–10 minutes performing some general warming up. This applies to *everyone* if it is cold. While a general warmup is still good sense for everyone even if it is warm when you train, it is compulsory for everyone over age thirty. Choose from *gentle* indoor cycling, skipping/rope jumping, or skiing or rowing, and preferably a full-body exerciser. The aim is to gradually raise your temperature a little and break you into a sweat.

16.12    The older you are, and the colder it is, the more time and care you should devote to the general warming up. In these circumstances it could even involve a little more than 10 minutes of low-intensity work.

16.13    Regardless of your age, experiment with an aerobic warmup of 20 minutes. If it enhances your weights workout that follows, stick with it. But if it detracts, drop to just enough to break you into a sweat.

16.14    The benefits of a general warmup prior to weight training include these three factors:

   a.   Making muscles more elastic and less susceptible to injury.

   b.   Reducing heart irregularities that may be associated with sudden exercise.

   c.   Priming the nervous system, and heightening coordination and mental preparedness for very rigorous training.

16.15    Spend this warmup time zeroing in on your training, and psyching yourself up. Switch off from the rest of your life. Cut out any frivolous thoughts, and do not get into any discussions. Practice ignoring potential distractions. Visualize the great workout you are going to have, and mentally go through some tough sets. Build yourself to a pitch of intense seriousness. Never mind that you may appear aloof. Treat the gym as a very serious work place.

16.16    After this general warmup period you can perform some ab work and back extensions. This will help to thoroughly warm up your lower back ready for the rigors of an intensive weights session.

16.17    Once you are sweating and ready to weight train, keep yourself warm. Stay well covered, especially between sets, and stay clear of draughts.

16.18    Do your serious stretching after you train with the weights and/or between sets, rather than before you start training. But *after* the general warmup work is over, do enough careful and gentle stretching of any muscles that feel tight and need loosening to their normal range of movement.

## 4. Specific warming up

16.19    Most people casually skip over warmup sets. As a result they are neither physically nor mentally prepared for the hard work sets to follow, and as a result very often mess up those sets.

16.20    There are at least four important reasons for warming up each exercise adequately:

a.  To get liquids pumped into your joint spaces and get the joints, tendons and muscles "oiled." This can be done without wearing yourself out by doing excessive work.

b.  To rehearse the form of each exercise. Take all warmup reps and sets *very* seriously. Do each rep carefully. Practice perfect exercise form. Only once you are *sure* you have the groove perfectly entrenched should you proceed to your work set(s). Add extra warmup work if you feel you would benefit from more groove rehearsal. This especially applies to the more complicated exercises, e.g., deadlift and squat.

c.  To practice concentration and mentally rehearse for the hard sets to come.

d.  To prime the muscles and body as a whole for heavy work.

16.21    On the heels of building up concentration during the warmup stage of a workout, is the sustaining of it throughout the session. Review Chapter 9, in the segment *Focus and Mental*

*Ferocity*, to help ensure you deliver the focus needed to train intensively enough to get terrific results.

16.22    When rehearsing the groove of each exercise prior to the work set(s), you probably cannot do a good job if you use very comfortable weights. You need 75% or more of your work set weight on the bar. This especially applies to low-rep work. Here you have no room for technique error if a work set is to be a success. Preparation must be 100%. For the exercises you use your biggest weights in, you need multiple warmup sets. The final one will be with up to 90% or so of your work set(s) poundage, but for just a few precision reps. It would be for only a single rep if you were doing very low reps in your work set(s).

16.23    If you do not warm up well enough, especially for low-rep work, you may find that your second work set (with the same weight as for the first work set) may actually feel no harder, if not a tad less difficult than that first set. This assumes that you rested well between the first and second work sets. Your body needs something fairly taxing in order to prime itself for the very demanding work set(s) to follow.

16.24    You may find that a warmup set with 90% or so of your work set weight will sometimes feel as heavy if not heavier than the first work set. This is part of the process of preparing yourself for your heaviest sets, so do not be too alarmed if your warmup sets feel heavier than you think they should. So long as your form is good, and you are feeling fine, all should be well.

16.25    Dropping too hurriedly into your heaviest sets, under the assumption that you are saving energy, can backfire. It can make the work sets harder than they would have been had you warmed up in a better way and spent more energy on it. Some individual experimentation and experience will help you to discover what *you* need to do to best prepare yourself for your work sets for each exercise. This will almost certainly vary among different exercises and rep counts.

16.26    How much warming up you need to do specific to a given exercise partly depends on the type of training you are doing. It is also influenced by any history of injury that necessitates more warming up for a specific area. Any muscle tightness that might be present would need to be eased by gentle but specific stretching, and maintained by stretching between sets.

16.27   If you are using very slow cadence reps you may not need to do any specific warming up unless you have a weak link that needs special care and warmup work. The general warming up and the early reps of the relatively light-weight work set will probably suffice, and you may not even need to do any general warming up unless it is cold.

16.28   If you are training with little or no rest between your work sets, and doing exercises back to back, you need to do all your warmup work prior to the workout proper, or else you will break the sustained intensity of the workout by having to do specific warmup sets prior to each work set. But this is not a practical way to train in a busy gym because it necessitates *several* pieces of gear being yours for a sustained period.

16.29   For more traditional training, each exercise is a unit in which warmup and work sets are completed before moving onto the warmup sets for the next exercise. Traditional training does not restrain poundages by having you move quickly between sets and exercises, or by reducing rep speed to a very slow cadence. Because the weights are heavier, more care needs to be given to ensure that sufficient warming up work is done.

16.30   The lower the reps you are performing, the more warmup sets you need. The higher the reps of the work sets, the fewer warmup sets you may need. But in either case you do not need to do lots of reps in each warmup set. About half a dozen deliberate and controlled reps for the first set followed by fewer for subsequent warmup sets will suffice.

16.31   For example, consider the same person and three different squat workouts: 250 x 20 (1 set of 20 reps), 320 x 6 x 3 (3 sets of

Many enthusiasts take aerobic activity to such extremes that they harm their bodies. A fit body is not necessarily a healthy body, and a healthy body is not necessarily a fit one. Fitness and health are not synonymous, but of course it is far better to be fit than unfit. Some people who were super fit also had serious heart disease, and died of that despite their high level of fitness. And many people who do not have heart disease are not at all fit.

6 reps), 360 x 1 x 5 (5 singles). The three different workouts, with warmup sets could be:

135 x 5, 200 x 5, *250 x 20*
135 x 5, 185 x 5, 235 x 5, 290 x 3, *320 x 6 x 3*
135 x 5, 225 x 5, 285 x 3, 320 x 3, *360 x 1 x 5*

16.32     If in doubt, always do *more* warmup work rather than less, especially if you have had an injury in the area being trained, but experiment with less warming up (especially in terms of fewer reps) and see how you get on. *But never put yourself at risk.* It is always better to do too much warmup work than not enough, even if it takes a few pounds or a rep or two off your work set(s).

## 5. Equipment check

16.33     Never plunge into an exercise without having first checked safety considerations. If you train at a home gym and are the sole user, and maintain your gear properly, you will not need to be quite so fussy, but it is much better to be safe than sorry.

16.34     Never use dumbbells without checking that the collars are securely fixed on. Never use a pulldown machine without checking that the cable is safe to use. If you are using a power rack, be sure the pins are correctly in place, and fixed there. Be sure the bench you are about to use is stable and not going to wobble while you use it, etc. All of this is common-sense advice, but this safety consciousness can prevent a nasty accident. Just one accident could put you out of training for a long time. You cannot be too careful.

## 6. Before each set

16.35     Double check that the poundage you have loaded is what you want—consult your training log. Then check that you have actually loaded what you think you have. It is easy to load a bar incorrectly. Leave no room for errors that could ruin a set.

16.36     Securely put collars on your loaded barbell. While most trainees usually do not put collars on their barbells, get into the habit of using them. Plates on one end of the bar sliding just a little can be enough to disturb the balance of the bar, and mar a set. Get yourself a pair of light-weight and quick-release collars if where you train does not have them. Take them when you train, along with your set of little discs, and perhaps chalk too.

16.37     If you use adjustable dumbbells, as against fixed-weight ones that have no adjustable collars, be sure they are securely fixed on before you use the 'bells. A dumbbell coming apart while in use, especially overhead, could prove disastrous. Be very fussy about checking all potential sources of accidents.

16.38     If between sets someone talks to you and disturbs you, politely but firmly make it clear you are there to train, not socialize. By anticipating the possibility of disturbance, and taking action accordingly, you can help avoid someone coming up to you during a set and ruining your concentration.

16.39     When you get in position for a set, pay attention to ensure you take the right grip and/or stance/body position. Do not charge into a set, grab the bar and then realize after the first rep that you took an imbalanced grip, wrong stance, are lopsided while on a bench, or whatever. Take the time, be conscientious, and get positioned right for every set you do. Mentally go through a few reps and establish that everything is in order before you take the bar and start the set.

## 7. Focus trigger

16.40     Immediately before each *work* set you may find it helpful to use a trigger that switches on focus and aggression. Use the same trigger, e.g., a tap on your forehead, a growl, or clap of your hands. Once your trigger has been activated, the battle has started and nothing less than your absolute best performance will do! Some people, however, find triggers distracting. Try it both ways, and see which way helps you the most.

16.41     Use mental imagery to help you train hard. Do not merely deadlift, but pull a vehicle off a trapped person. Do not merely bench press, but free yourself from being crushed by a huge boulder. Do not merely chin, but pull yourself up to save your life after dangling from a very high precipice.

## 8. During each set

16.42     Despite your having tried to ensure that you loaded the right weight and positioned the bar correctly, and adopted an even and precise stance or grip, mistakes still happen. If the first two reps do not feel right, stop and investigate to see if something is wrong. If you persist with a set that does not feel right, you will probably end up performing a bad set, being frustrated, and perhaps even getting injured. And despite your precautions someone may still disturb you during a set and ruin your concentration. Whatever the problem, stop the set and have a rest for a few minutes. Then, having corrected any error(s) you found in your concentration, weight loading, bar positioning, grip or stance, restart the set and this time perform it perfectly. Never be in such a hurry to get a set done that you accept compromises.

16.43    If you are performing singles, you have no second chance. If you get it wrong on the first rep, that is the whole set. The lower the rep count, the greater the need for no mistakes.

16.44    Always be under control in the negative portion of each rep of every exercise you do. Do not be in a hurry to get it over with. Take the extra second or two. Not only does this make your training safer, but it improves your form and position for the positive part of each rep. But avoid going to the extreme of making the negative excessively slow. Doing that will only weaken you for the positive phase. Use moderation.

## 9. Maintaining focus

16.45    Do not talk between sets. Cut yourself off from those who go to the gym to socialize rather than train hard. Talk after you have finished a workout. Avoid everything that diverts your mind from the rigors of intensive training.

## 10. Breathing

16.46    The usual tendency, especially when training hard, is to hold the breath during the hard stage of each rep. This can cause blackouts, especially if you are not used to intensive training. Even if it is just for a split second, a loss of consciousness could be enough to cause a calamity if you were squatting, bench pressing or pressing overhead. Though you may not suffer blackouts or dizziness, headaches are a common result of breath holding during intensive training.

16.47    Start now to breathe out during the positive phase of every rep, and it will soon become a habit. It does not have to be an explosive expulsion, but exhaling in an explosive way can help get the bar through a sticking point. *If you keep your mouth open, that should prevent you from holding your breath.*

16.48    If you train with intensity using very slow reps (five or more seconds for each positive or negative stroke) you will need to pant almost continuously during both the positive and negative strokes of each rep, especially at the end of a set when you are breathing heavily. Do not save the exhalation just for the positive stage.

16.49    Not holding the breath also applies out of the gym. Whenever you put forth a maximum effort, exhale as you do so.

16.50    During demanding exercise you will not be able to get enough air through your nose alone. Breathe through your mouth.

16.51    Always progressively and slowly build up the weights and intensity of your workouts, especially if you have been out of training for a while. Then your body will condition or recondition itself to the rigors of training. So long as you do not hold your breath while you train, you should not feel lightheaded even after the maximum-effort final rep of each set. If you do feel lightheaded, however, cut back your weights and restart the cycle. Build the weights back slowly, being sure to exhale as you drive through the hardest part of each rep.

## 11. Slaking thirst

16.52    Regularly hydrate yourself. Sip water between sets, aiming to drink at least one glass every fifteen minutes you are training. Use a quantity and temperature that is comfortable for your stomach. Drink between sets, but keep your mind fixed on your training, and get straight back into your workout. Avoid turning the visit to the water fountain into a social event. Immediately after training, have a big drink of water. Aim to drink enough water to produce *at least* one clear (color-free) urination after training.

## 12. Cooling down

16.53    Finish each workout with a repetition of the general warming up activity that preceded the workout. This will wind your body down after the rigors of an intensive training session, and help to get the recovery process off to a good start. It only needs 8-10 minutes, tapering off gradually after about the five-minute mark. And then is a good time to wind down further with a moderate and careful stretching program.

## 13. Post-training feeding

16.54    Shortly after your workout, and within half an hour, have a *liquid*, easily digested, protein-rich *and* carbohydrate-rich feed.

Consume about 30–50 grams of protein and 60–100 grams of carbs, depending on your size. Within the next two hours, have a meal of solid food, or another liquid feed.

## 14. Chalk

16.55    The chalk that is commonly used in the gym is magnesium carbonate. Properly used this is a great aid to a stronger grip. Though not support gear in the sense of something that is durable—e.g., straps, wraps, squat suits and bench shirts—the chalk is still a form of support tackle for weight trainees. Unlike all the other gear—with the exception of a belt, which is optional—chalk is a form of support equipment recommended for everyone.

16.56    Use chalk everywhere you need the help, especially in back exercises and upper-body pressing movements. In the latter, your grip is not going to give out like in the deadlift or pullup; but what often happens is that during the reps of the bench press, for example, the hands slip outward a little unless you apply chalk. Losing your grip, even just slightly, in any exercise may not only ruin the set in question, but can be very dangerous.

16.57    Experiment to find the right amount of chalk. Use too little and you will not feel much if any benefit. Use too much and your grip may slip. But use enough and your grip will be strengthened noticeably.

16.58    Get some chalk from an outdoor goods store that sells mountaineering gear, or from a general sporting goods store.

16.59    Chalk is not only for using on hands. For the squat, to help the bar not to slip, get someone to chalk your shirt where the bar is going to rest. If you are sweating heavily and are going to do some sort of pressing with your back on a bench, get someone to chalk your upper back. This will help prevent your torso sliding on the bench during the exercise.

16.60    Clean the knurled parts of your bar(s) with a stiff brush every few weeks to prevent clogging of the knurling.

## 15. Accurate weights

16.61    Unless you are using perfectly calibrated plates you cannot be sure you are getting what each plate is claimed to weigh. For example, a bar loaded to 250 pounds may really be 253 or 247 pounds. Then if you strip that bar down and load it to 250 pounds again, but with different plates, you are likely to get a different true weight than before.

16.62    This is an especially serious matter when you are moving your best poundages. An unbalanced or an overweight bar may ruin a set and perhaps cause injury; and an underweight bar will give you a false sense of progress. When you are using small discs to increase poundages by a pound or so a week, if your big plates are not what they seem, you cannot be sure you are getting a small increase relative to last time.

16.63    If you have calibrated plates available, use them exclusively. If there are no calibrated plates, try to persuade the management where you train to invest in some. Otherwise you need to do the next best thing. First convince the management of the importance of accurate weights. Then get permission to check all the plates and bars in the gym. The owner should be delighted you are willing to do this, but most owners will probably be resistant, especially in large facilities.

16.64    Assuming that the gym's scale is not already calibrated, you need to do some calibration. Take an object of about 20 pounds to a post office (or somewhere else that has a calibrated scale), and have it weighed. Next weigh the same object on the gym's scale and compare the two weights. Then make the adjustment that may be necessary to the scale, or make an appropriate allowance when you use it.

16.65    Weigh the gym's plates during a quiet time so that you do not disturb many people. Using permanent paint, and only whenever a plate does not weigh what it is supposed to, mark the actual weight on each plate (other than those on fixed-weight dumbbells). Also find the true weight of each bar and fixed-weight dumbbell you are likely to use.

16.66    Then when you train you will know precisely what you are putting on the bar. You will need to match equally weighted plates for balance (or use matching combinations), or use small discs to even out discrepancies.

16.67    If you are unable to mark inaccurate plates with their actual weights, manage as best you can. At least try to discover the plates that are the worst offenders, and avoid using them. Or find the brand that is the most accurate, and stick to that brand whenever possible, especially when you use big plates.

16.68     If you train at home, there will be no problem finding out the true weights of the individual items you lift.

## 16. Suppleness

16.69     A flexible body helps protects you from injury, so long as you do not perform your stretching exercises in a way that exposes you to injury in the first place.

16.70     As with all forms of exercise, it is much better you start out modestly, and be consistent with it, rather than start out with so much that you cannot sustain it for more than a few weeks. Better to start with 6–8 stretches on alternate days, than twenty stretches daily. Equipment is not needed and you can slot in at least some of your stretching while, say, you watch the evening news, thus not necessitating any time additional to what you are already investing in your exercise program.

16.71     Stretching between sets during your weight-training workouts is an economical use of time. Between-sets time is not used for much, so long as the equipment and weights are ready, so stretch then and you can get your flexibility work done without necessitating any additional exercise time.

16.72     See THE INSIDER'S TELL-ALL HANDBOOK ON WEIGHT-TRAINING TECHNIQUE for an illustrated step-by-step stretching program.

> Each rep and set of each workout is a chance for training perfection that cannot be had again. Each workout is a one-off opportunity to improve. If you do not get everything right at a given workout you have missed a chance to maximize your rate of progress. So get every component right so that each workout is another *full* step towards realizing your potential for muscle and might. When you train, switch off from everything else and "become" your training. Your focus must be that intense if you want to maximize your rate of progress.

## 17. Cardiorespiratory work

16.73    Weight training gives the cardiorespiratory system work, but
         just how much depends on how you train. To get into serious
         aerobic work you need to get specific.

16.74    Unless you are already fit, moderate *safe* aerobic training will
         increase your fitness, i.e., your cardiorespiratory efficiency
         and muscular endurance. Improved fitness will help you to
         weight train more intensively, and probably help your
         recovery processes.

16.75    Benefits from aerobic training can be obtained from just
         moderate work. Extreme dedication is not only unnecessary
         but actually counterproductive. Performing more than about
         thirty minutes of moderate-intensity aerobic work three times a
         week will probably have a negative effect on your weight
         training. Your gains in the gym may stall if not regress, you
         risk overtraining and, depending on the activities used, you
         may get injured.

16.76    Choose a zero-impact activity, e.g., stationary cycling (with the
         seat positioned so that your leg is almost fully straight when
         the pedal is at its bottom position, for knee care), or use a
         skiing, climbing or rowing machine, or choose a *very-low*
         impact activity such as brisk walking. The more musculature
         you can involve in the exercise, the better—for increased
         effectiveness and productivity relative to time invested—so
         skiing and rowing are superior to walking.

16.77    Millions of people have been injured from jogging, running,
         and road cycling, all in the quest for improved health. Some
         supposedly beneficial activities are very dangerous. Apply
         common sense and make sure you do not use an activity that is
         likely to produce either acute or chronic injury.

16.78    Just two or preferably three 25–30 minute aerobic sessions each
         week are fine, excluding the few minutes needed for a gradual
         warmup and another few minutes for cooling down, each
         session. Either perform the aerobic training after your weights
         workouts, on your off days, or a mixture of the two. Write a
         convenient and practical schedule, and stick with it.

16.79    *Moderate*-intensity aerobic training is important or else you will
         kill your gains in muscle and might. If you cannot talk, albeit

haltingly, while you do your aerobic work, you are training too intensively. You *should* be breathing much heavier than when you are at rest, but you do not need to be gasping. Always keep in mind that you cannot focus on getting a stronger and better physique if you are training like a competitive endurance athlete.

16.80 If you are currently not doing any specific aerobic exercise, and especially if you are over thirty-five years old, start pronto! But start out gently and take a month or so to progressively build up to the required duration and intensity. If you rush this process you may overstretch your recovery abilities, and overtrain. The body has a wonderful ability to adapt to imposed demands, but apply new demands gradually.

16.81 Start your aerobic session very easily and take a few minutes to work up to your intended level of effort—consider this as the warmup period. Your body needs a few minutes before it starts drawing most of its energy from the aerobic system.

16.82 This aerobic activity is for fitness, and help with fat control. Any possible benefits to health are additional. The health benefits from aerobic exercise are exaggerated by many enthusiasts. Because you are seriously working out with weights you are already getting tremendous benefits from exercise. But people who do not do any other exercise *are* going to get substantial benefits from even just modest aerobic training because that is their only formal exercise.

16.83 Many enthusiasts take aerobic activity to such extremes that they harm their bodies. A fit body is not necessarily a healthy body, and a healthy body is not necessarily a fit one. Fitness and health are not synonymous, but of course it is far better to be fit than unfit. Some people who were super fit also had serious heart disease, and died of that despite their high level of fitness. And many people who do not have heart disease are not at all fit.

## 18. Footwear

16.84 Running shoes and other types with a lot of cushioning (including air and gel) in them are not suitable for weight training. They distort and deform under heavy loads in exercises where you are standing, and can throw your balance and spoil your exercise groove. Get yourself some purpose-designed lifting shoes that minimize deformation when you are lifting heavy weights. You may even find that a pair of sturdy outdoor walking shoes will serve you better than regular training shoes.

16.85     Though an apparently small detail, even a small change in the size of the heel you wear, or the relative difference between the heel and sole thicknesses of your shoes, can mar your training. This especially applies to the squat and deadlift, though a change in balance factors can have a negative effect on some other exercises, e.g., the curl.

16.86     When your training balance is accustomed to a given heel height, you will disturb it if you change the heel height and immediately recommence heavy training. As little as quarter of an inch variation can make quite an impact. Once you have found a heel height that suits you, stick to it, though you may prefer to use footwear without heels for when you deadlift.

## 19. Chiropractic

16.87     If I was running a gym, every member—whether novice, intermediate or advanced—would be obliged to have a full examination by the best chiropractor I could employ, and get a thorough understanding of his or her physical structure and biomechanics, especially as it influences training.

16.88     I urge you to locate a competent chiropractor, especially one specializing in sports injuries. Some experienced and well-trained osteopaths and physiotherapists can also provide excellent service. Do not wait until you get an injury before you seek a chiropractor's services.

16.89     Of course, a competent chiropractor can greatly speed up recovery time, and should be used if you get injured. Skilled chiropractic adjustment may make you believe in miracles. But it is far better to know your body so well that you are unlikely to get an injury in the first place. And even if you do not have an injury, a checkup by a skilled chiropractor every few months can help to keep your body free of injuries. Some chiropractors, however, urge an excessive number of treatment sessions and checkups, and tarnish the reputation of chiropractic.

16.90     A UK-trained osteopath is much more similar to a chiropractor than is a US-trained osteopath. The training of osteopaths varies substantially between Europe and the USA. Generally speaking, the training of a chiropractor is more uniform throughout the world than is the training of an osteopath. This is *not* to imply that a US-trained osteopath is not a highly skilled specialist. It is just that osteopaths in different parts of the world can have significant differences in the techniques they use.

16.91    In addition, consult a foot specialist such as a podiatrist. Foot problems such as flat feet or bunions can seriously affect squatting and deadlifting form. A foot specialist may be able to help you to reduce if not eliminate the negative impact of a foot problem on your exercise form.

## Symptoms to respond to

16.92    If you experience one or more of the following symptoms, immediately seek the attention of a chiropractor or other qualified specialist.

    a.  Pins and needles in one or both legs or arms

    b.  Numbness in one or both legs or arms

    c.  Pain that goes down the back of a leg along the path of the sciatic nerve (sciatica)

    d.  Pain that goes down the front of the thigh to the knee (femoral neuralgia)

    e.  Any back pain or spasms

    f.  Hip pain or spasms

    g.  Neck pain

    h.  Headaches or migraines

    i.  Shoulder pain

    j.  Knee pain

    k.  Tennis elbow

    l.  Golfer's elbow

m. Hand and wrist problems

n. Foot and ankle problems

## Practical application

16.93    Many common and not-so-common conditions can influence
how well you tolerate certain exercises or specific variations of
them. What may be safe for most people may be unsafe for
you. Knowing your body well will help you to train with
safety uppermost in your mind. You cannot make any gains in
the gym if you are injured and unable to train.

16.94    Many people go through life, until they get injured, knowing
little or nothing about their physical irregularities. Conditions
including scoliosis, tilted pelvis, arms or legs that are different
in length, excessive lordosis, postural problems, spondylolysis,
and flexion imbalances between one side of the body and the
other, can all influence the exercises you select or avoid in the
gym, and how specifically you perform them.

16.95    Do not try to determine yourself (or with a friend/spouse)
whether or not you have one leg shorter than the other, and if
so, which one. It is easier than you probably think to make a
mistake, due to the body's compensatory adjustments. You
need an expert, e.g., a chiropractor, to do the assessment.

16.96    While any skilled manipulative therapist should be able to help
you with most injuries, only one experienced in weight
training will be able to help you with exercise technique,
selection and modification. The emphasis is upon getting
advice from an expert in biomechanics and manipulative
therapy who is familiar with weight training, or at least
sympathetic to it. The last thing you need is someone who
throws his hands up in horror at the thought of you lifting big

> The misinterpretation of muscle soreness has produced
> exercise distortions that have become part of the
> folklore of bodybuilding, and which are at the root of
> much pain and injury. Some of the resulting exercises
> have been harmful for many people, e.g., hack machine
> and Smith machine squats, and many exercises with
> exaggerated grips, stances and ranges of motion.

weights. Get acquainted with an expert professional before you get injured, so you are never in a quandary about where to go if you do get injured.

16.97    I have an unusual degree of congenital scoliosis (lateral curvature of the spine akin to the shape of an elongated letter "s"). I only found out about it after I injured my back in the summer of 1992. Had I found out about the scoliosis years ago, and been advised by a dark age orthopedic, osteopath, chiropractor or other therapist, I would have been urged to forget heavy lifting and may never have deadlifted 200 pounds for a single rep, let alone 400 for 20 rest-pause reps.

16.98    This scoliosis, together with my left leg being shorter than my right, influence my squatting and deadlifting form. There is no way I can avoid some lateral movement as I ascend. The vertebrae on the outside arcs of the lateral curvatures of my spine are less stable than are the other vertebrae. An asymmetrical push in the bench press or overhead press exposes me to much greater risk of malpositioning a vertebra (on the upper arc) than if my spine was of a regular formation. But knowing these faults, I modify my training accordingly to reduce injury risk, e.g., I never overhead press without being seated with my back supported by a steeply inclined bench.

16.99    If I was not aware of my in-built structural flaws, I would now be a wreck of one injury after another. As it happened, I only learned through pain and injury. I should have studied my body years ago, and learned the training modifications needed to reduce my chances of injury. Learn from my mistakes.

## How to find help

16.100    In HARDGAINER issue #36 the late Dr. Keith Hartman provided help for people trying to find a sports-orientated chiropractor:

> In the USA, you want to look in the Yellow Pages, and behind the doctors' names (that is where additional credentials are usually placed) may appear the initials CCSP, which stand for Certified Chiropractic Sports Physician. It denotes...the completion of 150 or more post-graduate hours in the diagnosis, chiropractic treatment and management of sports injuries...
> Additionally, in both the USA and internationally, you can ask the doctor over the telephone if he or she is a

member of FICS, which stands for the Fédération Internationale de Chiropratique Sportive. This is the international body that holders of the CCSP credentials belong to...

If you ask some questions of the staff person answering the phone, or the doctor him/herself, you should be able to determine if the doctor is orientated towards and knowledgeable in handling sports injuries. If the doctor is reluctant, or hesitates in the least when questioned about CCSP, I personally would be hesitant of seeing him. Another good source for sports-orientated chiropractors may be a local gym. The gym may know someone who is a CCSP, or a chiropractor who is good with sports injuries but does not have the CCSP credentials.

16.101    The professional you consult should know the basic weight-training movements, or be willing to learn from you, and ideally he should be a trainee himself. He should know the variations of form that need to be considered to fit an individual's structural uniqueness, and especially know the variations that should never be used.

16.102    Seek a sports-minded expert in biomechanics, injuries and manipulative therapy. You may need more than one person to cover these areas. But as with all professionals, standards vary. You may have to hunt around to find the quality of help you need. Make the effort, though, and you can add life to your training years, and years to your training life.

## 20. Responding to muscle soreness

16.103    Muscle soreness is a fact of life for everyone who lifts weights. It is one of the rewards from a hard workout, proving that you delivered the goods. Good soreness comes from intensive effort in exercises done in safe form, is purely muscular, and goes away after a few days. This is different from longer lasting soreness from injury due to abusive exercise form, from having started a cycle too heavily, or from having stretched too far.

16.104    Muscle soreness can be very misleading. Some muscle groups show soreness much more readily than others. That your shoulders, for example, may never get very sore does not mean they are not getting trained. And that another muscle may get sore very easily does not necessarily mean that it is going to grow faster than a muscle that is rarely if ever sore.

16.105　The misinterpretation of muscle soreness has produced exercise distortions that have become part of the folklore of bodybuilding, and which are at the root of much pain and injury. Some of the resulting exercises have been harmful for many people, e.g., hack machine and Smith machine squats, and many exercises with exaggerated grips, stances and ranges of motion.

16.106　Tendons attach muscles to bones via a sheath over the end of each muscle. The muscle under the sheath does not have as many blood vessels as the muscle away from the sheath. The areas where there are fewer blood vessels cannot clear waste products as well as areas that are well supplied with blood vessels. This is why the end of the muscle is more likely to be sore than the rest of the muscle. But this has nothing to do with more growth stimulation for the end of the muscle. The desire for soreness in the ends of muscles, e.g., lower quads and lower biceps, has encouraged exercise variations that produce exaggerated stress on the involved joints and connective tissue, leading to injury.

16.107　At the beginning of a cycle in general, and in particular when you are using a new exercise or one that you have not done for a while, take it easy. Pick up the intensity over a few weeks, never make any big jumps in training intensity, and then you will avoid getting any debilitating soreness.

16.108　When you are very sore you may be more prone to injury. Give yourself extra rest before you train the sore area hard again. You can do a scheduled workout that trains other areas of your body, unless you are wiped out systemically—in which case you need to recover more before you weight train again. On rest days, to help speed the easing of extreme soreness, do some additional low-intensity cardiorespiratory work, together with a carefully done stretching routine. Massage may also help to hasten recovery from soreness, as may a hot bath.

16.109　When you train a big exercise only once every 7–10 days, especially the squat, and train it intensively, you may get very sore. If so, and as noted elsewhere in this book, add a second but light squatting session later in the week. Do your regular warmup sets, but no top sets. This should be enough to substantially reduce any soreness from your next heavy squatting session.

## 21. Special note on hands

16.110    Your hands have a big strength potential. But few people get even close to achieving the strength potential of their hands and forearms because they rely on grip crutches and fail to train their hands properly.

16.111    Do not use gloves, wrist straps, or hooks that attach you to a bar. If you use grip supports you will eventually end up with underdeveloped hands on a well-developed body. You cannot lengthen your hands, but you can thicken them. As your grip strength increases, so will the muscle and connective tissue of your hands.

16.112    Appreciate the skin-on-metal contact of weight training, and the mental focus it provides. Toughen your hands with support-free training and use chalk as your only gripping aid.

16.113    By always performing the deadlift, pulldown or pullup, and shrug without grip support other than chalk, and becoming strong in those exercises, you will develop a pair of strong hands. If you have recovery "space" you can include a specific grip exercise once or twice a week in your exercise program, to further enhance your grip. Do not feel that you have to get into a great deal of grip work in order to build a strong grip. Just like with all weight training, you do not have to complicate matters in order to be successful. A few basic exercises done very well, and progressively, will do the job.

16.114    If you get *excessive* build up of calluses on your hands, control it by weekly use of a pumice stone after a shower or bath.

## 22. How to cope with sickness

16.115    Minor sickness—e.g., a cold, *slight* gastrointestinal problems, or influenza—should not mess up your training. Just stay out of the gym until a few days *after* you are back to feeling 100%, and then recommence your training. It should not be necessary to cut back weights and intensity and take a few weeks to get back on course. So long as no more than about 10–14 days have passed since you last trained a given exercise, and so long as you have felt 100% for a few days, you should be able to repeat your previous workout.

16.116    If you return to the gym when you know you have not fully recovered, then not only will you be unable to repeat your previous workout, you may hurt yourself in the attempt. Wait the extra day or few until you are truly 100% recovered.

16.117   If the sickness kept you out of the gym for a protracted time, then you must start back with moderate weights and intensity, and take two or three weeks (or longer, if necessary) to progressively build back to where you were before being struck down by sickness. Then return to the poundage progression scheme you were following pre-sickness.

16.118   If you drive yourself to train very hard despite being sick, even if just in the early stage of sickness, you are laying the ground for an infection taking a firm grip on you. You may even get something so seriously embedded that you cannot shake it off. It may keep returning on and off for six months or so, or even drag on for over a year, and thus devastate your training.

16.119   Never train when you are sick. Even a minor cold or sore throat, if trained through, could blow up into something serious. Wait until you are feeling 100% well, and then return to training. The older you are the more strictly you need to follow this advice, and the more heavily you will feel the consequences if you do not follow it.

## 23. Advanced training

16.120   As you grow bigger and stronger your training will evolve to meet your changing needs. As you become more advanced, i.e., once you are at or beyond the 300–400–500 numbers described in Chapter 4, or a comparable achievement relative to gender, age or bodyweight, you may need to try some methods of training different from those that took you to advanced status in the first place, in order to grow further. The training methods that took you to advanced status *may* take you to super-advanced status, but on the other hand they may not. Experimentation and experience will teach you which is the case *for you*.

> **The bottom line is poundage progression and muscular growth. If they are not occurring, you need to make changes until gains start happening. Results are what count. If you are progressing well on your current approach, stick with it. Do not change anything that is working well.**

16.121    Even at advanced-level training you have the same components to vary as you do do at any stage of training: exercise selection, different training intensity formats, rep cadence, single- or double-pause reps, one-and-a-half reps, use of partial reps, rep count, training volume, between-set rest periods, etc. You cannot vary all those components in any single program, but you can try different things in different programs, and compare the results.

16.122    The bottom line is poundage progression and muscular growth. If they are not occurring you need to make changes until gains start happening. Results are what count. If you are progressing well on your current approach, stick with it. Do not change anything that is working well.

16.123    Even when you are of advanced status you may not need to change anything in your training program other than your rate of adding weight to the bar. Make the increments so gradual that the poundage increases are so small and unhurried as not to be detectable.

16.124    Here are some specific suggestions to *consider* experimenting with if you have reached advanced status and still desire increased muscle and (especially) might:

   a.  Increased variety of exercise variations, either over time in *different* cycles, or even within the *same* program.

   b.  Use of specialization programs on a regular if not consistent basis, changing from cycle to cycle which exercise or body part you specialize on. For example, in a single shoulder specialization program you might rotate three different pressing workouts while training twice a week. You might spread these four exercises over the three workouts: overhead lockouts, dumbbell press, press from forehead, and full-range press from the bottom in a power rack. A few select big exercises and accessory exercises would be included to cover the rest of your physique.

   c.  Increased use of low reps (3–5), or even single-rep work.

   d.  Use of the method described in *Constant Working Poundages* in Chapter 7.

e.  Increased use of from-the-bottom double-pause reps. See Chapter 11.

f.  Increased use of partial reps. See Chapter 11. Partial-rep work does not have to include lockouts. Instead it could focus on the phase from the bottom of the rep to the sticking point, the phase starting at the sticking point and working till the lockout, or the middle phase, or a combination of all three phases spread over the two or three different routines rotated in a specialization program for a given exercise or body part.

g.  Increased use of ultra-abbreviated programs along with increased sets for each exercise.

h.  Possible increased use of brutally hard training, and even prudent use of to-eccentric-failure training. See Chapter 9.

i.  Moderately increased training volume. The use of extreme intensity techniques may be *counterproductive* at advanced status, depending on the individual. Moderately increased volume work may be a better option, but in the context of abbreviated training.

j.  Regular reacquaintance with the type of training that made you big to begin with. Do not lose touch with this proven training just because you are experimenting with more advanced training. A few months of intensive 20-rep squatting every couple of years, working up into new personal best achievements, may be enough to put into perspective all the supposedly advanced and superior approaches.

16.125  Whatever approaches you may experiment with, do not think that just because you have become big and strong you can productively use high-volume routines. While your capacity for work may have increased in some areas, and the interpretations of training open to you may have widened, you can still overtrain easily. Everything written in this book must still be considered when you put together your routines. Otherwise you will stagnate indefinitely, like most advanced trainees do. Never go copying the extensive routines of the drug-assisted and genetically blessed. Those routines will still overtrain you *even* when you are of advanced status.

## Finishing routines

16.126    When you are well developed you may move away from seeking ever-increasing muscle and might. If you are a bodybuilder you may seek a finished physique. If you want muscular balance, symmetry, detail, fullness of individual muscles, and unusual definition, you will need to make the appropriate changes to your routines. At least temporarily your focus will not be on getting bigger and stronger. "Finishing" is about refining the size you have already built. Without overdoing matters, because otherwise you will shrink in size, you may need to use quite a lot of isolation exercises. You will need to do whatever you can, short of surgery, to bring up lagging aspects of your musculature, perhaps detrain any parts that are excessively big relatively speaking, and emphasize certain parts of your physique in order to draw attention away from weak spots.

## Increased cardiorespiratory work

16.127    Though content with your size and strength you may not be interested in physique finishing. Instead you may now want to maintain what you have developed while giving increased attention to cardiorespiratory work. You would therefore maintain your strength by using the same sort of training that built it, but while using constant working poundages, and gradually and progressively build up the cardiorespiratory component of your exercise program. But the stress is on doing this gradually and while using safe zero- or minimal-impact aerobic activities. You would need to keep in mind that an exaggerated attention to cardiorespiratory training—as noted in section seventeen of this chapter, *Cardiorespiratory Work*—will conflict with your muscular size and strength, and cause a reduction in those respects.

16.128    Once you are truly of advanced status you will have an extensive understanding of productive training in general, and of how to train yourself. You need to draw on that wealth of knowledge and experience in order to devise the most productive training routines relative to the goals you have set for yourself.

## Examples of how to fine-tune a program

If your training program is not delivering progress, you probably need to implement *major* changes. Once your program *is* working, *rationally* experiment with fine-tuning to see if you can *increase* your progress.

Consider the bench press as an illustration, but change only *one* variable at a time. If a change improves progress—whether in strength only or strength *and* size, depending on your preference—stick with it. If not, drop the change.

1. Bench press on a Monday, Friday, Wednesday, Monday, etc., frequency for a couple of months. Then bench press just once a week for two months. Then compare the results of the different frequency.

2. If you perform just a single work set, try two or three work sets for a couple of months. If you usually perform three work sets, try two.

3. With a training partner's assistance, perform two forced reps at the end of your final work set once a week on alternate weeks. This *might* provide the stimulus needed to progress faster. Even if it does, however, do not use forced reps on a regular basis or else they will overtrain you.

4. Keep everything else constant in your training and nutrition, but get an extra hour of sleep every night.

Modify only one variable at a time, so you can account for any change in your progress. But once your progress is going very well, stick with it and change nothing!

---

That the use of anabolic steroids is so prevalent today, among bodybuilders and strength athletes, is testimony to the barrenness of popular training methods. Without steroids those training methods only work well for the genetically gifted.

## Summary of how to ensure a successful training cycle

16.129    Choose one of the six frameworks of program design given in Chapter 12, or something similar of your own conception.

16.130    Select exercises that are suitable for you—see Chapter 10.

16.131    Determine the set and rep scheme(s) you will be using (see the relevant parts of Chapters 7 and 13) and the intensity format (or formats, as some exercises may be trained more intensively than others) you will employ—see relevant parts of Chapters 7 and 9.

16.132    Determine a training frequency that is practical for you and which permits adequate recovery relative to the decisions you made in points 1 and 3 above. See especially Chapters 12–14. While finding this training frequency, through trial and error, you must be consistent with your volume and effort in the gym, and in delivering excellent rest, sleep and dietary habits out of the gym. All variables should be kept consistent other than training frequency. And when experimenting with weight-training frequency you need to consider the aerobic training in your program because that places a demand on your recovery abilities. Excessive aerobic training can kill your weight-training progress.

16.133    Adjust the individual components of the overall training program in the light of Chapter 13.

16.134    Put the program into practice and, if necessary, fine-tune it further in the light of the initial responses and reactions. Record your workouts and overall training cycle in a training journal.

16.135    Milk the training cycle dry—see Chapter 15—while looking out for signs of impending overtraining. If necessary, modify the program to avoid overtraining (see Chapter 14).

16.136    When the training cycle has ended, consult your journal, analyze the cycle, and compare its results with those from earlier cycles. Then review all conclusions accumulated from your most recent training cycles. While considering that wealth of data, repeat the training cycle design process.

## What if you are an *extreme* hard gainer?

16.137    First ensure that your recovery machinery is in good order:

      a.  Go to sleep early enough each night so that you wake naturally each morning. If you have sleeping problems, get them fixed—seek professional help, perhaps a sleep clinic.

      b.  Adhere to a nutrient-dense dietary program that provides *more* calories than you need to maintain your bodyweight, *at least* one gram of protein per pound of lean body mass, and six similar-sized *easily digested* feeds/meals each day. Poor digestion and assimilation will *kill* your progress.

      c.  Make weight training your *only* physically demanding activity. Perform no aerobic work. *Conserve your energy.*

16.138    Adopt a *bare bones* approach to program design. Follow a twice-a-week *super-abbreviated* program (Monday-Friday) built around the squat or *Trap Bar* deadlift, alternating two *different* routines with little or no overlap. See *Framework 5* in Chapter 12. *Do not add a single extra exercise.* Do warmups plus 2–3 work sets per exercise except the squat, where warmups plus 1 x 20 may work best. Apply all that this book teaches on effort and progression.

16.139    If after four weeks you are unable to add weight to the work sets of each exercise every workout you train it, try being more radical. Reduce your training frequency so that you alternate the two routines on a Monday, Friday, Wednesday, Monday, Friday basis, i.e., increase the rest days between workouts, and provide more recovery time.

16.140    If you do not start gaining now, and assuming you really are *fully* satisfying the recovery components, and are training very hard, add an additional rest day between workouts. Continue to increase recovery time until you start gaining.

16.141    Once you find the training frequency that works for you, stick with it for as long as possible, and milk it dry.

16.142    Commence a new cycle. Use the same format that worked well last time, but use two or three different core exercises. Add two different accessory exercises to each routine, one warmup and one work set for each. If they do not diminish your gains, keep them in. If your gains suffer, drop the accessory exercises. **BB**

*It does not matter how much your training may seem out of step with what others do. What matters to you is what works for you. Have the courage to swim against the training tide. Always keep in mind that popular training methods simply do not deliver the goods for most people. So why would you want to use popular training methods? Life is too short to waste any of it on useless training methods.*

# Section 3

## Special issues

*My audience was appalled, my wife was fearful for my well-being, and I was so possessed that NOTHING was going to stop me getting the full 20 deadlifts. This was the epitome of blood-and-guts and train-till-you-drop training. I was streaming with sweat and there was a pool of the stuff in front of the bar.*

*For years I tried to make the most of a relatively poor body for squatting, and neglected to apply myself to an exercise I am mechanically better suited to—the deadlift.*

# 17. A Real-Life Training Cycle for You to Learn From

17.1    This chapter is included for five reasons:

    a.  To show that a typical hard gainer, if not restricted by age or structural problems, can build up to respectable weights—in my case bent-legged deadlifting 400 pounds for 20 consecutive rest-pause reps—though the deadlift may not be the exercise that best suits your body structure.

    b.  To explain the real-life step-by-step practicalities of a training cycle, how a cycle is modified as it evolves, and how the ups and downs of life have to be accommodated.

    c.  To take you through the key lessons learned.

    d.  To confirm that I am no armchair instructor.

    e.  To show that abbreviated and basics-first training works.

17.2    This chapter is a revised and expanded version of an article published in issue #21 of HARDGAINER (November-December 1992). You are not going to get only the positive side of the training cycle. You are going to get the full story, to help equip you to avoid the mistakes I made.

## The background
17.3    The first requirements for realizing a very demanding goal are loads of resolve, heaps of persistence, and tons of effort. Whether your demanding goal is 300 x 20 in the squat, 350 x 20 in the deadlift, 300 x 5 in the bench press, or whatever, *you really have to want it*. There is no easy way to reach a demanding goal. If you do not want it enough to pay your dues, overcome expected and unexpected obstacles, and give

your pound of flesh, you will not get to your goal. The names of our game are effort and progressive poundages. While cycling training intensity does not mean full-bore effort at *every* workout, you *must* get into sustained periods of intensive workouts.

17.4    There are two crucial considerations to keep in mind when viewing my personal training achievements:

   a.  I have never taken bodybuilding drugs, and never will.

   b.  My genetic endowment is almost the opposite of what is needed to develop great strength.

17.5    While 400 x 20 is fine deadlifting for a hard gainer, it is not much in today's world where the genetically gifted elite grab the publicity and attention. But while some of these men are awesomely strong, more than a few of them are far less strong than their posed lifts (sometimes using fake plates) suggest. I did not use a lifting belt or any lifting gear other than grip support. I was 195 pounds—at 5-9, and about 15% bodyfat—when I did the 400 x 20, so I was pulling over twice bodyweight. This was in July 1992 when I was 33 years old.

17.6    When appraising my genetic endowment for lifting weights, there is nothing to marvel at. Two areas come out as better than average, i.e., calves and body structure for the deadlift and stiff-legged deadlift. Everything else ranges for average hard-gainer material to worse-than-average, with arms in particular being the pits for bodybuilding.

17.7    I had extensive work and parental responsibilities during the deadlift cycle. These prevented my resting and sleeping as well as I should have in order to recuperate speedily from training. I am a real-world person, not someone who can devote himself to his training with little or no thought for other aspects of regular life. As typical working hard gainers it is not just our genes that work against us. There are other out-of-the-gym factors as well.

## Reasoning for the deadlift focus
17.8    For almost all of my training years—right until this 400 x 20 deadlift cycle—I have always considered the squat *the* exercise to concentrate upon. While my deadlift poundage can almost

be depended upon to increase so long as I am injury-free, work very hard and infrequently, and eat and rest enough, the same cannot be said of the squat. For years I tried to make the most of a relatively poor body structure for squatting, and neglected to apply myself to an exercise I am mechanically much better suited to—the deadlift.

17.9    As it was I spent many years focusing on the squat while omitting the deadlift. The 1992 experience proved that while my back and knees would cave in from the squat, the deadlift could be kept moving.

17.10   I am not in a minority of one on this point; and I believe that the minority is a substantial one among hard gainers. *If you cannot get great results from the barbell squat*, and assuming you have put in some effort and investigated suitable modifications such as those described in THE INSIDER'S TELL-ALL HANDBOOK ON WEIGHT-TRAINING TECHNIQUE, then promote the bent-legged deadlift, *especially using the Trap Bar*, to at least equal status with the squat. (But not the stiff-legged deadlift, because it does not involve the quadriceps.)

17.11   If you cannot barbell squat but have access to a safe alternative that mimics the squat, e.g., the Tru-Squat, exploit it to the full.

17.12   Beginners and early intermediates should give equal priority to the squat and deadlift in their training. But once they have got to the intermediate stage—when they look like they lift weights—they should be able to see how they compare in the two exercises. Assuming the *same* degree of application to each exercise, if your squat is about the same or ahead of your deadlift, then you have a squatter's body structure. If your deadlift is well ahead of your squat, then it is the deadlift that is favored by your body structure. At this stage, at least some of the time, you should have specialization cycles in which you focus on the exercise you naturally favor. Make the most of whatever natural bias you have. While the very gifted can do very well in almost every exercise, the rest of us may have to settle for finding just one or two exercises in which to excel, but without neglecting other areas.

17.13   I started weight training in 1973. I got little or nothing out of most of those years other than lots of experience of what does not work despite single-minded determination and application.

I never got into any variation of the deadlift in a serious way until about 1988. Until then it had been the squat for my thigh, hip and lower back structure. I then got into low-rep deadlifting. After about three years of hard work in both the stiff-legged and bent-legged versions, but not both of them in the same cycle, I was capable of deadlifting 500 pounds. I was, however, still giving more focus to the squat, but was not getting results proportional to my application.

17.14    During the deadlift-focus period I am now going to describe I found I could progress on the deadlift akin to how the famous squatters did on the squat—train hard, rest a lot, eat well, and you can add weight to the bar almost every week, and do so for a long time. This was so very satisfying and made me wonder what I might have done had I clicked with this important reality early in my training life.

## Breathing, and deadlifting technique

17.15    When deadlifting heavily, whether in the stiff-legged or bent-legged version, I always used grip aids. I had neglected to do serious grip work and was paying the price by having to use the crutch of heavy grip support.

17.16    During the bent-legged deadlift the stress upon the body from holding the bar in the standing position while pausing to breathe is very great, and will increase fatigue. The alternative of breathing while the bar is on the floor or platform—while in the crouched setup position—is not satisfactory either. The legs and back tire from being kept in the setup position.

17.17    What I used to do was maintain my grip on the bar, though relaxing my hold, while the bar rested on the platform. I also maintained the positioning of my feet. But I did not keep my knees bent in the starting position. I straightened my legs, while keeping my hands and feet in position, and took a few quick and deep breaths with my legs and arms straight—my back would naturally round during this pause. Then I would bend my knees, get in position with a flat back once again, set the bar against my shins, and pull the next rep; and then repeat the process.

17.18    I always set myself up in a flat-back position, and the initial drive from the floor was with both thighs and back strength. But my legs quite soon locked out and the deadlift became a total back exercise. This became exaggerated after I developed knee problems—by taking more of the load on my back I reduced the stress on my knees. When my form got ragged, my back would round quite a lot at the top of a rep. While I absolutely do not recommend this round-back style of deadlifting, I got away with it for quite a long time. Even when I got injured at the end of the cycle I do not think the excessive rounding of my back was anything more than a contributing factor at most. But I urge you *not* to duplicate my deadlifting form. Use much more leg strength than I did, and keep your back flat.

17.19    Natural *squatters* usually use lots of thigh strength in their deadlifting. They are more able to maintain a flat back than are less-gifted squatters who use more back strength because of comparatively weaker thighs. Natural *deadlifters* have a tendency to want to bent-legged deadlift more akin to stiff-legged deadlifts (but with slightly bent legs) than the regular style that uses lots of thigh pushing strength. The great Bob Peoples—who, as noted in Chapter 12, deadlifted a stupendous 725.75 pounds at a bodyweight of just 189 pounds, and using the overhand hook grip—lifted with a rounded back and relatively little use of his thighs.

## The long cycle

17.20    I started the deadlift cycle on 21 November 1991, and peaked at 400 pounds for 20 reps on 9 July 1992. That was a cycle of nearly eight months. Prior to the November start I had done some preliminary work in the stiff-legged deadlift, building to sets of five reps with 300 pounds while standing on a platform so that the bar touched the laces of my shoes between reps. Today I neither perform this excessive range of movement myself, nor recommend others do. I do the stiff-legged deadlift on and to the floor, with 20-kilo plates on the bar.

17.21    To be sure to establish my deadlifting style, as I had not done the regular deadlift for about two years, and to get plenty of gaining momentum going, I started off very light—220 pounds. While I finished with 400 x 20, I only moved to 20 reps at the end of the cycle. For almost the whole cycle I was performing sets of 15 reps in the deadlift.

17.22    I could have started the cycle at a bigger poundage and tried to compress the eight months of relatively slow progression into

4–6 months of quicker progress. Patience and a slow rate of progress are imperative for success, however, so I resisted the urge to hurry. On hindsight, if I had been more patient I could have extended the cycle.

17.23      In the early part of the cycle, because the poundage was light, I did all 15 reps continuously—no short pause before each rep. The plates touched the platform between reps in what could have been considered "touch and go." This was a mistake because it was easy to touch only one side of the plates on the platform, lose the vital symmetrical pulling style, and jar myself into an injury. For continuous reps, only go down to a point an inch or so above the platform. This helps prevent possible torque and jarring. But as the cycle progressed, fewer of the reps were done touch and go. I gradually moved into a rest-pause style.

17.24      I always deadlifted with a pronated grip. I had found that a mixed grip (one hand supinated, and one pronated) exposes me to an increased risk of injury because of the torque produced. To hold onto the bar, and free myself from concern over losing my grip, I had to have grip support. I used metal hooks fixed onto adjustable wrist straps. By using these there was no way the bar could fall from my hands. But had I never used any assistance other than chalk, had I added poundage at a slower rate to give my grip a chance to adapt, and had I added some thick-bar holds for extra grip work, I could probably have managed without the crutch of the hooks.

17.25      I usually deadlifted once each week. There were two occasions, not late in the cycle, where I had to deadlift on the sixth day rather than the usual seventh day. Especially in the late stages of the cycle I sometimes took more than a week between deadlift workouts, to guarantee full recovery.

17.26      Each deadlift workout consisted of warmup sets—one to begin with, and three once the poundages became heavy—followed by a single work set of 15 reps. After a few minutes rest I would do 8 reps with 220 pounds in the stiff-legged deadlift while standing on a platform for a full range of movement. This remained at 220 pounds throughout the cycle. The only workout I did not do it was when I did the 20 reps with 400. Then I did not want to do anything but collapse, pull myself together, pick myself up, and go home.

17.27    Until I reached 330 pounds (150 kilos), I added 5 kilos (11 pounds) to the bar each week. I did 330 x 15 on 30 January 1992. At this stage I think I was doing 10 of the reps continuously and the remaining five in rest-pause style—do a rep, pause for a few breaths, do another rep, pause for a few breaths, etc. Once I had started a set of deadlifts, and was strapped in, my hands never left the bar until all the target reps were done.

## Workout schedule

17.28    During this deadlift-dominated cycle the other exercises were secondary and I would not have hesitated to drop anything that got in the way of focus on the deadlift. I would have dropped to a one-exercise-per-week schedule (deadlift only) if it became necessary in order to keep the deadlift progressing.

17.29    My basic schedule was this:

### Tuesday
   a.   Squat
   b.   Bench press
   c.   Bent-over row
   d.   Calf work

### Thursday
   a.   Deadlift
   b.   Military press
   c.   Calf work

17.30    Abdominal work opened most workouts, to warm me up. In the bench press, row and press I used a 5 x 5 set-rep format—a light and a medium warmup set followed by 3 work sets with the same poundage. I rested several minutes between sets to ensure that, with few exceptions, I made all the sets of 5 reps. So long as I made all 3 work sets of 5 reps for a given exercise I would increase the poundage a little at the next workout for that exercise. Calf work was a couple of hard sets in the standing calf raise, for about 20 reps per set. The squat was usually done for 20 reps a set though at above 250 x 20 it was denting my recovery ability for elsewhere. Had I not had to drop the squat due to knee problems I would have needed to have kept it under 250 x 20 so as not to mar progress in the deadlift.

17.31    My choice of training days was not ideal. At the time, I was employed as a school teacher three days a week—on Monday,

Wednesday and Friday. Tuesdays and Thursdays around midday were the best times to train in order to minimize potential disruptions and maximize concentration.

## Illness

17.32    I was ill during the first week of February, and could not train. I returned to deadlifting on February 13, with 286 pounds (130 kilos) for the usual 15 reps. On February 21 I used 308 pounds (140 kilos) and on February 27 I was back on schedule with the 150 kilos I used before getting sick. That 150 kilos felt heavier than the pre-sickness 150 did. On hindsight I should have worked back into it over an extra couple of weeks. I got away with it only because I was not maxed out at the time.

17.33    I moved to 160 kilos (352 pounds) over two weeks, using the pre-sickness 5-kilos-per-week increment schedule. I was now down to 8 continuous reps and 7 rest-pause reps per 15-rep set. At 352 pounds I reduced the weekly increment to 2.5 kilos (5.6 pounds) to help ensure that my form stayed tight and the gaining momentum was not killed by excessive weekly increments. On hindsight, the 2.5 kilos per week increments should have started earlier than they did, and the cycle lengthened accordingly.

## Injuries

17.34    I had a bad year in 1992 for injuries. Throughout late 1991 and early 1992 I had elbow problems caused by excessive zeal for specialized grip work, and not working into it progressively enough. This prevented all grip work and hampered me in all major exercises except the deadlift (because I was using grip supports). Due to an injury sustained while playing soccer in 1991, I had a problem with my right big toe until late 1993.

17.35    In late February 1992 I started using a hip belt for squats during the Thursday workout, for much regretted supplementary thigh work. This was an example of trying to improve on what was already a very productive schedule. When something is going well, leave well alone.

17.36    I started very light with the hip-belt squat—85 pounds—to get the hang of the exercise. It was awkward to begin with. I had to use a 2-inch board under my heels, though balance was still awkward. Being more mechanically suited to the deadlift than the squat probably exaggerated the awkwardness of the exercise *for me*. Plenty of people have prospered on the hip-belt squat but I am not one of them, at least not if it is done with a 2-inch board under my heels. My knees moaned from the first workout. The "moaning" was not enough to stop me. I mistook it for the discomfort of acclimatizing to a new exercise, and stupidly applied the "no pain, no gain" maxim. I persisted with the hip-belt squat for 5 or 6 workouts before I finally got the message that the exercise was damaging my knees, and abandoned it in early April.

17.37     To be fair, my knees were sensitive and quite easily irritated. Had I done the hip-belt squat in a power rack or from within the safety bars of a squat rack, holding onto the uprights to maintain balance *without* a board under my heels, I may have prospered on the exercise. I now vigorously oppose raising the heels while squatting other than by a regular heel of a shoe. (Raising the heels increases leg flexion and pushes the knees too far forward, greatly increasing the stress on those joints.) Never mind that some of the big physiques can apparently safely squat with their heels raised on a board, though they may pay the price in years to come. What matters is how *your* knees react. I paid a heavy price for my misjudgment.

17.38     With my knees injured from the raised-heels hip-belt squat, they now could not tolerate regular no-elevation barbell squatting. Even squats with light weights produced days of discomfort afterward. The soreness became unbearable and in June I dropped the squat.

17.39     While the knee problem ruined the squat, it did not mar the deadlift cycle. I was not using my knees a great deal in the exercise anyway. By taking my knees just a little more out of the movement the deadlift could continue to progress. The effect of this was that the stress upon my back was increased as my legs contributed less to the movement.

17.40     On 24 April I did 385 for 15 reps. I was down to 5 continuous reps and 10 rest-pause reps to get all 15 out. Then I got injured, but not while deadlifting.

17.41     While performing standing barbell presses I felt something "twang" in my upper back. The pain was immediate. I visited a chiropractor the next day and had two vertebrae in my upper spine adjusted. There was instant improvement and within a week my back was feeling 100%. From then on I did my overhead presses while seated and with my back supported against a high-incline bench.

17.42    Being cautious I did not deadlift again until 7 May, and then only with 330 pounds. A week later I did 363 for the usual 15 reps, and a further week later I did 374, and a week after that (28 May) I did the 385 I had done before the upper-back injury.

17.43    I then hurt myself again. While stretching at home, doing a familiar back movement, I got carried away and went for extra stretch. I felt another twang and regretted the enthusiasm for stretching. Great care needs to be given to stretching exercises because if you get carried away you will injure yourself.

17.44    Shortly after the second twang I went to the chiropractor again. Now I needed an adjustment in the lower spine. I did not think the problem was serious so I only took an extra few days off training before deadlifting again—twelve days of rest instead of seven. I felt fine so off I went. On 9 June I made the pre-injury poundage plus an increment of 2.5 kilos. Now I was up to 177.5 kilos (390.5 pounds).

17.45    It was about at this time that I foolishly bench pressed without a spotter or any safety device. I got stuck at the bottom. Alone I had to wrestle the bar down to my midsection before being able to sit up. In the process I damaged my right shoulder. With the use of ice, and tolerating the discomfort, I persisted with bench pressing till the end of the deadlift cycle, but the damage was done and would be with me for a long time.

> You may be wondering how I could have done some of the foolish things I did. "Didn't you know better?" you may ask. I did know better. I knew I was taking form liberties. But I was caught up in the emotion of a cycle that was going very well in some respects, and reveling in handling large weights in the deadlift. I was apparently getting away with the liberties I was taking, so I kept on at it. My heart was ruling my brain. But eventually I came to grief, and confirmed all that I teach in my writings—that taking liberties with exercise technique is foolish.

## Nearing the peak

17.46    I was now down to 3 continuous reps and 12 rest-pause reps, and the strain was extreme—actually, it had been very severe for some time now. I switched the workouts around so that the first exercise of the week was now the deadlift. On 16 June I did 396 pounds (180 kilos). The 396 was a very big moment because it meant that four 20-kilo plates could be put on each end of the bar. Eight 20-kilo plates on a bar for rep work, for a hard gainer who has really suffered over the years, was satisfying in the extreme.

17.47    People like me are the ones conventional bodybuilding throws on the trash heap. After many years of following the popular advice I finally discovered the information that can make even a hard gainer respectable. But the "respectable" is not relative to what the top competitive bodybuilders can do. Had I not finally pursued basic and abbreviated training I probably would not have gotten past 160 pounds bodyweight and a 300-pound one-rep deadlift.

17.48    On 23 June I deadlifted 182.5 kilos (401.5 pounds) for 15 reps, all of them rest pause. I was ecstatic.

17.49    Though I had been doing 15-rep sets, I had long harbored a thought that 15 reps would not be enough and that I would need to do the "magic" 20 to feel that the job was complete.

17.50    On 30 June I poured it all out and did 18 so-very-demanding reps with the 400-pound brute. Though it was summer we had a relatively cool and breezy day on the 30th—only 95°F (or 35°C). I could have done the entire 20 reps, but held back because I wanted witnesses other than the usual teenagers at the gym. Except for some local soreness and heavy systemic fatigue, I had no negative reaction to this 400 x 18 workout.

## The peak

17.51    Once there was around 370 pounds on the bar, the thought of the next deadlift session caused me considerable anxiety, even fear. I would have five regular days and then, 48 hours before the deadlift, my mind could settle on little else except for the deadlift. My intestines literally churned in anticipation.

17.52    On 9 July, just before midday, I was to peak. My wife and a photographer were there to witness the event, and activity in the gym ceased as I got into the set. I did not feel as strong as I was for the previous deadlift workout, and it was very hot, with no air conditioning, and zero breeze coming through the open windows of the third-floor gym. I was later to find out that 9 July was, till then, the hottest day of 1992 in Cyprus. The local meteorological office reported 107.6°F (or 42°C). All this took its toll because getting from rep 10 to rep 20 was hellish. My deadlifting style cracked up more and more with each rep—excessive rounding of my back and some asymmetrical pulling. My style had been much better at the previous deadlift session.

17.53    My audience was appalled, my wife was fearful for my well-being, and I was so possessed that nothing, and I mean nothing, was going to stop me getting the 20 reps. This was the epitome of "blood and guts," and "train till you drop" training. I was streaming with sweat and there was a pool of the stuff in front of the bar, having dripped there during the rest pauses.

## Appetite and the total gain

17.54    I did not make a conscious attempt to increase my food intake. My appetite took care of it once I was deadlifting about 330 pounds. At that stage, immediately after a bout of deadlifting, and the 2–3 days afterward, my appetite was almost insatiable. Then it dipped until the next deadlift workout. The deadlift-free workout had only a small impact on my appetite.

17.55    I ended the cycle about 5 pounds heavier than I was back in November 1991. Bear in mind that had I been working on 20-rep deadlifts a few years earlier—when I was successfully performing low-rep deadlifts—I estimate I could have done 20 reps with about 350 pounds. The net result of this 1991/92 cycle was a new territory gain of about 50 pounds on the 20-rep deadlift. I was not trained down at the beginning of the 8-month deadlift focus, only out of touch with the bent-legged deadlift. As a result I would not have expected a big bodyweight gain to accompany 50 pounds or so on the bar. Also, I am past the days of eating myself fat to produce big bodyweight gains. It is possible, however, that had I applied some of what is described in Chapter 21 I would have gained more muscle.

## The downside

17.56    For four days after getting all 20 reps I had severe muscular soreness, almost crippling. On the fifth day, the worst of the muscular soreness was behind me and I started to feel a twinge going down into my left buttock and leg. I thought it would fix itself. I had decided that I was now going to drop the sets of high reps and go to sets of 5 reps. On 21 July I was back deadlifting. I did 5 reps with 400 pounds. They felt very heavy and I knew that I was injured. When I did the 400 x 20 I had a feeling of indestructibility, but now I was beginning to feel like an invalid.

17.57    I cannot put my finger on the exact cause of the injury. There was the rounding of my back on 9 July that may have done it, or at least contributed. There was some asymmetrical pulling that cannot have helped. Perhaps neither did the damage but set me up for it from something else. Two days after the 400 x 20 I did my usual full-range bent-over barbell rows, while my back was still massively fatigued. Perhaps the too-vigorous bent-over rows with almost 200 pounds was the final straw that hurt my back. I will never know. But no matter what was the single or multiple cause of the problem, I was in for a long period before I could return to regular progressive training.

17.58    I am sure that had I had my witnesses and photographer in attendance on 30 June, I could have made the full 20 reps, wrapped up that cycle without injury, and then started the next cycle. As it was I made my goal but got an injury in return. I had, and still have, no qualms about trading the temporary back problems for the 400 x 20. The satisfaction of the latter was, and remains, massive.

## On hindsight

17.59    All the injuries I suffered could have been avoided. Here are the lessons I learned/had reinforced:

   a.  I should have been using the seated back-supported overhead press right from the start of the cycle.

   b.  I should never have risked my sensitive knees with any squatting that had my heels raised by more than the height of the heel in my training shoes.

   c.  I should not have overstretched.

   d.  I should have exclusively used the Trap Bar for deadlifting.

e. I should not have done the barbell bent-over row. The one-arm dumbbell row, prone row, or the pulldown would have been a better choice.

f. I should never have bench pressed without spotters or some arrangement to catch the bar should I have gotten stuck at the bottom.

g. I should not have used grip support, but should have released my grip between reps and stood upright in order to set myself properly for the next rep.

h. I should never have taken liberties with exercise form, no matter what training intensity I was using. But the greater the intensity, the even greater is the importance of using impeccable technique.

17.60     As well as preventing injuries, following the above would have spared me the wasted time recovering from the various injuries I sustained. That "saved" time could have contributed to the implementation of one of the other big lessons arising from this period—smaller poundage increases. I should have dropped to increments of 2.5 kilos per deadlift session earlier than I did, and I either should not have had a poundage jump every deadlift workout late in the cycle, or just made it 1 kilo at a time.

17.61     To accommodate a slower poundage progression scheme I would have needed to have increased the cycle beyond its actual eight months. Alternatively, I could have broken the very long cycle into two shorter ones. I could have peaked at about 370 x 20 in the first cycle, backed off for the start of the second cycle, built back to 370, and then slowly worked up to the 400 target.

17.62     The deadlifting form I used during this cycle, especially in the late stage, had my hips higher (and my back less upright) than a squatter's deadlift style, with my back not as flat. But I had a knee problem and weakened thighs to contend with, so getting my legs out of the movement and taking more stress on my back were the compensatory measures. I am *not* advising round-back, bent-legged deadlifting. Such a style of lifting is potentially very dangerous unless the subject has the necessary structure needed, as Bob Peoples had, to break such a cardinal rule of heavy deadlifting without apparent harm.

17.63     I should have deadlifted on the Tuesday each week right from the start of the cycle, and divided the two training days more evenly over the week.

17.64     Had I had no knee problems, and had I developed stronger thighs through Trap Bar deadlifting, and had I used the Trap Bar exclusively (rather than the straight bar I used, because there was no Trap Bar available), the improved form the rhombus-shaped bar permits, together with greater thigh strength and a slower poundage progression, would have produced much better deadlifting form. It would probably also have produced better overall gains (because the Trap Bar deadlift intensively involves more musculature than the straight bar deadlift).

17.65     On the 400 x 20 day I broke one of the key rules for safe deadlifting—"Keep the final do-or-die rep inside you." I broke this rule at least five times in a row, to get from rep 15 to 20. Not only that, but I was not feeling 100% on that day due to the high temperature. I should have left the Herculean effort for a day or two later when conditions would have been better.

17.66     Regularly during the cycle I should have had someone record my deadlifting form on video tape. Then I could have studied my form and corrected the flaws in my technique.

17.67     My being strapped in throughout each set of deadlifts was a major contributor to ragged form and the excessive stress on my lower back. I should have released my grip between reps, which is only easy to do if no grip support is used, and then I should have stood upright during the rest pause. After a few deep breaths I should have held the last one, flexed my lats, held my arms straight and crushed them against my lats. Then I should have quickly tensed my lower back, abs and hips, checked that my hips were in their natural alignment and not thrust out to the rear, dipped at the knees, and then lowered myself into position, grabbed the bar, and lifted immediately.

17.68     I was never getting into the proper lifting position because I was starting from a semi crouch. As a result I could not set the stabilizing muscles properly.

17.69     To be able to take the bar immediately without needing to look down to check hand placement on the bar necessitates special training. But with practice, it can be done so that the hands automatically go to the right position on the bar, so long as the initial standing position relative to the bar was correct. This is much easier to learn with a Trap Bar than with a straight bar. With a Trap Bar the gripping sites are determined by the handles (which need to be gripped in their centers, to prevent tipping), but with the straight bar there are no fixed gripping sites. (See THE INSIDER'S TELL-ALL HANDBOOK ON WEIGHT-TRAINING TECHNIQUE for how to take your correct deadlifting grip without having to look down to see.)

17.70    During the deadlift cycle I neglected to do some important accessory exercises. In particular I was not doing any side bends, back extensions or shoulder external rotator work. While doing those movements would not have prevented the foolish liberty taking I was guilty of, they may have helped reduce the severity of injury, and aided in the recovery process.

17.71    Finally, had I known in 1992 of the therapy I describe in the next chapter, I am sure I could have quickly erased the aches and pains I suffered in my lower back during the final stretch of the training cycle. BB

## Note on the Trap Bar and shrug bar

Where the Trap Bar® is referred to in this book, you may also read "shrug bar." The shrug bar came on the market after BEYOND BRAWN was first published. The two bars are produced by different manufacturers. Both are excellent training tools. The shrug bar provides more knee room because it has a hexagonal shape as against the rhombus shape of the Trap Bar. Please see page 481 for how to find more information on the shrug bar. You may, however, require a custom-made bar with gripping sites placed wider apart than the norm.

Never bemoan the discipline that must accompany serious training. Never bemoan the discipline that must be applied to your diet and other components of recovery. To have the opportunity to apply all of this discipline is a great blessing—appreciate it and make the absolute most of it because it will not last forever.

## More on rep speed

Several factors are involved in keeping training safe. Avoiding high-risk exercises, using excellent form (i.e., bar pathways), and having balanced musculature are all big factors. Highly skilled Olympic weightlifters are proof that it is possible to train explosively without getting injured. But I prefer to build a significant margin for error into training, hence why I do not promote explosive training or exercises that can only be done explosively. But I am not anti Olympic lifting. I am for Olympic lifting, but the proviso is that expert hands-on coaching is available, and the trainee concerned is suited to that type of lifting.

Different exercises have different "stroke" lengths. Some can be performed in smooth control a tad faster than three seconds for the positive phase. But three or more seconds for the negative is still a good rule of thumb, other than in very short-stroke exercises. Let rep *smoothness* be your guide, rather than rep speed per se.

Over the decades, with few exceptions, the safety aspect of weight training has been played down or almost ignored by the training world. Form has been given short shrift. Rep cadence and control have been given short shrift too. And "cheating" has even been encouraged by many people, in certain circumstances. It is no wonder that weight training has caused so many injuries, and produced so much dissatisfaction and disappointment. I am not going to be a party to this outrage, hence why I am so insistent on safety concerns and the prevention of injury.

Some men with more training and coaching experience than I—Dick Conner, Ellington Darden and Arthur Jones—also promote non-explosive training, and have seen terrific results from it. It is not the only way to train, but I believe it is potentially the *safest* way for most people, and one that can be *super* productive, *especially* for hard gainers and anyone who trains alone without a *truly* competent and alert coach to supervise every rep.

*Before I got injured in 1992 I had little or no interest in injuries and how to deal with them. This is how it is with most people. Until you start to suffer you do not learn much about how you could have prevented the suffering. Had I been interested before, and had I fully grasped the massive importance of good exercise form, I could have prevented the injuries from occurring. And should any injuries have occurred, I could have gotten over them without having to get detrained IF I had known of trigger point therapy.*

*The appropriate treatment at the right time can mean the difference between needing a week off training, or years off.*

# 18. How a Training Nightmare Was Silenced

18.1    If someone else had written this chapter I would probably be shaking my head after having read through just some of it, cynically muttering, "You expect me to believe this? What's in it for you?" But because I am the one who experienced the "miracle" I know the truth of what is written here.

18.2    Here is my effort to share a wonderful rehabilitation therapy. If what I came across only worked for me, I would be wasting time and space reporting it to you. But it has proven its miraculous-at-times worth for *many* people. And some people have benefitted from it in ways that make my gain look very modest.

18.3    This is a personal account, but how many detailed personal accounts of recovery from injury have you read? There are hardly any published. All people who exercise seriously and for long enough will experience injuries, and even people who do not exercise have lots of aches and pains. You can learn much from my account that will spare you from having to learn the hard way like I did. It was not until 1996 that I returned to my summer 1992 level of strength and development. Had I known in 1992 what I had learned by 1994, I would have avoided perhaps the most frustrating period of my life. Not only that, but I would have been able to continue building strength in 1992 despite getting injured. Injuries themselves are one thing, but how you deal with them is another. *Deal with them in the wrong way and they can become much more serious than they really are.*

18.4    I had better start by dealing with my own cynicism imagined in the first paragraph. I hope you will believe me because I *am* telling you the truth. But you cannot learn what I am about to reveal the results of without doing some studying of your own. For a one-time payment of $75.00 I got the three items—a book and two therapy tools—I needed to get the near-miraculous job done. You will need the same items, or similar ones, to give yourself the possibility of performing your own "miracle." This $75.00 was a pittance for the fantastic skill it gave me—information and a means of therapy I effectively administered myself independently of any professional therapist.

18.5    As a writer, author and publisher I am able to provide information to many people. I am taking advantage of this to help spread the word about what I have discovered. This can help make many people's training lives far less troubled by injuries, immediately increase short-term training productivity and, with time, greatly extend training longevity.

18.6    In answer to the question of what is in it for me, I have no financial or other type of vested interest in what I am going to reveal. I am totally independent.

## The injuries

18.7    In the previous chapter I detailed how I peaked with deadlifting 400 pounds for 20 consecutive rest-pause reps. Due to various factors, all avoidable, I incurred several injuries during that training cycle—all but one of them being unrelated to the deadlifting. These injuries combined to prevent me from training consistently for about eighteen months. The most troublesome injuries were to my right big toe (from playing soccer), my knees (the last straw for them being a few workouts of squatting with my heels raised on a 2 x 4 block), my right shoulder (from bench pressing without a spotter and getting stuck), and my lower back (from letting my mind push my body too far beyond what it was capable of tolerating).

18.8    The toe injury made even slow jogging an impossibility, and I could only walk for very short distances without pain.

18.9    The knee problems were so severe that I was unable to do a single freehand squat without suffering knee soreness the same day and for a few days afterward. Squatting with 400 pounds, 300 pounds, or just bodyweight on the bar was no longer even thought about. Just being able to sit up and down from/to a chair, discomfort free and while not using my arms and shoulders for assistance, became a dream.

18.10   In effect I became a semi-invalid. I would not have been able to run to save my life. I could not play the rough and tumble games my two young daughters liked to play. I could no longer carry even one of them down a staircase. I could no longer lift even very light boxes without having to be meticulously careful about a flat back and not bending over too far. I could not go up a staircase two steps at a time. I could only gingerly enter and exit a car. I avoided physical activity whenever possible. I delegated even very simple lifting tasks.

18.11   It was almost eighteen months before I got back into very light but *consistent* and progressive training throughout my body. Then there was the long haul of ups and downs before I returned to the strength level I had in the summer of 1992.

## What used to work

18.12   Until I got the rash of injuries—in the summer of 1992—my standard treatment for injuries, aches and pains always worked: Lay off the bothersome exercise(s) for a week or few, perhaps apply some ice over the first few days, skip some workouts if need be, ease back into training over a couple of weeks, and then all would apparently be well.

## The root of the injuries

18.13   Nearly twenty years of taking too many liberties in the gym, following advice from poor sources and not always following what I preached, finally piled up and I started to crumble. (The at-times extreme pressure and stress of work since starting HARDGAINER in 1989 probably also contributed.) A hard gainer is not only severely restricted in the type of training that will work, relative to an easy gainer, but is far less resistant to the ravages of exercise abuse.

18.14   I also believe that my four-year bout of veganism in my early twenties made a contribution to removing, *indefinitely*, some of the robustness of body structure I had before.

18.15   In July 1992 I was forced to give up hard training. I was riddled with so many injuries that there were no exercises I could do that did not irritate something. I applied the usual ice, a few weeks of reduced activity, and lots of rest, but there was no real improvement. Chiropractic care only helped my particular lower-back problem a little. The discomfort/pain down there, and the aching and tingling in my left leg (sciatica), were relentless. I hasten to add that chiropractic care is very helpful for many lower-back problems, and should not be discounted for lower-back problems based on my single experience. During the 400 x 20 cycle I had two upper-spine injuries that were very quickly healed as a result of skilled chiropractic adjustment.

18.16    The x-rays I had as a result of the lower-back problem revealed that I have a considerable degree of scoliosis. Efstathios Papadopoulos, DC, described it as "borderline serious." I had deadlifted 400 x 20 without being aware of the scoliosis. Perhaps it was as well I had been ignorant for so long. Scoliosis predisposes the spine to a greater possibility of injury relative to vertebrae of normal formation, and made a substantial contribution to making my recovery from injury so challenging.

## A year later
18.17    Over the course of the next twelve months I had several false training starts where my shoulder, lower back, sciatica in my left leg, and knees forced me to stop training. I was little or no better than I was in the autumn of 1992. I still could not train, jog, walk anything more than what was needed to do basic errands and general activities, sleep on my right side without discomfort, or play active games with my children.

18.18    In July 1993 I sought the opinion of an orthopedic surgeon. I had recently done about three minutes of laughably gentle work on a stepper, and had a terrible reaction. The doctor diagnosed severe chondromalacia patellae. He advised me never to squat or deadlift with anything other than very light weights—even after the arthroscopy which he deemed a must to get my knees somewhere back to normal. I was so desperate at the time that initially I decided to have the surgery. But I quickly changed my mind after consulting the chiropractor I use—Dr. Papadopoulos. He informed me of the probable negative effects of the arthroscopic surgery that the surgeon neglected to tell me about.

> **For a one-time payment of a mere $75.00 I got the three items (a book and two therapy tools) I needed to get the near-miraculous job done.**

18.19     In late July 1993, after a couple of weeks to recover from the
          mini bout on the stepper following a long layoff from leg
          work, I started performing some freehand squats to give some
          activity to my knees and thighs, but using a different stance
          to what I had used before. In August I started to squat with a
          bare bar over my shoulders. With a stance about 6 inches
          wider than normal, toes flared to about 40 degrees (as against
          the usual 20 degrees or so), and no inward travel of my knees,
          I found a more comfortable groove for my knees. I added 5
          pounds every week to the bar. My knees felt much better, and
          I could soon sit up and down without getting much knee
          reaction. This was great progress. But then I would have very
          low weeks when the soreness would reappear and I seemed
          back at square one.

18.20     During two weekend breaks in the summer of 1993 I could
          not dive into a swimming pool, and could not jump in no
          matter how carefully. I went into a pool once during both
          weekends, and the reaction from my knees made me regret
          that single entry.

18.21     Here I was, someone who had never smoked, never had a
          single beer, had not eaten meat for about fifteen years, had
          been very careful with his diet for twenty years, had been
          taking vitamins for supposed health benefits for many years,
          had exercised consistently all his life (except since July 1992),
          and still looked quite athletic and fit (but did not feel it). But I
          would not have been able to out-run my little daughters, or
          out-play a five-year-old at soccer, without incurring
          considerable discomfort for a week or two.

18.22     In the fall of 1993, well over a year since ending my last serious
          training cycle, my toe, shoulder and lower-back injuries were
          still incapacitating me. There was a bit of progress in my knees,
          and the discomfort in my left leg due to the lower-back
          problem had eased a little, but that was it.

18.23     I was now so desperate that I started to think my training days
          were now behind me, and retirement at age 34 was in order. I
          had long known that I was not genetically gifted to do great
          things with weight training, and I was never interested in
          using steroids to shore up genetic short comings. Perhaps now
          I should have given up the thought that I could ever get into
          even "keeping in shape" training, let alone hard training.

# The magic of trigger point therapy
## The genesis

18.24      In early 1993 John Leschinski urged me to investigate trigger point therapy (which is also called, among other names, acupressure, myotherapy, pain erasure, and shiatsu—though the precise techniques of each are not necessarily the same) in an effort to help my recovery from the injuries. Leschinski, when a very ignorant youngster, had abused his body with sloppy exercise form. He was now raving over the help he had received from trigger point therapy in enabling him to get back into training. It sounded almost too good to be true and my extreme skepticism, on top of a very heavy work load, made me procrastinate the investigation.

### October 1993

18.25      Nearly six months later, as a result of Leschinski's persistence, I bought the superb 350-page book, MYOTHERAPY: BONNIE PRUDDEN'S COMPLETE GUIDE TO PAIN-FREE LIVING, by Bonnie Prudden, and the most basic of the wooden hand tools called a "bodo." I received these in October. The Prudden book is not the only one on trigger point therapy. It just happened to be the one I found first. (See pages 388–389 for how to get this book.)

18.26      I read enough of the book in a couple of hours to give me the gist of what it was about—trigger point therapy. I found it very hard to believe that something so cheap, non-invasive, non-nutritional and not necessarily needing a professional practitioner could be so helpful.

18.27      Not only had I never known anything about how to de-activate spasm-causing trigger points until that time, I had never known that trigger points even existed. (Trigger points are highly irritable and very tender spots in muscles.) And despite being so wounded with injuries for well over a year I was not aware I had such chronic muscle spasms. But once I knew how to find them, I discovered I was absolutely loaded with trigger points. It was no wonder I was so plagued with injuries.

18.28      Be prepared for the discovery that you, too, at least in some areas of your body, are loaded with chronic muscle spasms that are causing you discomfort and pain. But you can quite easily control the muscle spasms, and thus control discomfort and pain.

## November 1993

18.29    In the first week of November 1993 I started to use trigger point therapy daily on most of my troublesome areas. Toe, knees and shoulders were easy to treat, but I could not get into therapy for my lower back until December when I got the right tool.

18.30    Improvement in my right toe was almost immediate—in the first few days. By now it was close to two years since I injured it playing soccer. *And I fixed it with a few applications of a single toe trigger point exercise that I held for about ten seconds at a shot.* Incredible, but true. Now you can start to see why I am raving over this therapy.

18.31    There was substantial shoulder improvement after a few weeks, and noticeable improvement over a mere few days; but my knees needed a few weeks before there was clear improvement. After less than a month of trigger point work lasting about 20 minutes each day I had made far more toe, knee and shoulder improvement than in the previous sixteen months. While that might not be a "miracle" in someone else's book, it is in mine. Much improvement was still needed.

18.32    From the start of the squatting with a bare Olympic bar in August 1993, adding 5 pounds a week, I persisted through the ups and downs of soreness and discomfort. The new squatting style made a big difference, but my knees remained very sensitive and bothersome. But with the trigger point therapy, my knees picked up, and I could squat with much less inhibition and discomfort.

18.33    At the end of November 1993 I was squatting 135 pounds for 20 reps, and experiencing less discomfort and reaction than I was with lighter weights during the previous three months. Just a few weeks of trigger point therapy made a noticeable difference. While 135 x 20 is very light squatting, if you keep in mind that a year earlier I could not do a single freehand squat without suffering considerable discomfort, then the 135 x 20 was terrific.

18.34    My shoulder was progressing well too. I had not been able to bench press without discomfort, even with only 135 pounds, since late spring 1992. Now I was able to bench press with much bigger poundages and *without* discomfort. This was tremendous progress.

18.35　　This was a terrific start to self-administered trigger point therapy. I started to feel there was hope for my own training, and that I would not become an armchair coach after all.

## December 1993

18.36　　I did not start lower-back trigger point therapy until the first week of December. The hand tool I got with the book was fine for everything I wanted to use it for except the lower-back and buttocks area. To apply pressure to the trigger points in that area I needed a different tool—a "backnobber" from Pressure Positive Co. I did not get this until December.

18.37　　Upon using the backnobber I discovered I was loaded with trigger points in an arc around my lower-back and upper buttocks area, especially the latter. Tackling the trigger points on a regular basis in my glutei was what made the most impact in controlling pain in my lower back. The glutei can take a lot of pressure during therapy. Like the ones I had in abundance in my upper back, thighs and shoulders (especially the right shoulder), the trigger points in my lower back and buttocks were almost painful to touch.

18.38　　There was immediate improvement in my lower back from the trigger point therapy, and after a few weeks I knew for sure I had struck gold for my lower-back problems. The discomfort there was reduced substantially, as was the sciatica down my left leg. Following the advice of Bonnie Prudden, most days I also did two specific stretches for my lower back. While these seemed to help with the back recovery, it was the trigger point therapy that was the big factor.

18.39　　At about this time I noticed that my knees suffered much less crackling and grittiness.

18.40　　I was very conscientious with the trigger point therapy, despite working 80 or more hours a week. If I could make time for it, then anyone can. I missed only a handful of days of therapy over the first three months.

## January 1994

18.41　　In early January my right shoulder seemed 100%, and I could add that to the complete success I had with the toe injury, and my knees continued to improve. I continued the trigger point therapy for maintenance purposes. By late January my lower

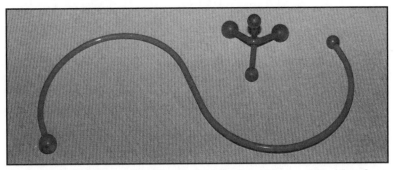

*Jacknobber and (bottom) backnobber tools, from Pressure Positive Co.*

back and the left leg connection felt nearly 100% most days, and actually 100% on some days.

18.42   In January I noticed that it was harder to find trigger points in all my former troubled areas, because I was no longer as loaded with them, and those that used to be very sensitive were now far less sensitive. Maintenance trigger point work for the right shoulder, for example, needed much less time than did the initial daily work needed to fix the problem.

18.43   I was now starting to feel youthful like I remembered in years gone by, giving me relative freedom to move around without having to watch out for this or that movement that used to bother me. I could now go down a staircase without my knees feeling rough and gritty. And I was able to carry my daughters down a staircase without discomfort—something I had not been able to do for nearly two years. It was a new lease on life.

18.44   For about eighteen months my knees would ache if I stood for more than half an hour or so. But in January 1994 I noticed that my knees did not bother me even if I stood for long periods.

### "Movie goer's knee"

18.45   Even from before the peak of the 400 x 20 deadlift cycle I had what is coined as "movie goer's knee," a condition that makes keeping knees bent at around a right angle very uncomfortable, hence making sitting in a cinema difficult unless the legs can be kept out nearly straight in the aisle.

18.46   It was around January 1994 that I noticed I could hold my knees bent without much discomfort. As the months passed, the ability to keep my knees bent became less of a problem.

The diagnosis of chondromalacia patellae and the need to "take it easy" I was given in summer 1993 by the orthopedic surgeon in Nicosia became increasingly suspect. This cast great doubt on the doctor's expertise and made me wonder how many people have been incorrectly treated by orthopedic surgeons. I am convinced that *many* people have written themselves off from vigorous activity when there was no need to do so—as long as trigger point therapy is practiced.

## April 1994

18.47   Come April 1994, the "miracle" had continued. Progress was slow but steady. I was now squatting 230 x 20, stiff-legged deadlifting 300 x 8 and bench pressing 230 x 5. All very modest lifting, but for someone who was so recently disabled by injuries throughout his body, and who was starting almost from scratch but with a very sensitive body, and doing it *drug free*, this was fine progress.

18.48   In April I bought and started using the "jacknobber" tool from Pressure Positive Co. The bodo I was using previously did the job I wanted, but I substituted the jacknobber because I found it more versatile. I was now almost exclusively using the backnobber and jacknobber as my therapy tools.

18.49   Much later that year I discovered that the jacknobber could also do the job of the backnobber. The jacknobber has a triangular base that enables it to be placed on the floor, with stability. I could lie over the device, positioning the upright prong where I wanted it to go on my back or glutes. Eventually the jacknobber became my sole therapy tool. This reduces to about $40.00 the total cost of a multi-purpose therapy tool *and* the book by Prudden, to enable you to apply trigger point therapy on yourself. That is even more of a pittance than the $75.00 I shelled out to begin with, to get started on the job.

## Anger with the orthopedic surgeon

18.50   I had now made sufficient progress, without surgery, to know that the diagnosis of the surgeon I visited in the summer of 1993 was way off the mark. I was already lifting weights way beyond what he would call "light," and my knees were doing fine.

18.51   I was angry that he could have been so wrong. And what makes me more angry is that the same man, and probably many others like him, so casually prescribe surgical measures that in many cases are not only unnecessary but, over the long term, may make matters worse. People like him, in private practice, are getting rich from their ignorance of non-invasive alternatives. (He was going to charge about $1,300 total for an hour or so of arthroscopic surgery on each knee, and one night in his clinic—a fee which is probably much less than it would be in the US for the same procedure.) That surgeons like him do what they do, with almost total impunity, is criminal.

18.52   As far as I am concerned, though of course I am not a doctor, never allow anyone to perform orthopedic surgery on you (unless it is reconstruction work following a serious accident) until you have thoroughly investigated non-invasive alternatives. Be sure you have pursued both chiropractic and trigger point therapy first. For serious problems you will need to go beyond treating yourself with trigger point therapy. See a chiropractor who has received training in this area, or a certified Bonnie Prudden myotherapist, both of which are available in the USA.

## May 1994

18.53   One Friday workout in May I was not feeling 100% but foolishly decided to push myself nevertheless, even to the point of breaking form a little, to get my planned 20 squats. This was an example of when it would have been better to have eased back for a workout rather than push hard, or to have postponed the session for a day or two. In pushing hard my form broke down and my lower back went into a crisis of spasms. It felt worse than it ever had. I was almost crippled.

18.54   I applied myself to lower-back and glutei trigger point therapy with extra vigor. I got my wife in on the act, to apply greater pressure with a bodo than I could by myself with the backnobber. At that time I had not discovered that the jacknobber could be used instead of the backnobber. Had I, I would not have needed the assistance of my wife. The usual trigger points were ultra sensitive now, more so than when I

> **Trigger point therapy could be some of the most momentous education you have ever had, or ever will have. It was for me.**

first started using the backnobber in December 1993. I had my wife use a pen with indelible ink to mark the key trigger points on my skin so she could apply pressure with a bodo at subsequent sessions without my having to direct her with, "Up a bit, left a touch, down a tad."

18.55    It all seemed in vain as I continued to be disabled. But I did not give up, and by Wednesday the spasms and pain had gone. I was back to normal and I returned to a regular level of trigger point work.

18.56    This got me to thinking that had I known about trigger point therapy back in July 1992 I may never have had to lay off from training for more than a week or so. The April 1994 lower-back problem was *much worse* than the July 1992 one. I fixed it in less than seven days in 1994, but the 1992 injury did not start to go away until I got into lower-back trigger point therapy nearly eighteen months later. All that getting detrained in the name of resting the injury, supposedly to permit recovery. It was not only a waste of time, but unnecessary to begin with, and even detrimental. *Oh for trigger point therapy in 1992.* Then I could have forged on in my training, building on the 400 x 20 deadlift instead of crumbling after it.

18.57    *The appropriate treatment at the right time can mean the difference between needing a week off training, or years off.* When you sustain an injury, seek expert non-invasive therapy *immediately*, and you may hugely hasten recovery time.

18.58    The May 1994 injury demonstrated that trigger point therapy had not corrected the root of the problem. Something was still seriously amiss—exercise technique. I injured my back again because my squatting form was not good enough. I was squatting too deeply *for me* (below parallel). This caused my lower back to round slightly. When I tipped forward excessively at the end of the set, the increased stress on my lower back caused the new injury.

18.59    The most devastating aspect of the 1992 injuries was that they forced me to stop serious weight training for a long period. As a result I lost a great deal of strength. I became very detrained, which in some ways made the problems worse. Rebuilding strength in a body that has more limitations than it had when the strength was originally built, is very difficult. But had I known in 1992 what I know now, I would *never have lost any strength to begin with*. It is *critical* to lose as little strength as possible while recovering from or managing an injury. Once the strength is lost you may never be able to gain it back. Of course in some acute injuries (broken bones, for example) you must have a period of immobilization. But with chiropractic and trigger point therapy, many injuries can be treated *without* an extended period away from intensive training, and thus without any significant loss of strength.

18.60    In May 1994 I started using the stepper that had given my knees such misery back in July 1993. While pushing through the balls of my feet made my knees feel gritty, pushing through my heels caused no bad reaction.

18.61    I had taken another step back to normality. The ability to do aerobic work had become but a fantasy for nearly two years. I could have been walking on flat terrain as soon as my right toe had been fixed in November 1993, but anything involving substantial flexion of my knees was out of the question until a while later.

## October 1994
18.62    In October I substituted aerobic work on a ski machine, partly because of the greatly reduced knee stress of the latter relative to the stepper, and also because of the superiority of the ski machine as an aerobic exerciser, because it involves much more musculature.

18.63    Also in October I started bent-legged deadlifting. I had tried bent-legged deadlifts once in late 1993, with a very light weight, but my knees gave me hell. Instead I kept to deadlifting exclusively with stiff legs but knees slightly unlocked. I started the 1994 bent-legged deadlifts using a Trap Bar, which is superior to a straight bar in a number of important ways. See the extensive technique descriptions of the Trap Bar deadlift in THE INSIDER'S TELL-ALL HANDBOOK ON WEIGHT-TRAINING TECHNIQUE.

18.64    I started the bent-legged Trap Bar deadlift with too much poundage. I used what was my stiff-legged poundage at the time—about 270 pounds. This was down from the 300 pounds of April, due to some unsuccessful training changes in the months in between. My knees were happy with it, but my back seized up and I was virtually crippled for a few days. After recovering, with the help of intensified trigger point therapy, I started again, this time with only 135 pounds, and worked up slowly, as I should have done to begin with.

18.65    The only bad experience I had with the Trap Bar was when I tried a single set with 135 pounds while standing on a 2-inch platform. I enjoyed the much greater involvement of my quadriceps, but my knees hated it. While I cannot do this deep deadlift, it is a terrific variation for those who can.

## November 1994
18.66    In November I dropped the policy of squatting to or below the point where my upper thighs were parallel to the ground. Having been imprisoned by the supposed virtues of such a depth of squatting I had been subjecting my lower back to stress that had been at the root of injury problems. Taking a few inches out of my squatting depth proved to be one of the most beneficial things I ever did to take care of my lower back. While this was a personal matter, there are many people who are squatting too deeply for their body structure and limitations.

18.67    Another training modification I made at this time was to stop bench pressing with my feet on the floor. By raising them on a 4-inch platform the lower-back stress arising from an excessive arch was eliminated.

18.68    Also in November 1994 I started to climb staircases two steps at a time, when the mood struck me. I had not been able to do this without discomfort for nearly three years. This was another memorable moment in my recovery.

## Completing the "comeback"
18.69    In summer 1995, rather than persisting with the squat and bent-legged deadlift, I switched to the Hammer Isolateral Leg Press and the Trap Bar stiff-legged deadlift.

18.70    A factor behind the shift from barbell squatting to leg pressing was advice from Dr. Papadopoulos that I should not put a bar across my upper vertebrae. From x-rays he discovered that my upper-thoracic vertebrae have an unusual semi-compacted formation, perhaps caused by years of squatting with a bar too high on my shoulders, at the base of my neck. Continued barbell squatting, even with the bar lower on my traps, would aggravate this abnormality. So I gave up barbell squatting for good.

18.71    In 1996 I returned to the strength level and development I had in early summer 1992. What a traumatic four years it had been. It was desperately frustrating on the one hand, but enormously instructive on the other. While everything I used to try to help my recovery has not been described in this chapter, and there *were* other negative experiences that delayed the "comeback," enough has been included to teach you about the most important factors. You can learn a lot from my experiences.

## The Tru-Squat machine

18.72    In 1997 I bought a Tru-Squat (from Southern Xercise, see page 481) and with it was able to return to intensive squatting. (Instead of the leg press and stiff-legged deadlift as my core leg and back exercises, I moved to the Tru-Squat, and stiff-legged deadlift from just below knee height.) The Tru-Squat mimics the barbell squat but with major differences and even some improvements. But it is not a barbell squat. If you can barbell squat safely and productively, then stick with that at least most of the time. There is no comparison between the Tru-Squat and Smith machine squat. The latter puts the lower back and knees at great risk. Used properly, the Tru-Squat spares the knees and lower back but while working the involved musculature to the hilt.

18.73    Here are the Tru-Squat's major differences and improvements relative to the barbell squat:

   a.   The resistance is applied through shoulder pads, akin to a standing calf machine. This is a far less uncomfortable way to bear weight than from a barbell. Additionally there is no contact stress on the vertebrae.

   b.   The back is supported.

   c.   During the descent there is no forward lean of the torso. The torso and hips actually move rearward during the descent. Despite the lack of forward lean there is still heavy involvement of the musculature of the lower back.

   d.   There is reduced forward travel of the knees relative to a barbell squat, reducing stress on the knees.

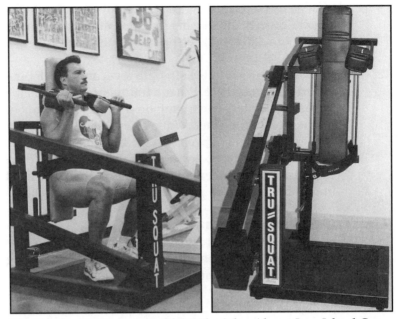

*The Tru-Squat demonstrated by Mike Schmeider at Iron Island Gym.*
*The stance used by Mike is closer than what works safely for me.*
                                    *Photo courtesy of Dr. Ken E. Leistner*

e.  There is an adjustable depth control.

f.  The user can squat to failure in total safety, *without* spotters.

g.  The leverages of the machine reduce, by around 30–40%
    (but varying according to the individual), the resistance
    needed to produce the same degree of muscular work as
    in the barbell squat. This makes loading and unloading
    weight easier because you need fewer plates.

h.  Breathing between reps is much less restricted than it is
    with the barbell squat.

i.  Once you have discovered the best setup for you, the
    guided pathway removes all concerns with balance and
    technique. When the reps become very hard you can focus
    on effort and not be distracted by matters of form.

j.  As a bonus, the Tru-Squat is an excellent calf machine—
    with the addition of a block for elevating the balls of the
    feet, if desired.

18.74    I can use the Tru-Squat without back or knee problems, and I can descend to the parallel position. My lower back is not put at risk at this depth, though it is in the barbell squat.

18.75    Though a costly machine it does not take up a great deal of space, and enables people who cannot squat safely with a barbell to be able to obtain the potential great benefits of the squat. Without it I would never have squatted again.

## Performance tips for the Tru-Squat

18.76    a.   Prior to use the Tru-Squat needs to be adjusted according to the height of the user. The heights accommodated range from 5-0 to 7-0. But the height settings can only be approximate. For example, if you have legs a little longer than the norm for your height, try the height setting immediately under your actual height. This will slightly alter the pathway your torso moves through, and reduce the forward travel of your knees. This may put you in a better position than you would be if at the setting that directly matches your height. Experimentation is needed to fine-tune the machine to best suit you. This should include adjustments of stance, to discover the optimum setup for you. For example, if you are 5-9, and set the machine at the 5-9 height, you may feel that you want to put your feet forward excessively. But set the machine at the 5-7 height and you may find that you are placed in a more efficient squatting groove, and no longer want to move your feet forward. Or you may want to use the 5-7 setting and a *slight* forward movement of your feet relative to where your feet would be if you stood with your legs perfectly vertical.

b.   With the resistance on your shoulders, stand upright like you would for a barbell squat. Do not elevate your heels. You may, however, find that moving your feet an inch or two forward puts you in a better position for squatting. Experiment! But do not move your feet forward by more than about 2–3 inches. Find the foot spacing and flare that best suit you by following the same guidelines as for the barbell squat—see THE INSIDER'S TELL-ALL HANDBOOK ON WEIGHT-TRAINING TECHNIQUE. (Depending on the individual, the Tru-Squat *may* allow more *safe* stance variations than the barbell squat.) "Dock" the resistance and use tape to mark the foot platform in such a way that you can easily adopt your optimum foot placement in every set you perform.

c.  Your lower back should not be pressed flat against the back board because this would weaken your back. The natural arch of your lower back should be preserved but *not* exaggerated. If the machine's belt is fixed tightly around the belt line it will flatten the arch of your lower back. The belt should be as low as possible without hampering flexion at your hips. Then your buttocks can be kept against the back support, and your lower back be free to adopt its natural arch. Lumbar support is recommended. A small rolled-up towel tied to the back board (e.g., by using a scarf), and placed in the hollow of your lower back, will suffice.

d.  Before being used as a calf machine, the height setting should be adjusted to the individual's height *plus* the height of the block used, to make getting in position easy.

e.  Avoid using it as a shrug machine. Shrugging with weight actually compressing the traps can lead to muscle tears.

18.77   While using the Tru-Squat I found that wearing knee supports (made of fabric, available from pharmacies) helps my knees. I *do not* use tight supports because they are crutches that can mask serious joint problems. The ones I use are sufficiently loose that they slip down when I walk, but stay in position for a set of squats. If I do not use the loose supports I experience a slight ache in my knees for a couple of days after training. The reason why the supports help probably lies in the temperature increase around my knees caused by the fabric.

## Inversion therapy

18.78   Gravity in general, and the stress of heavy exercise in particular, compress the joints of the spine, and the muscles and soft tissue of the back as a whole, but especially of the lower back. *This is at the root of many back problems.* But with the appropriate therapy this compression can be relieved, leading to a healthier and more injury-resistant lower back.

18.79   One of the simplest measures for taking care of the lower back is to take pressure off the lumbar spine. Not only is this inversion therapy a preventative measure, it can help during rehabilitation following injury.

18.80   I only started using inversion therapy on a regular basis in 1997. Before that I used it only occasionally, using makeshift

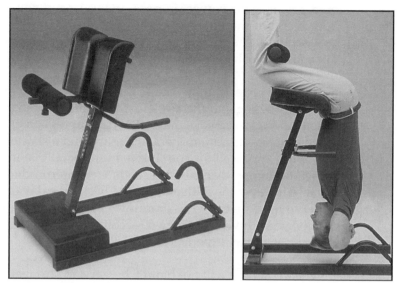

*The Back Revolution "anti-gravity" equipment.*
*Photos courtesy of Meyer Distributing Co.*

equipment. Once I got a proper setup that made inversion very easy to perform, I used it regularly. It has greatly helped me to maintain a healthy back free of injuries. Used properly, inversion therapy is an invaluable aid for maintaining a strong and healthy lower back—for everyone in general, but especially for people who lift weights.

18.81    Inversion therapy can be done using a back extension unit. Get in position ready to perform a back extension, but just stay with your torso hanging vertically. Do not twist, or take any action to exaggerate the decompression.

18.82    Alternatively there are several pieces of "anti-gravity" equipment commercially available for inversion therapy. I use "The Back Revolution®" unit myself. It was relatively economical, but safe, practical and very effective.

18.83    Without a back extension or "anti-gravity" unit you can use a home setup, with help from an assistant. Lie face down on a bench or any piece of furniture that is high enough for you to invert your torso without your head hitting the floor. Place a folded towel under your hips and shuffle forward until your entire torso is inverted, akin to if you were getting in position to perform a back extension. Take your weight on your hands on the floor while you get in position to suspend your torso. Your assistant should apply sufficient pressure to your legs to prevent your legs rising when your torso is freely suspended. Then take your hands from the floor and simply hang.

18.84    More is not better with inversion therapy (as with so much of physical training and therapy). Just one minute or so is all the time you need to achieve maximum decompression of your spine. A longer duration is not necessary, and a shorter time may work very well for you. I have even found that inverting myself for longer than 60–70 seconds is counterproductive because it leaves me with an irritated back for a day or two. Better to have several very short inversions per day rather than one long one. Invert for up to 60 seconds one or more times per day, and you may experience immediate benefits.

18.85    Inversion therapy will not build a bigger and stronger body. But it will help maintain the healthy injury-free lower back that is absolutely essential for intensive weight training—especially intensive deadlifts, stiff-legged deadlifts, squats and presses, which are major core exercises.

### Caution!
18.86    If any medical condition exists which might preclude the use of inversion therapy, such as high blood pressure, spinal problems, middle ear infection, or eye disorders, first consult your doctor. And never let children perform inversion therapy unsupervised.

## Other lessons
18.87    Until my back problems started in 1992 I could sit in any way I wanted, and on whatever surface, without any ill effect. I could slouch and have poor posture without suffering any bad effect. And I could sleep on a lousy mattress without much if any complaint from my back upon waking. After summer 1992, however, this "indestructibility" changed. I gave up sitting on soft chairs, always slept on a decent mattress, and gave attention to posture that had never been necessary before. If I cut any corners here, my back would irritate me. Trigger point therapy would relieve the irritation, but I had to stop the cause.

18.88    All that was necessary was for me to preserve the normal degree of lumbar lordosis, i.e., the inward curve of the lower spine just above the pelvis. I would sit up tall every half an hour or so of desk work or driving (or whenever I felt tension in my lower back), and very briefly exaggerate the lumbar lordosis. This was enough to preserve my normal degree of lumbar lordosis and prevent back pain.

18.89   Whenever I felt the need, I would do some neck stretching. Sitting for an extended period tends to cause the head and neck to protrude forward, even if a conscious effort is made to sustain good posture. This protruded position of the head and neck puts stress on the upper vertebrae that can lead to discomfort. Interrupt this protruded position regularly and the stress will be relieved. Retract the head while keeping the chin pulled down and in. Do this a few times and you should feel an immediate benefit. (See *Stretch H* in THE INSIDER'S TELL-ALL HANDBOOK ON WEIGHT-TRAINING TECHNIQUE.)

18.90   Even now, whenever I perceive any compression in my lower back, whether training related or otherwise, I do one or more of the back stretches described in the stretching routine in THE INSIDER'S TELL-ALL HANDBOOK ON WEIGHT-TRAINING TECHNIQUE, or perform some inversion therapy.

18.91   Prior to getting the inversion apparatus I would sometimes take most of my bodyweight on my arms while holding the arms of a chair (like in the top arms-locked position of a parallel bar dip), and gently relax my lower back so that the vertebrae there open slightly and the perceived compression is eased. But if I overdid it, it made matters worse. Proceed carefully if you perform this stretch.

18.92   While I used to stretch regularly even before the summer of 1992, it was not until 1994 that I substantially increased my investment in stretching. Prior to that it was more casual. Post injury I found an increased need to stretch very carefully any tight areas *prior* to training with weights. This helped to keep me supple during training and greatly reduced the chance of re-injury. I would only perform this pre-workout gentle stretching *once I was already warm*. A general warmup activity on a ski machine precedes every workout I take. I also found that trigger point therapy was sometimes helpful for easing tight muscles.

18.93   Give serious attention to following a sensible stretching routine on a consistent basis *before* you get a serious injury. Do not wait until after you have been injured to start to appreciate the benefits that are possible from following a good program of flexibility work.

18.94    I found the books TREAT YOUR OWN BACK and TREAT YOUR OWN NECK by Robin McKenzie excellent manuals for how to self-treat and prevent back problems. They helped me greatly. The lordosis and neck movements referred to in this chapter are from McKenzie's books.

18.95    In 1994, to prevent discomfort in my neck upon waking each morning, I took action. I started using a contoured pillow with a middle area lower than the top and bottom parts. This gave head and neck support and prevented the unnatural positioning of the upper vertebrae that a normal pillow usually causes. I fitted that particular contoured pillow but not everyone can fit the same contour. But it is worth a try if you suffer with post-sleep upper-spine discomfort. Consult your doctor, a chiropractor or other physical therapist for information on from where you can get a contoured pillow.

18.96    In summer 1995 I added reverse back extensions to my exercise program, against manual resistance. I found these to be helpful for keeping my lower back in good order. In the fall of 1995 I fitted a device onto my power rack to enable me to do reverse back extensions against progressive resistance. This proved to be more beneficial than the manual resistance.

18.97    Any back problem you may have, or get, cannot duplicate mine because your back structure is different from mine. Your injury history is also different. But you can learn from my experiences, and get insights that, when fine-tuned, may help you.

## Your aches and pains

18.98    If you are no longer in your teens or twenties it is almost certain you are carrying some aches and pains that you have learned to live with. You will have modified your training, cut out some exercises, eliminated some of the active things you did in your youth, and accepted it all as part of getting older.

18.99    Depending on the extent and type of damage you have, I believe you can partly if not wholly return to a relatively injury-free state. Investigate trigger point therapy yourself and apply it very seriously.

18.100   In her book, page 21, Prudden notes that only about 5% of people show no benefit from "myotherapy" (her name for the trigger point therapy she teaches). These are comforting and inspiring words for everyone, not just people who exercise.

> For the other 95 percent, we have found that we can alleviate all of the pain in most, most of the pain in others and at least control the pain in the rest; that is if they will continue with their exercises at home for the rest of their lives.

18.101   Before I got injured in 1992 I had little or no interest in injuries and how to deal with them. I had never needed to have an interest because it seemed academic, not practical. This is how it is with most people. Until you start to suffer you do not learn much about how you could have prevented the suffering in the first place. Had I been interested before, and had I fully grasped the importance of good exercise form, I could have prevented the injuries from occurring. And should any injuries have occurred, I could have gotten over them without having to get detrained *if* I had known of trigger point therapy.

## My mistaken view of injuries

18.102   Until I experienced the relief from pain and discomfort that results from using trigger point therapy I used to believe, like you probably do, that all pain meant some physical damage to muscles, joints, tendons or other tissues, and that the body needed rest and then a gradual return to activity.

18.103   Now I know that much if not most pain comes from muscle spasms caused by irritated trigger points, which can be treated with trigger point therapy. The muscle spasms then calm down and the pain disappears. What usually used to fix itself due to the relaxation following rest (but with age it takes longer to happen, if it happens), I can now often fix almost immediately with trigger point therapy I administer myself. And I am not an expert. I have learned a little about the therapy and how to find the trigger points in some of my own muscles, and yet I can perform little "miracles." You will likely need a few weeks of daily and serious practice before you can do something similar. But first you will need to study a book on the subject.

18.104   Prudden's book, for example, will give you a new perspective on diagnoses that doctors too quickly and inaccurately jump to, such as arthritis, chondromalacia patellae, carpal tunnel syndrome, and bursitis. Her book also gives a new meaning to headaches, "growing pains," back pain, and leg cramps. But as Prudden herself notes, start off on "easy" things—like the problems I handled quickly—get success there, and then move onto more serious problems if you have them. Her book provides the "maps" to find the trigger points you need to work on according to whatever problem you want to treat. Once you have some experience you can find the trigger points without having to refer to a text.

18.105     To be sure you are treating muscle spasms, get clearance from a medical or chiropractic doctor that you have no anatomical pathology. And consult a chiropractor so that any adjustment that can be done is done. Though unlikely, the sensitive bump in a muscle that you think is a trigger point could be a cyst or varicose vein. The evaluation by a medical professional is necessary because in some conditions any delay in professional treatment will cause deterioration of the problem.

18.106     Trigger points that are active can cause more than acute and localized pain, though it is the latter that is my focus in this chapter. Here is what Prudden says in her book, page 40:

> Active trigger points can do more than cause pain. Muscles in spasm can entrap nerves (sciatica), limit circulation (cold feet, slow healing and leg ulcers), pull muscles into a shortened state (spasticity in stroke victims), cause weakness ("the athlete's feet go first") and interfere with coordination. Even when they are so mild that they go unnoticed, they are dangerous. Given the right combination of physical and emotional stresses, they can magnify into a massive, tearing spasm that has the capability of ruining a career or even costing a life.
>
> Relief from pain is achieved by interrupting the spasm-pain-spasm cycle. Conventional medicine does that with medication, etc. [Trigger point therapy] does it with pressure.

18.107     Trigger point therapy is not something for just treating long-term injuries, but for preventing minor niggling aches and pains from developing into serious injuries.

18.108     Some physical therapists and chiropractors use trigger point therapy as part of their arsenal of tools. But it is kept within closed doors, so to speak.

# Chiropractic

18.109    Trigger point therapy cannot substitute for chiropractic
          (thrusting-type manipulations of the vertebrae) because there are
          injuries that only chiropractic or another manipulative therapy
          can treat. I am biased towards chiropractic because I have first-
          class experiences of its benefits, and because I know that
          chiropractic has standardized training for licensed chiropractors.
          The same cannot be said of osteopaths, however, where the lack
          of standardized training in all of its schools has produced major
          problems of inconsistency among practitioners—from the
          excellent to the bogus. (Physiotherapists, by the way, work under
          a doctor and are not qualified to diagnose, unlike chiropractors.
          Neither are physiotherapists trained in adjustments, though some
          "illegally" perform them, and some have produced severe
          damage in patients, and made problems much worse.)

18.110    There are injuries that are not usually in the territory of
          general practitioners of chiropractic. But chiropractors who
          have added adjunctive therapies (including trigger point
          therapy) from post-graduate training specifically for sports
          injuries will be able to help, e.g., a certified chiropractic
          sports physician. Examples of areas that may not be in the
          territory of a general practitioner of chiropractic are toe,
          shoulder and knee injuries.

18.111    In April 1993, before I was using a contoured pillow, I woke up
          one morning with my neck in a mess, and tilted. I could not get
          relief using the trigger point therapy I tried, but upon visiting a
          general practitioner of chiropractic I had an adjustment. I felt
          50% improvement immediately. The other 50% took place over
          the next two days. This was a graphic reminder of how
          powerful chiropractic treatment can be, and of how super-
          powerful trigger point therapy *and* chiropractic can be.

18.112    There is considerable overlap between trigger point therapy
          and chiropractic, with the former considered as a "nonforce"
          technique. To quote Cohen and Schneider[1]:

          > Within the chiropractic profession, there has been some
          > discussion about the role of soft tissue and reflex techniques,
          > or the so-called "nonforce" methods...Many chiropractors,
          > including ourselves, were only taught thrusting-type
          > manipulations in chiropractic school, where the emphasis
          > was on moving bones...

Although chiropractic has traditionally favored osseous manipulations as the mainstay of chiropractic treatment, many nonforce methods have become widely used in the profession...

Trigger point techniques are another means by which to restore joint mobility by removing the restrictive force of taut skeletal muscle. Because trigger points are sources of nerve irritation that disrupt the normal function of the spinal cord, their treatment fulfills the traditional view of chiropractic treatment as the elimination of interference within the central nervous system.

18.113    Some chiropractors know much about trigger point therapy and can practice it. It is a component in some chiropractic courses. But if the chiropractors do not share the basics of the skill with their patients, with guidance on how to use the skill in each patient's case, the patients are going to be dependent on the chiropractor for treatment. This would be prohibitively expensive for most people. If it was not for Prudden's book I would never have got to know about trigger point therapy and how to practice it myself.

## Training while you recover from injury

18.114    While you are following the appropriate therapy program it is very rare that some serious training cannot be pursued as well. Find those exercises and body parts that are not bothered by injury, and keep training hard there. In this way you can continue to derive some satisfaction from your training while you wait to get everything back in good order again.

18.115    For your recovery exercise program, so long as progress is happening, albeit slowly, watch out for trying to speed it up. Because you may feel ready for something more demanding does not mean that your muscles and joints are ready. Not coming back from injuries carefully enough is a major reason why people suffer from repeated injuries to the same area.

> **To be sure you are treating muscle spasms, get clearance from a medical or chiropractic doctor that you have no anatomical pathology. And see a chiropractor so that any adjustment that needs to be done, is done.**

## Trigger point therapy maintenance

18.116    For weight training to be effective, or any other type of
          exercise, you need to do it over the long term. To maintain
          myself in good enough working order to train I found, at
          least for several years, that trigger point therapy was a must.
          It kept discomfort and aches and pains at bay, so I could
          train progressively. Before I knew of the therapy, and before I
          had my debilitating injuries, I had ups and downs as I
          "recovered" from each minor injury that came along. I was
          not really getting injured, but was suffering from trigger
          point flare ups.

18.117    If, the morning after a training day, any of my sensitive areas
          were irritated, I would add an extra morning session of trigger
          point therapy for those specific areas. That got those spots in
          good running order immediately. Sometimes the trigger point
          therapy was like magic.

18.118    If my back was not 100% in the morning after waking, a little
          trigger point work would set me up for the day. The same
          goes if I am not 100% before training, or after. I slot in a little
          extra trigger point therapy whenever I need it.

18.119    Until November 1994 I still used trigger point therapy even if
          I felt no discomfort in the areas concerned. The areas that
          used to receive almost daily maintenance therapy were my
          knees, both big toes, both shoulders, lower back, elbows and
          fingers (especially on the day after a grip workout). Just 30
          minutes a day (I was thorough) kept me in good running
          order. From November 1994 onwards some trigger point
          therapy was done most days, but only according to what I felt
          my body needed rather than as a rigid schedule. I would still
          do some therapy most days, but not for the same trigger
          points each time.

18.120    In November 1994, after reducing my depth of squatting and
          sparing my lower back much unnecessary stress, I found that I
          needed to give less attention to posture and sleeping position.
          Not only that, but I found it unnecessary to do the McKenzie
          exercises as frequently as previously.

18.121    In 1997, injury-free, and as a result of no longer taking any
          liberties in my training, using the Tru-Squat, resting more
          between workouts, not overtraining, using a more controlled

rep cadence, performing inversion therapy daily, and stretching regularly, I reduced my need for trigger point therapy to only occasional occurrences.

## Practical application

18.122   Weight training is not about impact and collision like contact sports are, and thus its injuries are different and, relatively speaking, less likely to need medical or even chiropractic intervention. Therefore weight training's chronic and acute injuries are especially suited to care from self-administered trigger point therapy. Learn how to use this therapy and you will be able to keep yourself training very hard for long periods without needing a break. No longer will you be so much at the mercy of injuries. While injuries previously forced you to lay off training, under the impression that rest was what was needed to get over the pain, now you will know better.

18.123   But from another perspective chiropractic can be very valuable for weight trainees because it helps to decompress the joints of the spine, thus improving ease of movement and helping to prevent joint damage.

18.124   In my opinion, weight training and trigger point therapy go together perfectly. In fact, I think trigger point therapy should be an essential part of every weight trainee's arsenal of tools. It is cheap, you are not dependent on professional care unless you need to get into very advanced therapy, it needs no regular expense beyond the initial one-time purchase, and the more you do it the better you get at it. But you have to study up on it, apply yourself to regular therapy, and take it very seriously if it is going to work for you.

18.125   Trigger point therapy can help keep people training throughout their lives with far fewer obstructions from injuries and general aches and pains. I think it is one of the very finest discoveries, and it is available to everyone for a pittance of money plus a steady dose of personal application and persistence.

18.126   I am not guaranteeing that you will get the "miracle" I did, but I am sure that all who conscientiously apply trigger point therapy will get considerable benefit and be delighted they pursued it. I am not saying that all injuries can be successfully treated with this therapy, but I think most can.

# Warning!

18.127    Trigger point therapy cannot be used as a panacea for fixing persistent abuse of exercise. You must stop doing exercises and activities that are dangerous, and cease using poor weight-training form and uncontrolled rep cadence.

# Background on trigger point therapy
## Dr. Raymond L. Nimmo

18.128    Dr. Raymond Nimmo was a founding player in the development of trigger point therapy. Nimmo graduated as a chiropractor in 1926[1] and, as reported by Cohen and Schneider[2], "was one of the pioneers of a paradigm shift in chiropractic thought. [Nimmo] stated that the soft tissues of the body could also be the source of irritation to the nervous system, not just the spinal vertebrae." In another article[1], Cohen and Schneider noted:

> Nimmo coined the term noxious generative point to describe these areas of focal muscle tenderness that caused referred pain upon palpation... it is interesting to note that Nimmo had independently discovered what other researchers would eventually term myofascial trigger points.
>     Nimmo first became aware of the term trigger point in 1952, when he read an article by Dr. Janet Travell...

18.129    Janet Travell, MD, was another key figure in the development of trigger point therapy.

18.130    Nimmo developed the Receptor-Tonus technique for trigger point therapy, to which he "devoted over thirty years to researching and developing."[3]

## What is a trigger point?

18.131    According to Kle and Kreisman[3] a trigger point is:

> an accumulation of metabolic waste products (such as carbon dioxide, lactic acid, hyaluronic acid, etc.,) that concentrates at points in muscle. It causes local pain, as well as pain in other parts of the body. These metabolic accumulations cause pain by irritating nerve endings in the muscle, sending an excess of pain signals to the nervous system...
>     The muscles effected by trigger points can be tight and contracted, or weakened. When the muscles involved are attached to the spine, they cause spinal distortions and joint

problems. If the spine becomes misaligned, these problem
joints cause further irritation to the spinal nerves...This can
cause further problems such as sciatica, low back pain,
headaches, numbness, pain and tingling in the arms and legs.

18.132   Trigger points not only affect the vertebrae, but other joints of
the body. Instead of smooth and soft muscle pulling on the
joints, there is taut and lumpy muscle pulling incorrectly on the
joints and thus causing problems. Trigger point therapy returns
the muscle to its soft and smooth natural state.

## How to perform trigger point therapy

18.133   Find a trigger point by palpation (examining by touch) and
apply sufficient pressure to cause discomfort, hold it for about
5–7 seconds—or 10+ seconds if you can tolerate it—then release.
(According to what you have been doing to yourself, whether in
or out of the gym, the trigger points you need to concentrate on
the most may change from day to day. You will probably have
your "regulars," though.) Treat another trigger point or two,
and then return to the first one. Nimmo recommended two or
three sweeps on the same trigger point per treatment.

18.134   With my personal treatment—but remember that I am not
professionally trained in trigger point therapy—I do whatever
I need to do to feel the required easing of tightness,
discomfort or pain. Sometimes one application of pressure per
trigger point does the job, but usually two or three are
needed. Sometimes I temporarily had to be very aggressive in
a specific area, according to need.

18.135   According to Cohen and Schneider[2], though, Nimmo

...found that daily treatments are too much for the patient
to handle. He felt it was important to give the body time to
respond to pressure therapy by resetting itself and
rebalancing its efferent-afferent control. Also, since
mechanical bruising may occur after deep pressure therapy,
the muscles tend to be sore for a day or two.

18.136   Despite being *very* aggressive in my therapy, especially in
getting after the trigger points in my glutei, which were the
most bothersome ones for my lower back, I very rarely got any
bruising. Perhaps I would have gotten the great benefits I did
from treating a given trigger point only alternate days.

18.137    While it is best to get all the troublesome trigger points seen to in a given area, for quickest benefit, just fixing some of them has a knock-on effect in reducing the impact from the other ones.

18.138    This is only the *beginning* of the trigger point therapy, though it is the essence of the "quick fix" (as Prudden calls it) aspect of pain control. It is the quick fix aspect I have focused upon in this chapter, and that I concentrated on in my own early therapy—I was quick fixing myself almost daily. To do a permanent job, a more thorough approach is needed.

18.139    In Prudden's book there is more to pain control than the quick fix, despite the quick fix being so essential for immediate pain control. In Prudden's words on page 49 she says:

> The Purpose of this *Quick Fix* section is to first show you how to get rid of pain quickly and on the spot...The painlessness may last for hours, days, weeks or even for always. But if it doesn't, you must realize there was more work to do. See the *Permanent Fix* section to learn the next steps to take.

*Then on page 117 she writes:*

> The permanent fix is an extension of the quick fix. The latter is first aid for pain...like knowing where to walk in a minefield. Permanent fix gets rid of the minefield *and the enemy*.

18.140    Prudden details the "permanent fix" which entails an investigation of the deep-rooted causes of pain, trigger point therapy much more comprehensive than in the quick fix, and exercises (especially stretching). It is a very comprehensive yet cheap book. The Schneider manual is the Nimmo technique in great detail, aimed at the professional rather than the lay person.

18.141    Read one or both of these books. For expert hands-on guidance, link up with a chiropractor who has received

> **Injuries often need a multi-faceted treatment for full recovery. While trigger point therapy and chiropractic may be the most influential therapies in many cases, do not discount the potential benefit of some other therapies. Seek professional help.**

training in trigger point therapy, a Bonnie Prudden certified myotherapist, or any other therapist with experience in this area. Then find your own way from there. Unless you are very well off you will be unable to afford to have a professional therapist treat you several times a week. This is the reason why it is important to be independent but while being able to get professional help when you need it.

## Act, now!

18.142   Get in charge of your pain. You probably do not have to keep suffering. While I am specifically directing my writing at weight trainees, all people can benefit from trigger point therapy. All people experience pain at some times, and many people experience some pain all the time. Trigger points arising from accidents, sports, occupational hazards, diseases and operations—and activated by stress, thus throwing the muscles into spasm—account for a lot of the pain that people experience, if not most of it. Once you have proven on yourself what trigger point therapy can do, share it with others.

18.143   Human nature seems to procrastinate doing even beneficial things. Do not procrastinate. *Act now!* Get into some studying of trigger point therapy. You do not need to get into it in a big way to get started on your own therapy. I got started after spending only a couple of hours with the Prudden book, and then mixed practice of the technique with more study of it.

18.144   I urge you to learn about trigger point therapy, and then put it into serious, determined and consistent practice. It could be some of the most momentous education you have ever had, or ever will have. It was for me.

## How to avoid injuries

18.145   Adhere to the following and you will be able to train for a long lifetime, without suffering anything other than perhaps occasional minor injuries.

    a.  Use immaculate exercise technique—never cheat or use loose form.

    b.  Adhere strictly to a smooth and controlled rep cadence.

    c.  Even if your body can tolerate singles and very low-rep work, avoid using such high-force training for long periods. And use maximum-effort singles only very prudently. If your body is not suited to singles and very low reps, stick to medium and high reps. Use a rep count for a given exercise that suits *your* body.

d.   Only use exercises that are appropriate for you, and where appropriate modify them to make them safe for you. No exercise can be good for *you* if it hurts you.

e.   Stay clear of risky movements, e.g., behind-neck exercises.

f.   Use exercise poundages that are correct for you—only use a weight that lets you *just* squeeze out your target reps in good form.

g.   Avoid excessive ranges of motion.

h.   Respect your physical limitations.

i.   Personalize your training—only you can know your strengths, weaknesses and limitations. What works well for someone else, including a training partner, may literally ruin you.

j.   Avoid "rushes of blood" that lead to reckless training.

k.   Always be 100% focused and attentive while you train.

l.   Do not overtrain. For example, if you squat hard twice a week you may get sore knees. But squat hard just once a week and you may experience no knee soreness. Excessive training frequency causes injuries.

m.  Use alert and competent spotters.

n.   Always warm up *thoroughly*.

o.   Use robust and secure equipment.

p.   Keep yourself supple.

q.   Perform inversion therapy regularly.

r.   Avoid medium- and high-impact aerobic work.

s.  Self-administer trigger point therapy on a regular basis, and consult a trigger point expert for serious problems.

t.  Use a skilled and preferably sports-minded chiropractor to sound out whether or not a specific injury needs some related adjustment to hasten its recovery.

u.  Have a periodic checkup from a chiropractor.

v.  Eat healthfully.

w.  Do not cut corners with your rest and sleep schedule.

x.  Avoid extreme muscular soreness by *gradually* introducing changes in exercises and training formats.

## References

1.  Cohen, J. H., and Schneider, M., NIMMO RECEPTOR TONUS TECHNIQUE: A CHIROPRACTIC APPROACH TO TRIGGER POINT THERAPY, Aspen Publishers, Inc., 1992.

2.  Cohen, J. H., and Schneider, M., "Receptor-Tonus technique: an over view". CHIROPRACTIC TECHNIQUE, Vol. 2, No. 1, February 1990.

3.  Kle, J., and Kreisman, J., "Receptor Tonus Technique" (brochure article), 1988.

## Recommended books

1.  Prudden, B., MYOTHERAPY: BONNIE PRUDDEN'S COMPLETE GUIDE TO PAIN-FREE LIVING, First Ballantine Books Edition 1985. ISBN 0-345-32688-1. (Available through bookstores and Bonnie Prudden Pain Erasure– see the next page.)

2.  Schneider, M. J., PRINCIPLES OF MANUAL TRIGGER POINT THERAPY, published by Michael J. Schneider, DC, 1994.

## 2004 revision

*Here is the title of the most helpful book I have found on trigger point therapy:*
THE TRIGGER POINT THERAPY WORKBOOK (2001, New Harbinger Publications), by Clair Davies ISBN 1572242507.

## Sources of therapy tools

1. Bonnie Prudden Pain Erasure, P.O. Box 65240, Tucson, AZ 85728, USA (520-529-3979 and 1-800-221-4634), www.bonnieprudden.com
   *Also, instructional video tapes on trigger point therapy are available from here, as are Bonnie Prudden's books and a list of certified Bonnie Prudden myotherapists.*

2. The Pressure Positive Company, 128 Olberholtzer Road, Gilbertsville, PA 19525, USA (610-754-6204 and 1-800-603-5107), www.backtools.com

## Chiropractors trained in trigger point therapy

1. For a list of certified chiropractic sports physicians, contact the Fédération Internationale de Chiropratique Sportive, Inc. In English this is the International Federation of Sports Chiropractic. Write to Ch. de la Loliette 5, 1006 Lausanne, Switzerland.

2. For a list of other chiropractors trained in trigger point therapy, contact the national chiropractic association of your country.

   a. In the USA, it is the American Chiropractic Association, 1701 Clarendon Blvd., Arlington, VA 22209 (703-276-8800).

   b. In the UK, it is the British Chiropractic Association, 29 Whitley Street, Reading, Berkshire RG2 0EG, England (+441-18-975-7557).

   To find the national chiropractic association of your country, contact the World Federation of Chiropractic Secretariat, 78 Glencairn Avenue, Toronto, Ontario M4R 1M8, Canada (416-484-9978). BB

> Until I experienced the relief from pain and discomfort that results from using trigger point therapy I used to believe, like you probably do, that all pain meant some physical damage to muscles, joints, tendons or other tissues, and that the body needed rest and then a gradual return to activity.

*Regardless of how old or out of condition you are, it is never too late to take up exercise. Tomorrow is the first day of the rest of your life, so live for now and add years to your life, and life to your years.*

*Those who start training in middle age or later can achieve a near miracle in improvement of appearance and internal well-being, if only they would train appropriately, carefully and progressively, and make haste slowly. The older you get, the more that time is pressing and the more urgent it is not to make mistakes. Use it or lose it,* BUT DON'T ABUSE IT.

*The teenager is usually abundant in enthusiasm and energy, but deficient in effective instruction. Being so young, impressionable and gullible makes teenagers perhaps the most easily exploited group among want-to-be bodybuilders.*

# 19. How to Never Let Your Age Hold Back Your Training

## Aging

19.1    Aging will not be the bugbear for you that it is for most people, *if you know how to respond to its impact*. While there are age-based variations in goals, poundages and bodyweight, and food intake, this book was written to be useful for *all* adult trainees. Throughout this book the stress is on modifying training according to individual needs and limitations. The age factor is a big player here.

19.2    No one should ever feel too old to get into serious exercise. Keep Satchel Paige's words in mind: "Age is a question of mind over matter. If you don't mind, it doesn't matter."

19.3    Some inactive people have the attitude that, once past 40 or so, humanity is almost ready for the knacker's yard. With the right attitude, someone starting exercise in middle age or later can, if trained properly, hugely increase strength, physique and fitness. But someone who has been exercising seriously since he was a teenager cannot expect to be in the same condition at 65 as he was at 35. He can, however, expect to maintain a degree of condition that will make him a phenomenon for his age.

19.4    Weight training is no longer the domain of the young. Nowadays people are starting training late in life, and many others, though they started when they were very young, are continuing into their middle and later years. It is not a case of applying the cliché, "Use it or lose it." Much better is, "Use it or lose it, *but don't abuse it*." Of course this applies to all ages, but it especially applies as you go into middle age and beyond.

19.5    Older trainees, when compared on age alone, cannot be considered equally. Someone aged fifty who has been training consistently for thirty years cannot be compared to a fifty-year-old who is starting training. A forty-year-old weight-training beginner who has kept himself relatively fit from other activities cannot be compared to someone of the same age who has neglected his health and fitness for decades. Each individual is a unique case.

19.6    Regardless of how old or out of condition you are it is never too late to take up exercise. Tomorrow is the first day of the rest of your life, so live for now and add years to your life, and life to your years.

19.7    The benefits of exercise, even just moderate exercise, are *huge*, especially for older people. The older you get, the more important it is that you exercise.

19.8    Younger trainees are usually mostly, if not totally appearance and strength orientated. Many older trainees feel much the same way. But once beyond thirty-five years old, internal health and well-being from cardiorespiratory work should play an important part of a total exercise program. Then much later in life it should become even more important. But while strength training becomes less important as one ages, relatively speaking, it should always remain *very* important. Having strong and well-developed muscles does not merely have aesthetic benefits. Being strong produces critical health benefits and contributes greatly to reducing the ravages of Father Time. Exercise truly helps you to stay young for your years.

19.9    Especially if you are in middle aged or older, you *must* get a physician's clearance before starting an exercise program. Even minimal exercise can be extremely stressful for someone in poor condition.

19.10   While progress in strength, muscular development, flexibility and cardiovascular fitness can be made at any age, the possible negative side of exercise (aches and pains, and injuries) is greater as you age. The potential beneficial value of exercise also increases as you age. But without care being given to an appropriate, careful and progressive exercise program, the negative side will dominate and lead to terminating the exercise program. Remember, "Use it or lose it, *but don't abuse it.*"

19.11    The older you get, the more careful you need to be with making changes in your training load, and in your program as a whole. The room for error for the young person is much greater than for the older person.

19.12    The ability to recover from injury, at least at a physiological level, is usually greater for younger people. But an experienced and wise trainee should be more knowledgeable about how to hasten recovery than is a much younger but lesser experienced person. (Consider my experiences described in Chapter 18.) So an older but savvy person may be able to recover faster from injury than a much younger but naive trainee. What a shame it is that wisdom and youth rarely coincide.

19.13    With age you must be even more sure to perform adequate warmup work prior to doing work sets. This is just one example of the "less room for error" maxim that applies to older trainees. *Never* skimp on warmup work, and never make poundage jumps of more than 50 pounds between sets of a big barbell exercise as you work up to your top sets(s) for the day. Whenever you feel that an extra warmup set seems like a good idea, *always* do it. Never be in such a rush to finish a workout that you take shortcuts. Take your time, and get it right, always. If the first rep or two of a set feel(s) wrong, stop the set, discover what was amiss, correct it, rest a few minutes, and then do the set properly. And always keep yourself warm while you train.

19.14    It is not just warmup work specific to a given exercise that you need to give more attention to as you age. There is the general warmup work prior to touching a weight. This becomes increasingly important as you age. Take 5–10 minutes to gradually raise your temperature and heart rate, and break into a sweat. Do not skip this important period in order to reduce your total workout time.

19.15    With age usually comes a reduced ability to sustain full-bore training for long stretches, and possibly an increased need for intensity cycling.

19.16    You may find an increasing preference for medium and high reps as you move into your late thirties and older, rather than lower reps. Especially in the barbell squat, for example, you may move away from both low- *and* medium-rep work, and elect to use very high reps with a fixed weight. Rep progression would become your primary focus, not weight progression. Whether or not this move could apply to you will, at least in part, depend on your structural individuality, overall training experience and expertise, and whether or not, in your youth, you abused your body through overtraining, excessive use of singles and very low-reps, and poor exercise technique.

19.17    An older body cannot tolerate repetitive stress like a younger body can, all other things being the same. You must become especially attuned to the warning signs of overtraining (see Chapter 14). Be sure to take action before you get worn down by overtraining. Manage your training intelligently. Heed the advice that the older you are the more rigorously you should avoid overtraining, and the more heavily you will feel the aftermath if you do not avoid overtraining.

19.18    The older you get, the greater the need for consistency in your training. While a young person can lay off training for a couple of months and get back to previous best strength and fitness levels quickly, it takes more time for the older person, and the chance of incurring problems along the way is usually much greater. And if you lay off too long, you may never make it back to where you were previously.

19.19    Older people often have parts of their bodies that do not work with the unrestricted range of motion of youth. There may be damage from injuries or accidents of years ago. While ranges of motion can be improved, for some people there will always remain limitations. It is essential that older people do not imitate youngsters, but modify exercises to accommodate their own limitations. Not only do some exercises have to be modified, but some exercises need to be avoided. Anything that hurts should not be done. You must exercise without pain. Exercise-induced discomfort of the good kind is one thing. Training through pain due to a body that cannot co-operate is another. Application of the "no pain, no gain" maxim will kill your training, so forget that cliché.

19.20    Without selling yourself short, keep your goals realistic. Focus on the next 5–10% improvement, and then the next, again and again and again. That is the way to go for safe and sure progress, whether in the strength, muscular development, flexibility or cardiovascular component.

19.21    Exceptions to the former point are *long-term and very-advanced trainees*, as opposed to people starting their training in middle age or later. These already-very-experienced trainees, once over fifty or so years old, may no longer be interested in getting stronger still. They have already achieved very close to their absolute potential, and thus have been super strong. They have accepted that, with the passage of time, their absolute strength has to wane. At this time in their life they may never try to increase their poundages. Instead they might maintain a high level of strength by using taxing but not overly demanding poundages. Alternatively they might pursue different fitness goals altogether.

19.22    Heavy weights are *not* the privilege of only young people. A well-trained person who has trained most of his life may be able to lift heavier weights in his fifties and sixties than nearly all drug-free gym members of almost any age. Rise to the challenge of training yourself to do more late in life than most people ever do in their youth.

19.23    Your value judgements may change as you age. You will probably strive for different things during different phases of your life. You will not be young forever, but the beauty of exercise is that you will never cease setting new goals. If you set challenging but realistic goals, and set about realizing them in an intelligent way, you will be lined up for a life of achieving goals with all the accompanying excitement and satisfaction.

19.24    If you start training in middle age or later you can achieve a near miracle in improvement of appearance and internal well-being, *if* you train appropriately, carefully and progressively, and make haste slowly. Over a year you can transform yourself. But try to do it in just the spring to get ready for the summer, and you will be on a road to ruin.

19.25    While you cannot improve indefinitely, if you train well you can continue to improve long after you probably think you can. And even when regression starts, by holding as much strength and conditioning as you can, you will continue to improve relative to your peers who are deteriorating from an already much lower base point.

19.26    The older you get, the more that time is pressing and the more urgent it is not to make mistakes. While the young person has plenty of time for mistake making, the older trainee does not have that luxury. The older you get, the smarter, more knowledgeable and careful you need to be.

19.27    Choose specific exercises, style of training, and aerobic work that you enjoy. You may, for example, be a power person interested in short cycles, and balancing out your exercise program with some regular walking at a fast clip, and stretching on alternate days. On the other hand you may prefer medium and high reps, and long cycles, and prefer performing your aerobic work on a ski machine while watching TV, and feel better from stretching *every* day. The key is to find something you can do safely and enjoyably *over the long haul*.

19.28    While attention to exercise is very important, do not neglect the vital role of nutrition. Additional to this are factors that greatly influence your health at any stage of life—job satisfaction, quality of relationships, financial state of affairs, environment you live and work in, whether or not you smoke, alcohol intake, state of mind, etc. While you can shrug off many harmful activities when you are young, and without any apparent harm, they take their toll later in life. Get in charge of your life before it gets in charge of you.

19.29    Being strong and fit does not necessarily mean you are healthy, though of course it is *much better* to be strong and fit than weak and unfit. Exercise is not a panacea that can compensate for abuses and neglect in other areas. Exercise can only be a part of your overall strategy for external *and* internal well-being.

## Training the very young

19.30    In BRAWN there is a segment on the training of teenagers. Here is a revised version of it:

19.31    Teenagers are usually abundant in enthusiasm and energy, but deficient in effective instruction. Being so young, impressionable and gullible makes teenagers perhaps the most easily exploited group among want-to-be bodybuilders.

19.32    Teenagers who have read the conventional instruction will likely find it impossible to believe that progress in the gym is not the product of long and frequent workouts, wondrous sounding food supplements, use of sophisticated machines, and dedication to the point of fanaticism.

## The maturity factor

19.33    Youngsters should not be rushed into intensive weight
         training. Due to great variations in structural maturity there
         can be no standard starting age. Other than for especially
         immature individuals, most teenagers of age 14 should be up
         to benefiting from an intelligent, safe and organized resistance-
         training program, but not necessarily formal weight training.

19.34    Rather than trying to determine physical maturity by
         chronological age, determine it according to maturity as
         indicated by secondary sexual characteristics. While some boys
         can grow a beard before they are age 14, and some girls have
         started menstruating by age 11, others have to wait a few years
         yet. Chronologically young but sexually mature youngsters
         may benefit from training procedures suitable for adults, while
         older but less sexually mature youngsters cannot.

19.35    Consider the 15-year-old boy who still looks like a 10-year-old.
         Compare him with a classmate who is visibly as physically
         mature as a man. Though the same age, one is a boy and one is
         a man. The "boy" cannot benefit from the hard and heavy
         training that the "man" may be able to, but he *can* damage
         himself by using adult training methods, and erase whatever
         interest he has in training.

19.36    But keep even this maturity factor in perspective. A 13-year-old
         boy still has a 13-year-old skeleton, even if his musculature is
         well developed for his age.

19.37    The necessary maturity needed for serious weight training is
         not just physical. Serious weight training is a very regimented
         and disciplined activity. Before starting systematic weight
         training the teenager needs to be sufficiently mature to be able
         to deliver *of his own volition* the required discipline.

19.38    All youngsters will benefit from safe and practical training,
         especially those involved in competitive sport. By
         strengthening muscles, joints and ligaments the youngsters will
         achieve greater resistance against injury. But this safe and
         practical training does not have to be formal weight training.

## Some general guidelines

19.39    The very early teenager, both pre-adolescent and adolescent,
         can derive abundant benefit out of exercises that use the

bodyweight as resistance. Pushups, dips, chins, crunch situps, and slow back extensions without any hyperextension will thoroughly work the upper-body. High-rep step-ups holding dumbbells (or stair climbing) together with regular running activities can round out the program.

19.40    Once in the later teens—15 or 16 for most—comes the time for more serious training. As long as low reps are avoided and exercise execution is safe and controlled, regular squats and deadlifts should be included.

19.41    Maximum-effort low-repetition work is out for a long while yet. Maximum singles *do not even come into consideration*, and neither do forced reps, negatives and the like. If competition is wanted, have it for high reps—"Who can do 12 chins with the most weight?"

19.42    Explosive lifting, and exercises that compress the spine and apply shearing forces, should not be used by youngsters. Movements that are especially potentially dangerous for the early teenager include barbell squats, vertical and 45-degree leg presses, deadlifts and plyometric exercise. (Plyometric exercise is a type of training for explosive power that involves very sudden and highly stressful loads.) Plyometrics are potentially very hostile to anyone, regardless of age.

19.43    Teenagers should learn the priority importance of using proper exercise form. They need the discipline to do things correctly, regardless of what others around them may be doing. Many teenagers use sloppy form in order to hoist bigger poundages. Form comes first, not numbers. The benefits from this hierarchy are that the teenagers will suffer fewer injuries, get better results, create good habits, and thus be likely to train for life rather than a fleeting fancy.

19.44    Unless teenagers are unusually blessed genetically, are very mature physically for their age, or are fooling around with steroids, they cannot build substantial size and strength until in their late teens. Expectations have to be kept realistic.

19.45    The very skinny teenager who "eats like a horse" is not unusual. Adding a lot of size and strength demands determination and application at all times. For the hard-gaining teenager, the usual formula needs to be followed with special attention. More calories and nutrients need to be consumed, an abbreviated routine followed, physically demanding activities outside the gym severely curtailed or temporarily eliminated, late nights avoided, and a clean lifestyle followed.

19.46    Like the rest of us, teenagers have to spill hard earned sweat in the gym, and do so for a long and sustained period. The poundages used should slowly inch their way up. Progressive poundages in good form are the name of the game.

## Supervision

19.47    Supervised workouts are usually a must with teenagers, to keep them on the given program and prevent unsafe training. Regular reassurance concerning the appropriateness of the program needs to be provided. The temptation to follow irrational and potentially dangerous programs has to be countered.

19.48    I have intentionally been conservative in my recommendations for the training of teenagers. The value of good supervision is so great that I would remove *some* of my proscriptions if *hands-on* and *expert* coaching is available. But very few people have that sort of good fortune, and of those who do, probably most are getting it from fathers who are long-term trainees. The latter will probably have spent a chunk of their lives training incorrectly, but can finally get it right—for the training of their children. Here is when youth and wisdom can be united in a training situation, so long as the coaches do the job properly and do not repeat their own mistakes.

19.49    A child should not be pushed too much too soon. Premature pressure can kill a youngster's enthusiasm, and risk destroying a good parent-child relationship. *Haste makes waste.* [BB]

You can train full-bore on squats, deadlifts and a few other great exercises, but if you are not adequately consuming the building materials your body needs, you can forget about making good gains.

If you cannot get the basic combination of training, ordinary food and adequate rest to deliver good steady gains in muscle and might, you should not even consider taking any non-nutritional bodybuilding food supplement.

The studying of practical and effective nutrition and training is great, and needed, but the purpose of it is to help you build a stronger and better developed physique, not just educate you for the sake of it. Apply the learning with every ounce of drive and desire you have got.

# 20. Your How-To of Practical Bodybuilding Nutrition

## The percentage factor

20.1    There is a lot of hokum about nutrition being 50% or as much as 80% of bodybuilding success. Would you rather train very hard, including going through the near agony to get the final few reps of an intensive set of squats or deadlifts, or sit down in comfort and eat a nutritious meal of food that you enjoy? Which of the two is really most responsible for weight-training success?

20.2    Even though nutrition is not 80% or even 50% of weight-training success, do *not* become casual about its role. Good nutrition is vital! Some trainees have their training in good order but persistently short-change themselves with their nutrition. It is a total package that delivers gains for hard gainers. You need to be methodical and conscientious about *all* the components that contribute to weight-training success.

20.3    If you cannot be bothered to keep tabs on your total caloric intake, your training will suffer. If, for example, you need to average 3,100 calories a day to gain muscle (assuming you are training and resting adequately) but do not get them, do not blame your training when you start to lose size and strength.

20.4    Nutrition matters a heck of a lot if you are on a poor diet while training well. You can give your all to squats, deadlifts and a few other great exercises, but if you are not adequately consuming the building materials your body needs, you can forget about adding iron to the bar every week or two, and making good gains. Some easy gainers progress well despite following an appalling diet; but for hard gainers a good diet is critical. If you are living on a deficient diet but training and resting well, your lack of progress will be totally due to poor nutrition.

20.5    I always assume, but perhaps I should not, that anyone who
        trains very hard on an abbreviated basics-first program also
        has the desire and conscientiousness needed to eat a basics-first
        and sound diet, in sufficient quantities and *on a consistent basis*.

20.6    Getting enough calories and nutrients can be a problem for
        some people due to day-to-day circumstances, in which case
        you need to depend on liquid feeds to plug the nutritional
        gaps. But this is a darn sight easier to fix than it is to drive
        yourself to get the final couple of reps in a tough set when
        your body is screaming that it has had enough.

20.7    The contribution of nutrition to bodybuilding and lifting
        success is not the same as the contribution of nutrition to your
        visual appearance. Once you have some muscle on your frame,
        the most visually striking feature of a physique, except for
        hugely developed bodies, is the amount of bodyfat covering the
        musculature. And as far as controlling the amount of bodyfat is
        concerned, nutrition is the most influential factor. From *this*
        point of view, the "80% nutrition" opinion does have validity.

20.8    The contribution of nutrition to bodybuilding and lifting
        success is not the same as the contribution nutrition makes to
        your state of health. You can have an *unhealthful* diet that is
        adequate for getting bigger and stronger, and for altering body
        composition in a desirable way. On the other hand you can have
        a *healthful* diet that is not compatible with intensive, serious
        training. What you need is a healthful diet that *is* compatible
        with serious bodybuilding and strength training.

## The bottom line

20.9    Never forget that the role of nutrition is purely to help you to
        maximize your recovery and rate of progress while sustaining
        good health. Always keep this in mind. Then you have a simple
        reality check to apply when you experiment with adjustments
        to your diet. If *you* can steadily but consistently add weight to
        your exercises while maintaining consistently good form, your
        nutrition must be in good order for building muscle and might.
        This applies even if you do not consume as much protein or as
        many calories, micronutrients and supplements as some
        trainers and writers advocate. As a bonus your food bill will not
        cost so much. But if you are not progressing well, and assuming
        that your training, rest and sleep *are* in good order, you are
        almost certainly being held back by nutritional shortcomings.

20.10    Nutritional guidelines can be very helpful, but only through
         personal practical experience will you find what delivers the
         goods for *you*. Find what works best for *you*, using what follows
         in this chapter as a guideline. Always evaluate dietary changes
         by their effect on your training progress, body composition and
         health. If a change does not help your progress, or improve
         your health, it has no practical value for you.

## Dietary needs

20.11    You need a diet abundant in nutrients, and sufficient in
         calories so that you can gain size, unless you are looking to
         lose bodyfat and thus need to cut calories so that you are in an
         energy deficit. The fewer calories you need to consume, the
         more critical it is to ensure that your calories come from
         nutrient-dense foods. Calories, by the way, are units of heat
         energy. One gram of protein or carbohydrate yields 4 calories,
         and one gram of fat yields 9 calories. So you need over twice
         the weight of protein and carbohydrate to provide the same
         number of calories as pure fat.

20.12    Your caloric requirements depend upon your lean body
         mass, age, activity level and goals. The basic rule for gaining
         in muscle and might is to consume as many calories and
         nutrients as you can, but while not getting fat; and to have
         feeds frequently enough to prevent your getting very hungry.
         Many hard gainers who follow the eat-and-drink-your-way-
         to-size advice just become fat as a result. Excessive attention
         is given by some people and companies to getting hard
         gainers to eat and drink way too much. We are after lots of
         muscle, not lots of fat. A little fat accompanying a lot of
         muscle is acceptable, and often even necessary, but do not
         overdo matters and line yourself up for a lot of fat
         accompanying only a little muscle.

### Determining maintenance caloric intake

20.13    First you must accurately record your bodyweight. Every
         time you record your bodyweight you must use the exact
         same conditions—same time of the day and relative to the
         same activity of your bowels and bladder, and while
         maintaining approximately the same intake of fluids (so as
         not to be dehydrated).

20.14    The best way to determine the caloric intake that maintains your
         bodyweight is to keep your food intake steady for a period *without*

trying to gain or lose weight. While doing this, calculate your
daily caloric intake. Get a kitchen scale, a book that gives you the
caloric and macronutrient value of each food and drink item you
consume, a calculator and notebook. Keep a log of the caloric
value of everything you consume, together with how many grams
of carbohydrate, protein and fat you take in. At the end of a period
of three weeks, compute your daily average caloric intake.

20.15    If your bodyweight is constant over this three-week period,
you will have discovered your maintenance intake. If you lose
or gain weight, make an adjustment to your daily caloric intake
and carry out a further test period. Continue this process until
you find your maintenance intake.

20.16    Once you know how many calories you are targeting each day
for maintenance purposes, you should only need a week or
two of weighing and computing to familiarize yourself. Unless
you are always changing your food selection, or are making
very fine adjustments, you can quickly get to grips with sizing
up your food for its caloric value without having to weigh and
compute every item. But you will need to check on foods you
add to your diet that are not regular inclusions. To make it very
easy, you could compose several dietary schedules that meet
your needs, and rotate them. To keep tabs on your caloric
intake—to see whether or not you are straying from your
target—keep a dietary log on a sporadic basis.

20.17    All this numerical work is time consuming, and involves some
hassle. But it is necessary because without it you will never
really know where you stand nutritionally.

## Gaining muscle
20.18    Many hard gainers simply do not eat enough. On top of that,
they overtrain *and* focus on the wrong exercises. No wonder
they do not build any muscle. Almost any male who is
consuming fewer than 2,000 calories is never going to build

> **The harder and more seriously you train, the greater
> the need to satisfy nutritional requirements. Better to
> oversupply on the nutritional front than undersupply.
> Do not give your all in the gym and then sabotage
> your progress by cutting corners with your diet!**

himself up. Many hard gainers actually think they eat "lots of food" and a "high-protein" diet. But if they would keep a food log for a few days they would discover that they never consume more than 2,000 calories or 100 grams of protein per day. And no amount of amino acid capsules, creatine, vitamins, HMB or whatever-else supplement will help you if you are deficient in the big factor—sufficient quality food. Keep a food log yourself, and see where you *actually* stand rather than where you *think* you stand.

20.19   In summary, if your training is in good order as measured by the guidelines of this book, and you are sleeping well and not running yourself ragged out of the gym, you are almost certainly not consuming enough nutrients or calories. It *is* that simple.

20.20   To gain *muscular* weight there are three fundamental factors which you must satisfy *before* increasing your caloric intake. And you must consume excess calories—you cannot build muscle out of nothing.

   a.   You must consume a healthful diet of nutrient-dense food.

   b.   You must know the baseline caloric intake that maintains your bodyweight.

   c.   You must train intensively and appropriately to stimulate growth without overtraining.

20.21   Add 100 calories to your maintenance daily caloric intake. After a few weeks, determine if you have increased your bodyfat. Use fat calipers to keep tabs on your bodyfat. (Your technique must be consistent each time you use the calipers.) If your bodyfat does not increase, add another 100 calories and monitor your bodyfat. Continue this gradual process until you reach the point where you can detect a (slight) bodyfat increase. Then stick there for as long as you continue to gain weight. When your gains plateau, and assuming that your training and recovery are in good order, increase your daily intake by 100–200 calories.

20.22   This gradual increase in calories will enable your digestion to adapt to increasing demands, and let you determine the most you can eat without getting fat. If you just eat "a lot more," how will you know exactly how much you are consuming, and at what point you went overboard? And big increases in caloric intake will produce digestive tract distress in most people. Make the increases incremental and gradual, and your digestive system will adapt.

20.23   When increasing your caloric intake, get the calories where you seem to need them most. If you currently eat little protein, then get all your extra calories from protein-rich food. If you currently eat a very-low-fat diet, add oil-rich natural foods to your daily fare. For example, add seeds, nuts, avocado and oily fish such as sardines, and put virgin olive oil on your salads. If you currently eat few carbohydrates, then increase your consumption of grains, fruits and vegetables.

20.24   If adding additional calories is difficult, concentrate on consuming calorie-dense foods. For example, eat dense cereals rather than puffed up ones, bread rather than potatoes, dried fruit and bananas rather than juicy fruits, and foods high in healthful fats rather than low-fat everything. And use liquid feeds if you find getting extra calories through solid food to be a problem.

20.25   Only stay at your gaining caloric level if you are training hard. If you are in the early stage of a training cycle, back off a little in your caloric intake because at that stage you are not stimulating growth. Increase your calories as you move up the intensity gradient of a training cycle.

20.26   As your muscular mass increases, so will your maintenance caloric intake. As your muscles grow, gradually increase your maintenance caloric intake. If you hold your caloric intake steady, gains will slow and bodyfat will decrease.

20.27   As you age, all other things being equal, you will probably be able to gain on gradually fewer calories. Caloric requirements are reduced approximately 3% per decade after the age of thirty. So a sixty-year-old will need about 90% of the caloric needs of a thirty-year-old of the same gender and the same *lean* body mass. Lean body mass means total bodyweight less fat weight.

## Can you gain muscle while losing fat?

20.28   Gaining mode (anabolism) and losing mode (catabolism) are opposite conditions for the body to sustain. To combine them is nigh on impossible for most drug-free typical trainees, other than perhaps raw beginners, and formerly well-developed athletes returning to training following a long layoff.

20.29    In the old "bulking up" days, there was no concern with fat gain while building muscle. Most bulkers used to gain more fat than muscle; and some used to blow up like whales, gaining up to 100 pounds at a shot in some cases. Then they used to go to the other extreme, adopting a meat and water diet in some cases, and end up losing a lot of muscle as they dropped huge amounts of fat. This is very costly, both to the pocket and health.

20.30    When in muscle-building mode, minimize the fat you gain (but you almost certainly will have to gain some fat). If you overdo fat gain while building muscle, switch to a fat-loss program for a few months, to reduce your bodyfat to no more than 12% (for a male). Then get back into gaining mode, assuming you want to build bigger muscles. But adjust your caloric intake so that you add muscle but less fat than before. Whenever you hit 15% bodyfat, change modes and trim back to 10–12%. If done properly, each time you trim back your bodyfat you will have more muscle than the previous time. When you know what you are doing, it is easier to lose fat and keep your muscle than it is to build muscle in the first place. Getting bigger muscles is the hardest part.

## Number of feeds

20.31    A caloric intake that permits muscular growth is not purely about a number. How you consume the calories is very important. It is what your body digests and assimilates that counts, not just what you swallow. The quantity of food consumed at any given meal is a major factor influencing how your body handles the food.

20.32    Perhaps you need 3,100 calories a day in order to grow. But if your body cannot process those 3,100 calories, you are not going to get the nutrition you need. If you have three poorly digested meals of about 1,000 calories each, that will not do the job. But if you have five well-digested meals of 600–650 calories each, then your body is more likely to get the nutrition it needs.

20.33    If you do not find the quantity and combination of food at each meal that you can handle, then when it is time for your next meal your stomach will still be processing the previous meal. Putting in a meal on top of a partially digested meal will give you digestive tract distress, make you feel sluggish, give you gas, and just plain hinder your recovery and training.

20.34     Initially target five meals a day, spread evenly over the waking hours. For example, feed at 7AM, 10.30AM, 2PM, 5.30PM and 9PM. That means you would be feeding every three and a half hours. I say "feeding" rather than eating because some of the feeds can be liquid meals rather than solid-food meals.

20.35     But a desirable regular feeding pattern will only work if you can handle food at that frequency. Smaller and more frequent feeds are only part of the task. You need to find the mixtures of different foods that suit *your* digestive system. What suits one person can cause digestive tract distress for another person. You could assemble a basic outline of five daily feeds that agree with you, and that you can handle well so that your stomach is ready for each feed as it comes time to have it. And make each feed of similar caloric value so that the processing load per feed is similar. Then stick rigidly to your feeding outline excepting if you have some digestive tract upset that delays digestion. In such a case you would be better off delaying a feed until you have some appetite rather than put in more food on an undigested previous meal. Then perhaps catch up with the skipped calories over the next day or two, by adding 50 or so additional calories per feed.

20.36     Once you can comfortably process five feeds per day on a regular basis, progress to dividing your daily caloric needs over six meals a day. Do this by reducing the between-feeds spacing to just three hours, to squeeze in the sixth meal.

## A reminder

20.37     Even the very best food and supplements will make you fat, if you consume too much. And even the "right" quantity will make you fat if you are not training properly. You have to deliver intensive training and progressive poundages on a sensible weight-training program if you are to use the nutrients to build muscle. You must provide the stimulus to grow before you can turn any nutrients into muscle. There are plenty of people whose diets are more than adequate for growth, but because they do not train properly they do not have a chance of building much if any muscle.

20.38    Whether you can gain 10, 20 or even 30 pounds of muscle in a year depends on many factors including age, your genetic endowment, how underdeveloped you are before the period of assessment, how you train, how well you rest, and how dedicated you are. Rather than putting an arbitrary number on it, dedicate yourself to doing the best you can both in and out of the gym, and let the results take care of themselves.

# Macronutrients
## Protein

20.39    How much protein do you need? Who *definitively* knows, really? There is no need to go overboard with protein when you are not training full-bore. A gram of protein (mostly from animal origin) per pound of *lean* bodyweight should be in *excess* of what you need. If you are eating 4,000 calories or more each day, and including generous amounts of animal products, then it is almost impossible not to get lots of protein in your diet. But if you are on fewer than 2,500 calories a day (for a male), and in hard training, then you will probably have to make a deliberate effort to get enough protein.

20.40    When you are training at your most intensive and are close to or in new poundage territory, play it safe and get as much protein as you can comfortably digest—more like 1.25–1.5 grams per pound of lean bodyweight. You will probably not need this much, but without this amount you *may* be limiting your gains. Experiment and find out for yourself. Put theory and "research" aside and get down to some personal empirical investigation. There is, however, a chance that you might overdo protein intake, which could limit your progress. You need to experiment to see how your training progress is affected by changes in protein intake.

## Protein experiment

20.41    Using a reference book that provides a breakdown of food constituents, i.e., how much protein, carbohydrates and fat are in each item of food, discover how much protein you consume on average each day. When in the *intensive* stage of a training cycle, carry out this protein experiment. Increase your protein intake by 100 grams per day for the duration of the cycle. Do this by deducting 400 calories total from your fat and carbohydrate intake, and replacing them with the additional 100 grams of protein. (One hundred grams of protein contains 400 calories.) This will give you a big protein boost.

20.42    If you detect a noticeable improvement in your recovery, rate or progress, or in the length of time that progress is sustained, then adopt the protein boost every time you are in the intensive stage of a training cycle. But if you add the 100 grams of protein on top of your regular food intake, i.e., *add* 400 calories to your diet, you will be unable to determine whether it was the protein or extra calories that did the trick.

20.43    When increasing your protein intake, spread it out over five or six small feeds per day rather than pack it into two or three large meals, to avoid overloading your digestive tract.

20.44    While boosting protein intake is important when you go into new poundage territory, it is not just for that stage. If you are making a comeback following a long layoff, you will probably need to boost your protein intake long before you are back handling your previous best poundages.

## Carbohydrates

20.45    You do not need a treatise on carbohydrates to know what to eat. You will have heard and read enough over the years. But be sure you are putting the good advice into practice!

20.46    You need to focus on unrefined cereals and grains, fresh and dried fruit, and raw and minimally cooked vegetables. Make it a rule to include, daily, one large raw salad, one large bowl of fiber-rich cereal, four or more servings of fruit, several servings of non-salad vegetables, and wholegrain bread and/or pasta. Then you will have carbs covered together with obtaining a lot of valuable micronutrients—because your carbs will be found in nutrient-dense foods. Totally skip sugar and other junk carbohydrates, or at the very most only have them in small quantities on an occasional basis, say once a week for a treat.

## Fat

20.47    Some people seem to do well on very-low-fat diets but others do badly, with gains in muscular size being impossible to make. Find a balance of protein, fat and carbohydrates that suits you and makes you feel well. Just because some people appear to do well on a very low-fat diet, i.e., fewer than 10% of calories from fat, does not mean everyone can do the same.

20.48    Mere caloric value and percentage of your total caloric intake that fats comprise is only part of the story.

20.49    Fat has received a lot of bad press over recent years, largely because all types of fat have been grouped together and given the "bad" tag. Not only are some fats *not* bad, they are actually *essential* for good health. Without them you would seriously damage your health over the long term. Study the monumental book by Udo Erasmus, Ph.D., FATS THAT HEAL FATS THAT KILL, and you will get a new perspective on fats and their role in health. For sure some fats are very harmful, and should be avoided, but some fats (especially foods rich in the essential fatty acids) are very healthful and essential for your well-being.

20.50    Getting most of your ration of fats from fish (especially those high in essential fatty acids, e.g., sardines, mackerel and salmon), avocados, olive oil, raw nuts and seeds, *boiled* eggs, and low-fat dairy products is *vastly different* from getting the *same* quantity of fats from pizza, fried food, margarine and shortenings (i.e., hydrogenated oils), high-heated (fried) oils, refined oils, omelettes and scrambled eggs, and *full-fat* dairy products. The overall caloric value might be the same, but the impact on health would be vastly different.

20.51    Having lived in Cyprus for many years I have come to appreciate the very high esteem with which virgin olive oil is held in Mediterranean countries. Use it daily on your salads and elsewhere that is appropriate, e.g., on fish, and dip bread in it rather than use margarine or butter.

20.52    How you prepare food can determine whether or not the fat in it is healthful or unhealthful. The body can handle some oxidized fat, oil and cholesterol, but give it too much and it cannot cope. Reduce the consumption of fats which have been heated while exposed to air, and processed fats and cholesterol. Cured, processed and aged foods should be avoided, e.g., sausages and some meats and cheeses. Eggs should be boiled, not fried or scrambled. All fried food should be avoided. And butter should be used (sparingly, though) instead of margarine.

20.53    Check out the ingredients of convenience foods and snacks, and see how frequent shortenings, shortening oils, and partially hydrogenated vegetable oils appear. Avoid those foods. And even be careful with oils that have the potential to be very healthy, e.g., flax and hemp. These oils must be fresh and in their natural state. If they are exposed to light during processing, storage or display, or if they are exposed to heat during processing, or if they are used for frying in the kitchen, they turn into harmful oils.

## Macronutrient percentages
### Discovering your current macronutrient intake
20.54   Using the data compiled from the test period(s) described under *Determining Maintenance Caloric Intake*, determine the balance you typically have between the macronutrients, i.e., carbohydrates, fat and protein. Total up the grams of carbs, fat and protein for each day. Calculate your daily average. Then calculate how many calories came from each macronutrient, and the proportion that number is of your total intake.

20.55   For example, and purely for illustration purposes, over three weeks you may have averaged 2,900 calories daily, and 140 grams of protein, 50 grams of fat, and 470 grams of carbs. The 140 grams of protein equals 560 calories (4 x 140), which is 19.3% of your total caloric intake (560 divided by 2,900, multiplied by 100). If you do the same operations for fat, you get 15.5% of total calories; and for carbs it comes to 65.2%.

### Optimizing your macronutrient percentages
20.56   Nutritional fare for weight trainees has fashions, and bodybuilding in particular is notorious for extremes. For quite some years the low-carb diet was fashionable, even for gaining size; and huge amounts of protein and fat were consumed by some people. Then there was the fat-and-cholesterol-are-evil phase. Then cholesterol started to lose some of its "bad guy" image, and in some quarters there was a move back towards lower carbs and more fats, but selected fats.

20.57   Stick to dietary moderation with no extremes among fat, protein and carbohydrates. Fine-tune the proportions according to how many calories you need and what balance of the three food constituents makes you feel your best. As a general recommendation, and as a starting point for individual fine-tuning, consume 20% of your calories as fat, a sufficient percentage to supply your protein needs, and the balance as carbohydrates. And within each macronutrient, get what you need from quality healthful food. Percentages are only a part of the picture.

20.58   As an example, suppose you weigh 190 pounds with a bodyfat of 10%. That gives you a lean body mass of about 170 pounds.

And suppose you are targeting 1.25 grams of protein per pound of lean body mass, and 3,100 calories. If you get 20% of those calories from fat, that means 620, leaving you with a balance of 2,480. For protein, multiply 170 by 1.25, which gives 212.5 grams of protein daily. Multiply that by 4 to convert to calories, i.e., 850. So the total fat and protein caloric intake comes to 1,470, leaving a balance of 1,630 calories to be covered by carbohydrates. These particular numbers come out as 20% fat, 27% protein, 53% carbohydrates. With less fat, the other percentages would need to be higher. But going below 15% fat could jeopardize your muscle-building progress and possibly even your health.

20.59    On a lower caloric intake, to get 1.25 grams of protein per pound of lean body mass will produce a higher protein percentage. Suppose the same example person, of 170 pounds lean body mass, is consuming only 2,500 calories daily. To get the target 212.5 grams of protein, i.e., 850 calories worth, it will come to 34% of total intake. That increase in the proportion of calories from protein needs to be compensated for by a reduction in the fat and/or carbohydrate percentage(s).

20.60    If you eat a lot of fatty foods, even if they are all healthful, you may find that your appetite is so well satisfied that you can go long periods without getting hungry. Then you will be unable to have five or six feeds a day without force-feeding and suffering the almost inevitable digestive tract distress. You need to fine-tune the proportion of dietary fat so that you can comfortably satisfy your caloric needs over five or, even better, six feeds a day.

## Dietary fiber

20.61    If you eat adequately of unrefined carbohydrates, and do not abuse your body with junk food, you should get plenty of fiber in your diet. Fiber is *crucially important* for good bowel habits. You should have at least one bulky bowel movement each day. Adjust your fiber intake until this regularity is the norm. This

Fat has received a lot of bad press over recent years, largely because all types of fat have been grouped together and given the "bad" tag. It is critical to understand that not only are some fats *not* bad, they are actually *essential* for good health.

regularity is essential for getting waste products out of your digestive tract quickly, before they can do any harm.

20.62    Some itemized high-protein diets published in bodybuilding magazines and books are terribly low in dietary fiber, and are going to wreak havoc on the elimination systems of those who follow them. A large serving of a wholegrain and perhaps bran-enriched breakfast cereal in the morning, and legumes, salad and wholegrain bread or pasta for dinner (as well as your evening protein), on top of some fruit and whatever else you consume at other times during the day, should provide sufficient dietary fiber. But dietary fiber will not do its important work if you are dehydrated.

## Water

20.63    Adequate water intake is *critical* to your health and well-being. Merely not being thirsty does not mean that you are necessarily properly supplied with water. Most people do not appreciate the value of water. Coffee and tea (unless decaffeinated) and alcoholic beverages do not count in water intake. Drinks containing caffeine or alcohol can even *increase* your need for water because of their diuretic effects.

20.64    There are some serious consequences from long-term water deficiency (dehydration). These include kidney and urinary tract problems, e.g., kidney stones.

20.65    It is much better to be oversupplied with water than undersupplied. The negative consequence of excessive water intake is merely more visits to a toilet. The negative consequences of inadequate water intake are major.

20.66    Ensuring adequate water intake is easy. Consume enough water evenly distributed over the course of each day to produce at least four *clear* urinations each day (in addition to colored urinations). Until you produce your minimum of four clear urinations a day, gradually increase your intake of plain water, juicy fruits, fruit juice, and perhaps even milk. (If you already drink a lot of milk, your water intake may already be adequate.) Liquids need to be pleasant tasting if you are to drink more of them. Get a water filter if your tap water does not have a pleasant taste; or drink bottled water that tastes good. Reducing or, better, eliminating coffee, tea and alcohol consumption will make a big contribution to net water intake.

20.67    During and following training you need additional water, and during hot weather you need to greatly increase your water intake. Stick to the four clear urinations rule, and modify your liquid intake according to the climate and your activity level.

20.68    If you take a lot of vitamin supplements you may find that your urine is colored even though its volume and frequency of production are high. In such a case you will need to judge your hydration by the volume and frequency of urinations rather than by their lack of color. But the discoloration caused by some vitamin supplements will only occur within a few hours of supplementation, not all day. If your vitamin intake heavily discolors your urine that is probably a good reason to reduce your supplementation because a lot of it is going to waste.

## Micronutrients

20.69    If you are deficient in a vitamin or mineral it could have a harmful effect on your training and recovery. The deficiency could be the result of following an obviously very poor diet, and thus be easily corrected. Alternatively it could be because you have some increased need for a given nutrient, or even several nutrients. Some people apply a shotgun approach and try to mega-dose on every known micronutrient in the hope that any possible deficiencies would be corrected. This strategy assumes that the supplements taken are actually used by the body.

20.70    Swallowing whole tablets is no guarantee that they will be used by the body. No matter how supposedly good a tablet is, if it passes out of your body whole, it will do you no good. Chew your tablets before you swallow them.

20.71    Suppose that you have truly applied the training and rest advice given in this book, and *all* the nutritional advice given in this chapter. If you still cannot gain, it would make sense to investigate whether you are deficient in some nutrient(s) that is/are inhibiting your gains. Get yourself tested for nutritional deficiencies by an appropriate professional, perhaps an orthomolecular nutritionist (ask your physician for a referral), and then take any necessary corrective action.

## Making the most of milk

20.72    Milk is a concentrated source of nutrition. If you stick to low-fat or, better, skim milk, you can get a lot of protein, carbohydrates and water in a very convenient and economical form. To eliminate milk and its products from your diet when you are trying to build muscle and might can make meeting caloric requirements tricky, especially if you have well-above-average caloric needs.

20.73    Whether you drink milk will largely depend on your ability to digest it. If you suffer from gas, bloating or diarrhea after drinking milk or eating a dairy product such as cheese or ice cream, you are probably lactose intolerant. This means that your small intestine does not produce enough lact*ase,* the enzyme needed to digest lact*ose.* Lactose is the natural sugar found in milk and other dairy products.

20.74    Lactose intolerance is a common condition, though the extent of the intolerance can vary a great deal. While some people do not produce enough lactase to handle even a couple of mouthfuls of milk, other people need to consume a couple of pints of milk before they exhaust their immediate production of lactase. You may find that your tolerance of lactose decreases as you age.

20.75    *2004 revision: I used to drink a lot of milk, but no longer. Especially due to how milk is produced today, it has shortcomings. Now, I prefer to recommend milk products—kefir, and cheese, for example—rather than liquid milk, and more solid food from other sources, to provide one's caloric and nutritional needs.*

### Dealing with lactose intolerance
20.76    If you are lactose intolerant, and still want to include milk in your diet, here are some suggestions:

a.   Drink milk by itself two hours after a meal. Later that day have the same quantity of milk with a meal. Compare the way you feel after each, and plan your future milk consumption accordingly. The milk may digest well when apart from a meal, but not when taken with a meal.

b.   Due to their reduced fat content, you may find low-fat and skim milk easier to digest than regular (full-fat) milk.

c.   Have a week off all dairy products and then add them to your diet but do it in a very gradual way, starting with very small quantities. Only choose the products that produce little or no negative reaction. Consume some dairy product(s) each day and try to build up your tolerance by adding just a little more each week until you get to a satisfactory quantity you can handle comfortably.

d.   A few mouthfuls of yogurt each time you drink milk may help in the digestion of the lactose. This is because the organisms contained in yogurt will break down the lactose.

e.   If the yogurt does not help enough with the digestion of milk, eliminate milk and substitute with yogurt, cheese and cottage cheese. Comparing the same quantity of protein and other nutrients, yogurt, cheese and cottage cheese come with much less lactose, and in some cases even no lactose.

f.   Add the lactose-digesting enzyme when you consume dairy products. In the USA, try tablets and drops you can get over the counter at pharmacies, e.g., Lactaid®. Through trial and error you can determine how much you need relative to the type and quantity of dairy product you consume after it. Consume milk that has already been treated with the enzyme—for example Lactaid 100% Lactose Reduced 1% Lowfat Milk.

20.77   If you still cannot handle milk after trying all the above suggestions, then one of the substitutes you should consider is a lactose-free protein powder such as whey. Then settle for getting the rest of your caloric and nutrient needs from food free of lactose. As convenient as milk is for bodybuilders and strength trainees, you can manage well without it. You just need to be more creative in your meal and drink design.

20.78   Whether you drink milk will at least partly depend on the caloric intake you need. If you are weaning yourself off regular milk, do it progressively. Move to low-fat milk for a while, and then consider going to skim milk. In this way the big taste difference between regular and skim will not be so noticeable. And different brands of skim milk can have different tastes.

## Meal schedules

20.79   Invest an hour or two composing some basic meals and whole-day feeding schedules. Compose at least ten alternatives for each of the solid feeds you have each day. List the foods,

portions and the resulting caloric and macronutrient ratings for
each meal. Do the same thing for liquid meals. Then put the
feeds into daily schedules so that you have a variety of ways of
meeting your caloric and protein targets each day.

20.80    Nancy Clark's SPORTS NUTRITION GUIDEBOOK, second edition, has
well over a hundred recipes, with macronutrient and caloric
values given for each. Refer to those recipes if you need help
with putting together healthful meals and drinks. The book is
also packed with lots of practical and sensible advice on
nutrition in general, though its focus is on endurance athletes.

20.81    For gaining muscle and might, five or six meals a day, rather
than three large ones, is the ideal. Due to your daily schedule it
may be very difficult to get so many solid-food meals a day,
but with an abundance of desire it can still be done.

20.82    If you eat a solid-food breakfast and evening meal, you could
depend on drinks for your in-between feeds. Then you can get
your five or six feeds per day with minimal interruption of
your daytime activities. How much trouble is it to have a drink
out of a flask? Use a blender for the smoothest multi-ingredient
drinks. Make up enough of a nutritious drink at breakfast time,
or the night before (and store overnight in a refrigerator), and
take it with you to work or school in a thermos. You may need
two flasks, depending on the quantity of the concoction you
make up, and the flask size. Blend together ingredients that
you can digest easily. For most people, the base item will be
milk. Enrich it with things that are usually compatible, e.g.,
skim milk powder, yogurt and cottage cheese.

20.83    Raw eggs can kill people, due to salmonella poisoning. Do *not*
take a chance on eating raw or undercooked eggs. Cook your
eggs well, even if you are using them in blended drinks.

20.84    Perhaps you will want to eat solid food three times a day—
breakfast, lunch and dinner—and have three liquid feeds in
between. Perhaps you will prefer four solid-food meals and
two milk-based drinks. Perhaps you will prefer six similar-
sized solid-food meals each day. Perhaps you will mix it up
from day to day. No matter what, get organized so that you
have ready-made daily dietary schedules that satisfy your
caloric and nutritional needs. Find what works best *for you* as
far as your digestive, culinary and practical limits permit.

# Special meals
## Breakfast

20.85    Especially when in hard training, always eat breakfast. After eight
or more hours since you ate last, your body needs a quality meal.
If you skip breakfast you will miss one feed a day, and extend the
fasting period. This will start your day in catabolic mode rather
than anabolic mode. Your first meal of the day does not have to
be a traditional cereal-based one, though breakfast is a common
time to have a fiber-rich meal. Make breakfast any quality food
you want, and include a good portion of animal protein. But do
not overeat. You want to be feeling hungry within three hours, for
meal number two. Make time for breakfast. If you are pressed for
time in the morning, prepare your breakfast the night before.

## Pre-workout meal

20.86    As noted in Chapter 16:

> Through trial and error, discover the food types, balance
> and quantities that will carry you through an intensive
> workout without any waning of energy. It may, for example,
> be a bowl of wholegrain pasta topped with grated cheese, or
> a couple of baked potatoes and a couple of scoops of cottage
> cheese. Find what works best for you, and then stick with it.

20.87    You need to be able to handle the food well enough so that you
can train 90–120 minutes after the meal. Then following your
workout you can still make your next scheduled meal. If you
eat too much before training, or eat some mixture of foods or
specific food item that you do not handle well, that may ruin
your workout, or cause you to postpone it. That will disrupt
both your training and your feeding schedule.

## Post-workout meals

20.88    Also as noted in Chapter 16, you need to have a protein-rich *and*
high-carbohydrate meal almost immediately after training,
preferably a liquid one for easier assimilation. (Protein alone is
not adequate after training; you need lots of carbs too.) A quart
of skim milk will do a reasonable job, and you can add skim
milk powder or other enrichment. Be sure to take in plenty of
water too. Drinking enough to produce two *colorless* urinations
during the period after training will ensure you are hydrated
following working out. About two hours after the post-workout
meal, have another quality meal. But you may not have time for
two post-workout feeds if you train in the evening.

## Can you gain on a vegetarian diet?

20.89    A vegetarian diet means different things to different people. For some it means a diet that only excludes meat and fowl; for others it excludes fish, too; and for some it means the exclusion of *all* animal products. The latter is what I will refer to as a vegan diet, and is the purist's interpretation of the vegetarian approach. These different interpretations are important because each defines what protein sources are consumed. For example, a vegan diet is greatly different from a lacto-ovo vegetarian diet (one that excludes flesh but includes dairy products and eggs).

20.90    I thought it was possible to gain on a vegan diet. I believed it so strongly that I was a vegan for four years during my early twenties. Not only did I find it impossible to gain strength and development on a vegan diet, I found it impossible to maintain what I already had. I persisted with training as well as I could, and I ate sufficient calories to even gain bodyfat (so I was not deficient in calories), and I paid attention to balancing the shortcomings in amino acid profiles. But it still did not work.

20.91    Veganism was a calamity for me, and on hindsight I wonder how I persisted with it for four years before coming to my senses. I had tried to convince myself that size and strength were unimportant, that health was where it was at, and that shrinking to about 130 pounds was okay because I was "healthy." That "health" precluded any demanding exercise because of the severe soreness I suffered in some joints following any heavy work. Activities which used to be very easy became impossible, even in a watered down form, e.g., I could not jog very short distances on a giving surface without suffering severe joint soreness, let alone actually run.

20.92    Perhaps I was an extreme example, but adding animal protein—initially just a few eggs a day—made me feel like I had been given a new body. It was miraculous. Almost

> Comparing the *same* quantity and quality of food, consuming it over two or three meals cannot provide the benefits for muscle building that five or, even better, six meals can. Eating many evenly spaced meals a day is one of the big components of bodybuilding success. Do not underestimate its importance.

immediately I could do what previously was impossible, and do it without any negative reactions. I was slowly but gradually able to build back size and strength. I believe even to this day that I still suffer from some reduction in the hardiness of my joints as a result of the four-year period of veganism.

20.93    I have known of no one who, on a vegan diet, was able to gain (not *re*-gain) a *large* amount of muscle and might. But I know of a number of vegans who woefully failed to build any significant size and strength. I would never advise anyone to combine veganism and intensive weight training. They are diametrically opposed, at least for the huge majority of people. But a lacto-ovo vegetarian should be able to build size and strength without problems if he trains properly and includes enough animal protein from eggs and/or dairy products. Some fish in the diet is a wise addition, especially fish rich in essential fatty acids, but meat and fowl are not necessities. I have not eaten meat or fowl for nearly twenty years, but during that time I was able to build considerable strength, including deadlifting 400 pounds for 20 rest-pause reps.

20.94    As important as a mixed diet is for successful weight training, this does not mean that you should go to extremes and live almost totally on animal foods. Some bodybuilders and lifters go to this extreme and have very unhealthful diets as a result.

## Beyond food

20.95    If you can mix almost any foods with no negative reaction, continue as you are. But if you experience digestive tract distress or *any* negative reactions to what you eat, this segment will apply to you at least to some degree.

20.96    No matter how nutritious a meal may be on paper, and no matter how well it may work for someone else, it may not be good for you. If you cannot digest it comfortably, and if it seems to "sit" in your stomach for the rest of the day, and you do not get hungry until many hours later if at all that day, then that meal should not be repeated. Through experimentation, find meals you can process so that you start to feel hungry within three hours or so of each. Experiment by changing one variable at a time, altering components and quantities.

20.97    The timing of the return of your appetite following a meal is likely to be related to the intensity of your training, and your training days. Following a meal on the day after training your appetite may return faster than it does following an identical meal three days after working out. And your appetite may be slower in returning following a meal in the early stage of a cycle than late in a cycle.

20.98    Get "in tune" with your stomach. If putting some fruit spread on your toast at breakfast time delays your digestion of that meal, do not use fruit spread in that way. If having a drink of milk after a meal hinders the digestion of that meal, do not have milk with other food. If milk drank by itself well away from a solid-food meal digests easily, but when you blend in a banana, honey or peanut butter it becomes difficult to digest, then stop adding things to the milk. Drink more milk instead. If cucumber or onion in a salad disagrees with you, eliminate the offending item(s).

20.99    Discover what mixtures and timings of different foods agree and disagree with you. Then organize your feeds so that you only consume combinations of foods you digest well. If your digestive tract is in a mess, then even eating only healthful food is not going to help your gains in the gym. It is what you digest and assimilate that matter, not just what you put in your mouth.

20.100   Much of the rest of this segment is based on personal experience. This is not to discount academic study and honest anecdotal reports from others. While my experiences are not the same as yours, I want to relate mine so that you can see the importance of individual adjustment. Your needs will be at least partially different from mine, if not substantially different, but what is important is that you recognize any special needs you have.

20.101   I used to be obsessively fussy about ultra-strict food combinations during my four-year stint with veganism. My digestion seemed to be impaired during that period as a result of the radical diet. Strict food combinations were a necessity then to minimize digestive tract discomfort. But strict food combining did not work for me once I was training intensively and including some animal products. This was because I could not get enough nutrition in a single day if I kept to the strict combinations. But I found that strict food combinations no longer seemed to be a necessity. My powers of digestion improved noticeably when I stopped being a vegan. While dismissing food combining rules altogether would cause a lot of digestive tract discomfort for me, a compromised version works very well.

## Milk

20.102    If I mix milk with anything other than dairy products, my stomach gives me distress. I do not mix milk with anything other than dairy products, and I keep a milk-based meal well away from any other meal. I never have milk unless I am feeling hungry from my previous feed. But I am fine if I have another type of food an hour or so after a large milk-based feed.

## Fruit

20.103    I never mix fruit with anything. I have it by itself and *at least* half an hour before consuming any other food. That gap is enough for my digestive tract to be able to comfortably deal with both the fruit and whatever comes after it. If I put the other food in on top of the fruit, or follow the convention of fruit after a main meal, my stomach would torment me.

## Protein and starch

20.104    I do not mix concentrated starch foods with concentrated protein foods. I know that some foods have a fair bit of both, but I categorize all cereal/grain foods, legumes and potatoes as starch foods. I separate them from concentrated protein foods (eggs, fish and dairy products) by having a gap of about 20 minutes between the protein and the starch. For example, I will have fish, eggs and green salad followed 20–30 minutes later by a mixture of bread, legumes, potatoes and pasta.

20.105    On a rare occasion I am forced to break my rule of separating protein and starch (but I never break the milk-by-itself and fruit-by-itself rules). I can get away with only minimal "protesting" from my stomach if I mix protein with potatoes, but to mix protein with grains or legumes is disagreeable.

# The age factor

20.106    In my teens I used atrocious combinations by my standards of today, but still I could be downing something substantial every 2–3 hours. At that time I could down a heavy breakfast of juice, liver, eggs and cereal, and shortly afterward get earnest about a milk-based concoction, such as a pint of milk with lots of yeast and even soya powder stirred in. I would hold my nose and pour the terrible-tasting stuff down, but my stomach would process it without complaint. If I was to drink one of those "bombers" today, my stomach would be in a mess for the rest of the day, and perhaps the following day too.

20.107    As you age, generally speaking, the sensitivity of your stomach increases. Do not force your body to try to do what it only could when you were much younger.

## AM and PM foods

20.108    You may find that certain foods are better suited to certain times of the day. To some extent this may be due to individual habit, but I think there is more involved. Find what you seem to handle better at certain times of the day, and schedule your nutritional intake accordingly. For example, I cannot easily handle solid-food meals (except fruit) other than at breakfast or dinner, and have not been able to for many years. During the day I stick to milk-based drinks, and fruit.

## Further enhancement of digestion

20.109    As simple as proper mastication of food is, many people do not chew their food adequately before swallowing it. Always chew your food until it is a complete paste, prior to swallowing.

20.110    Avoid eating on the move. Slow down, sit down and calm down before you eat or drink. Take a break from whatever you are doing, to focus specifically on each meal. Eating on the move can impair digestion.

## Digestive aids

20.111    *After* you have sorted out combinations of nutritious foods that best suit you, and have eliminated items you cannot handle well, then use of digestive aids *may* be an option to pursue.

20.112    There may, however, be a possible downside to digestive aids, so if you pursue this avenue do so with caution. Natural production of enzymes and hydrochloric acid may be reduced if you take digestive aids that you do not really need. This could produce a dependency on the digestive supports and create a problem. Play it safe and do not use digestive aids unless:

    a.  there is a critical food item you cannot digest and,

    b.  a doctor has determined that you are deficient in a specific factor involved in digestion.

20.113    Follow any specific medical advice you may be given in this area. You may find one specific digestive aid or a combination of them helps you to digest and assimilate your food. This will make you feel better, make your meals feel lighter, and help to maximize your recovery abilities. You may even find that, with digestive aids, some of the foods or combinations that did not seem to suit you no longer bother you as much.

## Psychological factors

20.114    If you are angry, extremely excited, or otherwise agitated or churned up at a feeding time, delay that meal *unless you have hypoglycemic tendencies*. Generally speaking, if you eat while mentally distressed or worked up, your body will not process food well. The meal may "sit" in your stomach for many hours, cause digestive tract distress, and mess up the rest of your eating schedule for that day. Better to delay that meal, or even skip it altogether. Then add a little to each of the following few feeds to regain the nourishment that was "lost."

## "Listen" to your body

20.115    *In moderation*, satisfy food cravings you may experience. Depriving yourself of a food you crave may even harm you. You may also have an intuitive feeling that a certain food is not good for you, though in theory it is a good food.

## Food supplements

20.116    You should not be anti food supplements, but you should be anti anything that distracts you from a 99% focus on the fundamentals of basic training, basic rest, and basic nutrition through food. All the maybes of nutrition, and supplements especially, take up way too much of most trainees' attention.

20.117    The use of food supplements is part of the common image of a weight lifter, and something that gives a feeling of membership. The reality is that *some* (but "some" does not mean all) food supplement companies are guilty of:

    a.    Deceitful claims that their products can never deliver.

    b.    Listing fictitious ingredients and quantities (usually in order to offer a "quality" product at a low price).

    c.    Making up research studies; selecting research that has nothing to do with healthy hard-training humans; and drawing on research that is based on methodology utterly devoid of any scientific credibility whatsoever.

20.118    Once people swallow the "nutrition is 80% of bodybuilding" belief (or even the "mere" 50%), and the "magic bullet" way to bigger muscles, they become marketers' dreams—prime candidates for any food supplement doing the rounds.

### Conditions to satisfy before trying "bodybuilding supplements"
20.119    You must have the fundamentals in place before you go experimenting with only *possibly* useful extras. No supplement will compensate for a diet deficient in a major component. Here are the fundamentals to get in place:

    a.  Daily satisfaction of your caloric needs.

    b.  Satisfaction of your daily caloric needs through five or six evenly spaced, evenly sized, easily digested meals.

    c.  Daily satisfaction of your full sleep requirements.

    d.  Production of muscle and might gains through the combination of a–c plus intensive training. Get this basic formula working in practice, and actual muscle growth happening, to prove you have a successful program and that you really can train and recover properly.

20.120    I am not saying that some of the new supplements will not help you. What I am saying is that none of them will help you as much as will getting the above in 100% good order. So get the above in perfect order *before* you tinker with your rate of gains by experimenting with supplements.

20.121    Absolutely no food supplement can produce muscular gains like steroids can. People who claim that a food supplement works like steroids are taking liberties with the truth, possibly in order to convince trainees to buy the supplements concerned, which the advocates happen to sell.

20.122    If or when you experiment with bodybuilding supplements, do not use a shotgun approach. Try one supplement for a month or so, during an intensive period of training. Only buy a minimum supply for the test period, and choose a reputable company that offers a money-back guarantee. If the supplement helps, keep it in and possibly add another. If that helps, keep it in. If a supplement makes no difference, drop it (and get your money back!) Do not use year round supplements that you find helpful. Save them for periods when you need a boost, i.e., at the end of training cycles. But still remember to keep 99% of your focus on the basic combination of training, rest and food.

## Nutritional supplements

20.123    Vitamin and mineral supplements, unless you are seriously deficient in something, cannot make an immediate impact on your training, other than perhaps the placebo effect in some cases. But what they may do, over the long term, is benefit your health which in turn increases training longevity. A good potency and well-balanced vitamin and mineral formula all the time is sensible for everyone. I strongly recommend beta-carotene and additional vitamins C and E, selenium, bioflavonoids and other anti oxidants because I believe they may be helpful for long-term health.

20.124    As noted in Chapter 15, taking a multi vitamin and mineral supplement may not be enough. There are micronutrients that are not available in supplement form. *You must eat a good diet.* Be sure, in particular, that you consume daily green leafy vegetables, yellow/orange vegetables and fruit, and regularly consume seeds, e.g., pumpkin and sunflower. And be sure you have a significant quantity of raw food daily.

20.125    Using an easily digested quality protein supplement when you are training very hard is the basic bodybuilding supplement to experiment with. If you are on a very tight budget, make your own protein drinks by adding skim milk powder (if you can digest it well) to milk.

20.126    Watch out for weight-gain products. While they may provide a big boost of calories (some of which come through protein), they can be difficult to digest. And some of these products grossly overdo things and are more accurately described as "fat-gain products."

20.127    Always remember that no matter how nutritious *anything* is, if you cannot digest it easily and comfortably it is not going to do you much if any good, no matter how expensive or hyped up it may be. Experiment with a *small* purchase of any food supplement to test how well *you* digest it. Some people find that skim milk powder stirred into fresh milk is easier to digest than expensive protein powders. The protein supplement that is the easiest of all for many people to digest is an increased quantity of fresh milk spread out over the day.

20.128   Even expensive "engineered" protein supplements can cause digestive tract distress for some people. And despite the advertising hoopla there is absolutely no guarantee that expensive cross-filtered, lactose-free whey with digestive enzymes and whey peptides will be easily digested.

20.129   Some of the advertising hype that goes with weight-loss products gives the impression that the special sachets and formulae do the fat-reduction job. What does the job is the user's combination of desire, exercise, calorie-reduced diet, and persistence. The meal replacement may contribute to the dietary part of it, but that is all. The success of a fat-loss program is not measured in terms of how much fat is lost in the short term, but by how much is kept lost over the long term. If you depend on anything for the short term—such as a meal replacement formula, and depriving yourself of real food—but revert to your usual eating and a lust for real food over the long term, then it has all been for nothing.

20.130   When mixing powder into a liquid, especially by hand, adding the liquid to the powder is usually more efficient than the other way around. Warm liquids produce better mixing than cold ones.

## Non-nutritional supplements

20.131   A long catalog of much-hyped but useless products (including "steroid replacements") have come and gone over the years, and plenty more will come and go in the future. When I wrote BRAWN, back in 1990/1991, some of the fashionable supplements were octacosanol, cytochrome C, beta-sitosterol, smilax officianalis, gamma oryzanol, inosine, yohimbe bark extract, cyclofenil, dibencozide and ferulic acid. How many of those do you see heavily touted today? None!

20.132   Some of these products did hang around for a few years even though they did not work. If enough people try something, just once, that is enough to make the scam worthwhile for manufacturers. And notice how often an "improved" version of an original scam is promoted, to get more mileage out of it.

20.133   One or a few of the current crop of vogue non-nutritional
         supplements will hang around for long enough to produce
         enough positive feedback to prolong sales, but nearly all of
         them will fall by the wayside as people discover that they do
         not work. Of course, this will happen only after a lot of money
         has been wasted; money that could have been better spent on
         quality food. So the supplement manufacturers will have to
         come up with other products. Hence, in a few years from now,
         different supplements will be touted to those that are doing
         the rounds today.

## Growth hormone and testosterone elevating compounds

20.134   A number of "supplements," e.g., androstene, androstenedione,
         pregnenolone, insulin growth factor derivatives, GABA, tribulus
         terrestris, and acetyl-carnitine, are each *claimed* to produce
         significant elevations in growth hormone or testosterone
         production. A lot of the advertising claims are plain dishonest,
         and some are based on non-human studies. If any of the
         hormone elevations are truly substantial, then the product
         concerned will soon become a prescription drug. No product
         that produces substantial hormonal changes is going to remain
         as a bodybuilding food supplement for long.

20.135   If you take hormone boosters for extended periods it is likely
         that your natural production of the hormone(s) concerned will
         be reduced or even impaired. Any substantial increase in
         hormone output beyond normal levels—other than for
         correcting deficiencies, and strictly under medical supervision
         (and even then it is a risky business)—is potentially dangerous.
         Just look at the havoc that steroids and growth hormone cause!

## Creatine

20.136   Creatine in its numerous forms has become perhaps the most
         popular bodybuilding supplement of the nineties (together
         with whey protein). For many users creatine does produce a
         fast gain in bodyweight over the first week or two of
         consumption, during the "loading" phase. But when they go

---

> **You should not be anti food supplements, but you should be anti anything that distracts you from a 99% focus on the fundamentals of basic training, basic rest, and basic nutrition through regular food.**

off it, they experience a *loss* of bodyweight. So what sort of weight did they add? Certainly not "solid" lasting muscle. To keep that water-weight people have to keep taking creatine.

20.137   Creatine *does not* work for all users, even the genuine creatine, and even when used exactly as directed by the manufacturer. Creatine has greatly distracted many people from the priorities of proper training and food-nutrition. Rather than learning about and then applying proven strategies of how to add 10–20 pounds of solid muscle yearly, for consecutive years, many people have got caught up in the excitement of the possibility of gaining 5–10 pounds of water weight over just 1–2 weeks. But then there is the downside—the impossibility of holding *all* that weight while going off creatine for a long period, and the impossibility of repeating the 5–10 pounds gain experience on a *cumulative* basis. *And of greatest importance is the fact that long-term creatine supplementation has not been proven as safe.*

## Closing words on food supplements

20.138   Never see food supplements as panaceas. Never get distracted from satisfying the fundamentals of sound training, and sound nutrition through ordinary food. Never look at supplement displays for answers to your training woes. The answers lay elsewhere, though prudent and rational use of quality supplements from reputable companies may help you on your way once you have a productive combination of training, food-nutrition and rest happening.

## Fat loss

20. 139   Many people who want bigger and stronger muscles also need to lose bodyfat. The fat and undermuscled hard gainer has a bigger mountain to climb than has a skinny hard gainer. Hard gainers are usually better off focusing on one type of body composition change at a time. If you have a lot of fat to lose, focus for a year or so on fixing that, while at least maintaining your current strength. Then switch your focus to building muscle without adding fat. But if you are a novice starting out fat, initially focus on gaining muscle—muscle is needed for fat burning.

20.140   Better than getting rid of excess fat is not getting fat in the first place. Some advice directed at skinny hard gainers encourages too rapid weight gaining. Do not go the mega-calorie trip. Too many people switch from weight-gain to weight-loss products.

20.141    While hard gainers can rarely stay extremely defined and still build muscle, it is possible to stay on the lean side so that you always look like a bodybuilder when you are not covered up.

20.142    There is lot more to looking good than being visibly big when dressed. Big arms, deltoids and chest do not look so good when the shirt comes off and there is a flabby waist underneath it all.

20.143    The waist pinch should be an essential marker of any weight-training program, so that you can keep close tabs on what sort of weight you are gaining. If your bodyfat is increasing too much, then you are eating too much. If your weight is going up and your fat pinch is staying constant, then you are gaining what you want—muscle. Accurate waist measuring can be a good indicator of body composition, but keep in mind that developing your lower back and oblique muscles will increase your waist measurement without increasing your bodyfat.

20.144    To keep closer tabs on your bodyfat, get some skinfold calipers. Calipers come with instructions for use that involve taking one or more skinfolds from specific sites on the body. By following the instructions you can estimate your total bodyfat percentage. You can use this to evaluate the composition of any weight gain (or loss), rather than rely on the more crude but still effective waist fat pinch.

**Body hardness**
20.145    The average adult male has about 13–17% bodyfat and the average adult female about 7% more, i.e., 20–24%. These are too high for showing muscular definition, so aim for 10% for men and 17% for women if you want to look well defined by the standards of non-competitive bodybuilders. To become "ripped" like a top-level competitive bodybuilder of today, men need to get down to no more than 5% bodyfat, and women to under 12%. The body *must* have some bodyfat. The essential fat for a man is about 5%, and for a woman about 12%. To get below those numbers is extreme, and fraught with possible health hazards. It demands obsessive behavior and may necessitate harmful drug assistance.

20.146    These percentages assume the use of an accurate method of testing. The accuracy of bodyfat determination varies according to the method used, and the expertise of the tester. Using the same subject, but different methods of fat determination, and different but experienced operators, percentages of several points difference may result.

20.147   If possible, seek out someone with considerable expertise at measuring bodyfat, and discover your current bodyfat percentage. Then compare that to the reading you get using your own skinfold calipers. Then you will get an idea of whether or not you are over- or under-calculating your bodyfat count. But more important than whether your particular technique produce accurate measurements, is the consistency of your technique and the *changes* in the percentage you measure over time.

20.148   A well-lighted mirror and a discriminating eye will tell you when you are defined enough. But keep in mind that your body has a "set point" for bodyfat. To go below that set point will probably involve extreme discipline and measures, and perhaps a heavy price in terms of lost muscle and might.

20.149   What is fat, what is smooth, what is lean, and what is very lean partly depends on your perspective. The "ripped-to-shreds" condition of top competitive bodybuilders is the extreme, and very unhealthy. A pinch of skin and subcutaneous tissue at the waist of these men taken in contest condition may be less than what most lean adult men have on the backs of their hands.

20.150   For general training purposes I suggest you keep yourself between lean and smooth, or approximately 10–13% bodyfat for a man, and 17–20% for a woman. Any less bodyfat than that and you may inhibit your muscle building. But going under 10% and 17% respectively is a necessary temporary condition if you want to look your best for a contest, photography session or other special occasion.

20.151   Some hard gainers, however, are naturally very lean, i.e., below 10% (male) and 17% (female). This is their natural condition which they do not have to discipline themselves to maintain. These people do not necessarily need to increase their bodyfat in order to gain muscle.

20.152   Bodyfat more than 15% may mistake you for a fat man rather than a muscleman, especially when you are dressed, unless you have huge muscles.

20.153    Before you apply yourself to getting a very low level of
          bodyfat, make sure you have enough muscle. Never forget
          that if you want better muscle shape you had better apply
          yourself to getting bigger muscles. Ideally, spend a few years
          getting big and strong while keeping your bodyfat level at no
          more than 15%, for a man.

20.154    Once you are satisfied with your development, at least for the
          time being, you can concentrate on detail, symmetry, definition
          and the full aesthetic package—if you are so motivated. If so,
          you may need to spend the necessary cycles on a sequence of
          specialization programs to correct apparent symmetry
          deficiencies—see *Framework 6* in Chapter 12. Then you will need
          to follow this specialization period, which could last as long as
          a year, with a fat-loss program in order to become very lean.

## Goal setting

20.155    Accurately calculate how much fat you need to lose to get
          yourself to a given bodyfat percentage, say 10%. For example,
          if you are 20% fat at 200 pounds, you have 40 pounds of
          bodyfat. To reduce to 10% fat you will have to lose 20 pounds
          of fat. You can then calculate how many months you need to
          get to your target. Knowing so specifically where you stand,
          and the map of progress to your goal, will help rivet your
          attention. If you are holding your muscle mass while losing
          bodyfat, your gross bodyweight will decrease in line with your
          fat loss. But if you are a beginner you may be able to maintain
          your gross bodyweight, or perhaps even increase it if you gain
          more weight of muscle than you lose of bodyfat.

20.156    Very importantly, lose bodyfat at no more than a pound a week,
          and preferably more like a pound every two weeks, so as not to
          risk altering your metabolism in a negative way. The body gets
          more efficient on a diet, especially if you make excessive
          reductions in your caloric intake. This needs to be avoided! This
          is why I urge moderate caloric reductions, along with a
          moderate increase in energy output, and the acceptance of a
          slow but gradual weight loss. The slow rate of weight loss is also
          necessary to minimize the risk of losing muscle. Scale weight is
          only part of the picture. The composition of the weight loss is
          the other major part. You want to lose fat, not muscle.

20.157    It took time to get smooth or fat in the first place, and it will
          take time to get lean. How long it will take depends on how

much fat you have to lose, how receptive your body is to losing fat, your age, and your degree of application to the program. Success will breed success. As you see the fruits of your dedication you will find it easier to maintain your discipline to produce further success.

## Desire

20.158   The most important deficiency among those who want to be lean is insufficient desire to get the job done. Sensible fat-loss programs work. But good advice counts for nothing unless you act on it with determination, diligence and persistence. Sensible fat-loss programs do not fail. It is the lack of consistent application of the program that causes the failure.

20.159   Because you are already a believer in the value of exercise, and are actually a regular exerciser, you are already well ahead of inactive people who want to lose bodyfat.

20.160   Whatever type of body you have got is all you are going to get. That a friend may be able to lose fat on 3,200 calories per day and without doing any aerobic work, while you need to drop to 2,200 *and* do moderate aerobics, is not important. What matters is doing what *you* need to do to get the job done.

20.161   Calorie counting may appear to be a chore, but quite quickly you will get to know how many calories you are eating *without* having to weigh everything and refer to a calorie breakdown book. Like with so many things, once you get in the swing of it, it becomes much easier than it appeared initially. Get to it—you can achieve a near miracle if you really want to do it, and if you have a good plan.

## Program for bodyfat loss

20.162   You will find gaining strength and muscle very difficult while losing bodyfat. But you can hold onto almost all of your muscular size (though gross size will be reduced), and nearly all of your strength, if you set about it properly. If, however, you are returning to training after a long layoff, or are a beginner, you may be able to increase muscular size and strength while simultaneously dropping bodyfat.

20.163   To hold onto your muscle, train as you would when gaining it in the first place—intensively, briefly and while focusing on the big exercises. If you switch to overtraining by increasing your training days, exercises, reps and sets, you will encourage your body to drop both muscle and fat, and perhaps *more* muscle than fat. To hold onto your muscle you have to impose the demands upon your body that will force it to keep what it has already developed. Train hard and briefly, and then get out of the gym and rest, recuperate fully, and then come back for another dose of hard and brief training. Before you start to lose bodyfat it is best that you have had the actual experience of gaining a substantial amount of muscle. Then you will know *first hand* what to apply to at least maintain your muscle mass.

20.164    Do not start a fat-loss program during the initial part of a training cycle. Wait until you have picked up the poundages and thus are training hard and providing the stimulus to retain all your muscle. Intensive weight training is an *essential* part of a fat-loss program. It is not merely optional.

20.165    Use a weight-training program from this book. If you are not quite at your previous strength best, then strive to get there week by week. Once there, strive to get stronger still, but if the bodyweight loss causes you to lose some strength, then focus on holding as much of your strength as you can. You do not need lots of sets and reps to do this strength maintenance work, just as you do not need them to get strong in the first place. One or two warmup sets per exercise followed by 1–3 hard work sets will do the job, if the work sets are intensive.

20.166    Because you are not going to feel at your strongest on a fat-loss program, select your training program accordingly. Do not get involved in 20-rep squats or deadlifts. These are brutal even when you are at your strongest in a gaining cycle. Also, avoid very low rep work because a little loss of strength will be very noticeable there. Stick to medium reps where you are more in control if or when your strength drops a little as you shed fat.

20.167    Before starting the fat-loss program, measure your waist girth and fat pinch and/or body composition, and your bodyweight. You will be taking these parameters regularly through the program. Be sure to take them at the *same* part of the day each time, and use the *same* method. Even if the bodyfat determining system you are using with calipers is not perfect, and even if you (and an assistant—depending on the instructions that accompany the fat calipers) cannot carry out the instructions perfectly, so long as you keep doing things the same way each time, that is all that really matters. This will give you the comparison, and that is what you need. Keep accurate written records in a book, not on pieces of paper that are easily mislaid.

20.168   Follow the guidelines given earlier in this chapter to find out how many calories you need to maintain your bodyweight.

20.169   Reduce your energy intake by 200 calories a day relative to your maintenance caloric intake. Any greater reduction risks causing the body to alter metabolism in a way that will hurt your fat-loss plans—the last thing you need. Drop the calories from refined and heavily processed food, should you be eating any. If you are only eating healthful food, and thus have no junk to cut out, trim the caloric reductions across the board by slightly reducing helping sizes. With some intelligent planning you can still eat a filling amount of nutrient-dense food without going to extremes like a very-low-fat diet.

20.170   For the macronutrient composition of your caloric intake, follow the same basic framework as given earlier in this chapter: about 20% fat, enough protein calories to provide at least one gram of protein per pound of lean body mass, and the balance of calories as complex fiber-rich carbohydrates. You could even try a higher fat intake, up to 30% of total caloric intake (all good fats, of course), and a corresponding

A modified dietary program, and a small energy deficit is one thing, but severe diets are another. Severe diets do not work over the long term because they produce denial, and binge eating. They can also alter the metabolism in such a way that fat loss becomes an even harder task to accomplish.

Your body has a minimum "set point" as far as your bodyfat is concerned. To try to get lower than that is extremely difficult to achieve. You may have to accept a bodyfat level a little higher than your ideal, because the price to pay for getting a lower bodyfat level may be extreme measures, loss of muscular bodyweight, and a negatively altered metabolism.

reduction in carbohydrate intake. Some people get better results with a moderate fat intake than a lower fat intake. The additional fat helps to keep hunger pangs at bay, and provides more eating pleasure, together with some possible biochemical benefits.

20.171   Take a quality broad spectrum vitamin and mineral supplement to be sure you are not short on micronutrients—the less food you eat, the greater the chance of not getting enough nutrients. Be sure to chew the tablets before you swallow them, or else they may leave your body as they went in—whole, and wasted.

20.172   Do not make your fat-loss diet into one of deprivation and extremes. You want to be able to keep to your new dietary program for the long term, not just stick to it for a month or two and then return to normal. There are *plenty* of tasty, filling and satisfying meals you can eat if you do some investigation and use your imagination.

20.173   Visit a bookstore and pick up a title that provides tasty and satisfying meals, while keeping calories in check. Nancy Clark's SPORTS NUTRITION GUIDEBOOK is a title to check out for help with recipes.

20.174   Along with the revised dietary schedule, increase your energy expenditure. Do this to enable you to eat enough to satisfy you both nutritionally and enjoyment wise, but while keeping you in energy deficit. You must be in energy deficit so that you draw upon your fat stores for the balance of your energy needs. Avoid vigorous aerobic activities because you do not want to hurt your ability to recover from your weight training. Covering a mile "burns" about the same calories whether you walk it, jog it or run it. The only difference is the speed of covering the distance. Add walking to your weekly schedule. Start with three walks a week for 20 minutes each, preferably on the days you do not train with weights. Without getting carried away and turning the walks into competitive races, pick up the speed of the walks a little as the weeks go by so that you cover more distance in the same time period, and increase the duration of your walks to 30 or more minutes at a time. If you are grossly fat, then walk for an hour or more every day until you have your fat level under control. Aerobic exercise that works more musculature than walking, e.g., use of rowers and ski machines, uses more energy for the same time investment and perceived effort, and is thus a better choice. If you have access to this machinery, use it several times a week.

20.175   Religiously maintain your bodyweight maintenance caloric intake minus 200 calories for four weeks, along with the stepped up energy output. A 200 calorie reduction in input, together with, say, an increased average output of 200 a day (approximately equivalent to walking two miles a day), totals a 400 daily caloric deficit (2,800 per week). That will produce adequate results for many people, keeping in mind that a pound of fat contains 3,500 calories. But if no bodyweight loss is registered, reduce your caloric intake by a further 100 and test again a few weeks later. Continue this process until you discover the caloric intake that produces a gradual but steady loss of no more than a pound a week, preferably a pound every two weeks.

20.176   The absolute minimum caloric intake you should have is 12 calories per pound of lean bodyweight. If you go lower than that, assuming you are fairly active and doing the minimum aerobic exercise, you are going to lose weight too fast, strip off more muscle than fat, and risk messing up your metabolism. Most people should be able to slowly but steadily lose fat by consuming their maintenance caloric intake minus 100–200, together with an *increase* in their energy output. If you do little or no aerobic activity, you need to trim more calories from your food intake. It *is* possible to lose fat while doing no aerobic activity, so long as you adjust your caloric intake accordingly and maintain or increase your muscle mass. The main advantage of increasing your activity level is to permit you to consume more calories. Without getting into extreme levels of activity, the more calories you can consume and yet still lose fat, the better. Then you are physically and mentally better sated, plus you are more likely to meet your needs for nutrients.

20.177   Whenever you get the urge to consume something you know you should not, see in your mind two images—the lean body you want, and your current physique. Remind yourself that you want the "new" body, and discard the offending food item. Unless you are unusually strong willed and can say no to anything, go through your kitchen and get rid of everything that is going to tempt you to break your new dietary schedule.

There are probably others in your household who would also benefit from dropping some bodyfat, so you can all get in on this together. If not, then the others around you should be understanding and eat at different times or in different locations. No matter how it works out in practice, try to make matters as painless as possible. But the bottom line is that you need willpower to stick to the new program for month after month after month.

20.178   Stay clear of food temptations! Keep your eyes and mind off food. At parties, socialize away from the food area. Keep out of the kitchen when at home. When out shopping, steer away from the most appetizing food. But keep in mind the adage, "A little of what you fancy does you good." Occasionally satisfying a craving is better than denying yourself and then finding you cave in and open the floodgates to lots of "forbidden" food. But if you do not have any cravings, then there is nothing you need to treat yourself to. And should you go overboard on any given day's calorie quota, compensate for it by adding a couple of long walks to your usual activity for that week.

20.179   Reward successful dieting with something that is not food. For example, buy yourself an item of clothing, a compact disc or a book upon getting to a specific target.

20.180   Avoid letting yourself get very hungry. There are two approaches to try, to see which gives you the best control over hunger. Either have three medium-sized meals a day, or five or six small meals. With both options, avoid eating heavily late in the day. On a fat-loss program, finish your last regular meal by 7PM. But just before you go to sleep, have an apple, a raw carrot, or something else that is bulky but low in calories, *together* with some protein, to help prevent muscle loss.

20.181   Eat some raw and bulky food with each meal to help fill your stomach and satisfy your appetite. Start with a salad. And drink lots of water over the course of each day.

20.182   Eat slowly. This will help to sate your appetite. Sit down to eat. Do not eat on the move. Take your time. Take small mouthfuls and chew each thoroughly. Not only will this more likely sate your appetite than fast eating, but you will enjoy your food more even though you are consuming less of it.

20.183   To close this section, a reminder to lose fat slowly. A steady loss is easier to sustain mentally and physically, and lets you train with the effort you need to hold onto your muscle, and recuperate from this training. If you lose weight too quickly, you invite a loss of energy, a substantial loss of strength, and a tendency to loosen your form in the gym to compensate. This brings injury and the ruining of your training.

## Switching to a gaining program

20.184   When you are at a satisfactory level of bodyfat, keep yourself there, or thereabouts. To switch to anabolic mode, increase your caloric intake enough to get gaining but *without* your bodyfat increasing much if at all; and increase the number of times you eat unless you are already eating five or six times a day. Up your daily caloric intake by just 200 for the first few weeks. If your fat pinch is steady after a few weeks, add another 100 calories. Continue until you find the maximum number you can consume without increasing your bodyfat. Keep close tabs on your caloric intake and body composition, and adjust the former accordingly if or when necessary. But as noted earlier in this chapter, gaining a *little* fat while you build a lot of muscle is fine, and in many cases it is actually *necessary*.

20.185   If you adjust your energy expenditure, this needs to be reflected in your energy intake. For example, if you reduce your aerobic work you need to trim your caloric intake accordingly.

20.186   For as long as you want to stay lean you will need to control your eating very carefully. This means a life-long dedication to dietary control. It should never mean extremes and deprivation if it is to be successful, but for sure you need to be in firm control. The better your physique becomes, and the more satisfied you are with how you look, the easier it will be to exert the control you need to keep yourself looking good.

### Further reading

20.187   The fat-loss strategy given in this chapter is neither very-low-fat nor very-low-carbohydrate, but built on calorie control. Two opposing opinions in the bodybuilding world regarding losing bodyfat are represented by Clarence Bass and Jay Robb. Bass advises a high-carbohydrate and very-low-fat diet together with lots of aerobic work, while Robb recommends (relative to Bass) a low-carbohydrate, high-protein, moderate-fat diet (but "friendly" fats not "garbage fats like margarine, hydrogenated oils, high heated oils, processed oils or palm kernel oils," to quote Robb), plus a moderate amount of aerobic work. Both approaches can work, but some people are more suited to one than the other. Another option is the middle-ground approach given in this chapter.

20.188    For detailed counsel on the Bass and Robb approaches, write to:
a.  Clarence Bass, 528 Chama NE, Albuquerque, NM 87108, USA
b.  Jay Robb, 1530 Encinitas Blvd., Encinitas, CA 92024, USA

## You are not just what you eat

20.189    "You are what you eat," says the cliché. But there is much more to it than that. For a start, what you actually eat is only the beginning. What you digest and assimilate is what counts, not just what you swallow. But you are so much more than that. You are also a reflection of your lifestyle, activity levels, working environment, relationships, emotions, and more. As important as nutrition undoubtedly is, your health is the result of a composite of many factors. Even if your nutrition is "perfect," your health will be severely compromised by major emotional stress on the domestic or work front. Much more important than worrying about whether you are getting a few calories of fat too many, or too little of a given micronutrient, is removing the major sources of stress from your life. **BB**

## How to avoid catabolism

Going too long between meals puts you in catabolic mode, which is the antithesis of what is needed for muscle building. This is why you should have feeds every three hours or so. Short workouts are needed for two reasons—to minimize the chance of overtraining, and to prevent excessive delay between feeds. An easily digested liquid meal 90 minutes before training, a general warmup followed by a 60-minute workout, followed very soon by another easily digested liquid meal, will mean about three hours between those feeds. That should keep you in anabolic mode.

A liquid meal does not mean a glass of water or juice with a food supplement stirred in. It means something much more substantial and nutritious—e.g., a large milk-based drink, or solid food liquefied in a blender.

So far in this book, the maxim of "build strength to build size" has been promoted. This is, however, a SIMPLIFIED maxim. Though it has great practical value for most of the training of most people, the maxim does not apply in all cases at all times—depending on the individual, set-rep format used, current training experience and development, and other factors. Some methods of building strength do not, at least in some cases, build much if any size. The "build strength to build size" simplification may need to be modified, depending on the individual. This chapter describes interpretations of abbreviated training that should be tried if you find that required gains in muscular size do not accompany strength gains— assuming, of course, you want to build more size.

# 21. Additional Important Training Information

*This is an important supplementary chapter for the revised edition of* BEYOND
BRAWN. *It contains information not discussed in detail in the initial edition. The
information comes from a three-part series of articles published in* HARDGAINER
*issues 72, 73 and 74, revised for use in this book.*

21.1    The ideas in this chapter are *strictly* for trainees who are *already*
        converted to the merits of abbreviated training, and who are
        *experienced* in applying it and finding out how their bodies
        respond to it. Considering bodybuilders and strength trainees in
        general, most of them need to *reduce* their training volume and
        frequency. But of those who *have* followed abbreviated programs
        for a good while, some may benefit from *prudently* increasing
        their training frequency and volume *as described in this chapter*,
        but while *still* staying in the scope of abbreviated training.

## Strength, mass and training frequency

21.2    This book has already provided different interpretations of
        abbreviated training. This chapter provides additional ideas, to
        help you find what works best *for you*, or at least what works well.

21.3    If your sleeping and nutritional habits are in a mess, no amount
        of experimenting with exercise program design will make much
        difference. I am taking it as a given that the major components
        of recovery are in *excellent* order.

21.4    Some trainees and trainers are adamant about the need to train
        each exercise, or at least most of them, every 4–5 days, and
        report examples of folk who detrain if they work the exercises
        on a lesser frequency. Then there are other trainees and trainers
        who are equally adamant about the need for less frequent
        training of individual exercises, and they report examples of folk
        who stagnate or even lose strength when using the greater

frequency. Both groups cannot all be all right, but at the same time both groups cannot be all wrong. Truth be told, both approaches work for some people, and both groups have probably disregarded the trainees who did not do well on the regimens that the reported success stories used.

21.5    I am adamant about the need for a *range* of interpretations within the overall framework of abbreviated training. Many variables, at least in part, can explain why one interpretation works well for some people, but not for others. These variables cannot be identified and quantified so that we can say we are comparing like with like when considering different groups of trainees. These variables include training intensity, genetics and individual recovery potential (even if nutrition and sleep are optimized), age, strength level, length of routine, and exercise selection.

21.6    No one can know your individual situation as well as you, and no one can train you as well as you can *providing* you know enough about training and all the related components. You need to combine this information with an understanding of your own unique situation, tailor it to suit you, experiment to find what works best for you, and adjust your lifestyle in order to enhance your recovery and thus improve your response to training.

21.7    Response to substantial strength increase varies. Some people get substantial increases in size when they achieve substantial increases in strength, while others get only modest increases in size from substantial increases in strength. Some people do not want to get a lot bigger, and desire maximum strength at only a modest size. Others are far more size and appearance focused, and see strength gains purely as a means for building bigger muscles.

21.8    Infrequent training—i.e., hitting each exercise once a week, or less often—at least for some people, builds a lot of strength but not much size. I have even heard reports from some people who have reduced their training frequency and volume to extreme levels—like a single work set per exercise every three weeks, or even less frequently—and yet have *still* managed to increase their strength, *but with no increases in size whatsoever.* For these trainees, just moving to a more common interpretation of abbreviated training whereby each exercise is worked once a week, may yield the required size gains. *But for trainees who are not making required size gains on the once-a-week training of each exercise, trying the ideas detailed in the rest of this chapter makes sense.*

21.9    More frequent training, *within reason*, may build the same strength increases and produce more size; or, it may yield greater strength and size gains. In some cases, the greater frequency of training may build less strength but more size, *relatively speaking*. You need to experiment, sensibly, to find the right balance for you. Naturally, if you increase training frequency too much, your progress in all respects will stagnate or even go backwards. There can be a fine line between enough, and too much.

21.10   *Your level of strength and development can affect the effectiveness of a given interpretation of training. While more frequent training may better suit novice and some intermediate bodybuilders, it may be a negative step for advanced power men.*

21.11   If you are steadily getting stronger, and strength is your priority, stay with what you are currently doing. If you are getting stronger from abbreviated training, but not seeing the size increases that you think should accompany the strength gains, I suggest you try the following.

## Twice-a-week divided program . . . *modified*
21.12   The additional Framework I want to include is a modified version of Framework 2 in Chapter 12. Framework 2 has a full-body list of exercises divided into two groups, and each group or routine is typically performed once a week.

21.13   For the "Twice-a-week divided program . . . *modified*," split the full-body (but still abbreviated) list of exercises into two routines with no serious overlap, then alternate the routines over *three* workouts per week, rather than the two workouts per week as in Framework 2. In this way, instead of each exercise being hit once per week and thus two times every two weeks, each movement is now hit three times every *two* weeks, i.e., every four or at most five days. Here is an example:

### Monday
   a.  Squat or squat equivalent
   b.  Stiff-legged deadlift from just below the knees
   c.  Calf raise
   d.  Ab work

### Wednesday
   a.  Dip
   b.  Chin or pulldown

    c. Overhead press
    d. L-fly

### Friday
    a. Squat or squat equivalent
    b. Stiff-legged deadlift from just below the knees
    c. Calf raise
    d. Ab work

### Monday
    a. Dip
    b. Chin or pulldown
    c. Overhead press
    d. L-fly

21.14   Rotate the routines on subsequent workout days. I have included the "big five" movements here, plus three important accessory exercises. Recovery "space" permitting, an additional accessory movement could be added to each routine—perhaps back extensions or side bends, and curls or neck work.

21.15   *The deadlift in particular (though not included in this illustrative program), and perhaps the squat and stiff-legged deadlift too, may still be best trained only once a week, depending on the individual.* So you may need to fine-tune the training frequency of those exercises.

21.16   As far as sets and reps go, use what you have found work well for you. If you do not know what this is, please follow the guidelines given in Chapters 9 and 13.

21.17   *Do not increase volume of training along with an increased frequency, or else you may undo the possible good of the additional frequency.* If, for example, you normally use warmups plus 2 or at most 3 hard work sets per exercise, stick with that. If you normally do warmups plus just a single very hard work set, stick with that.

21.18   While alternating the two different routines over three workouts per week rather than two may not appear a big change, it is actually a major increase in training frequency. It is a 50% increase, and may make a noticeable difference in the muscular development you experience while you build strength. Instead of training each exercise every seventh day, now it moves to every fourth or fifth day. This is a sensible experiment, but for it to be a positive change, there are three *essential* requirements:

a. Full satisfaction of the components of recovery. This is easily said, but not so easily achieved. It means, primarily, a high quality diet every day that provides a caloric and nutritional surplus, spread over five or preferably six feeds each day, and a full night of sleep *every* night, which means sleeping till you wake naturally each morning. It is not just for this program that you need full satisfaction of the components of recovery. *But if you cut any corners on a three-days-per-week exercise program, the negative impact will probably be greater than on a two-days-per-week program.*

b. If you are not gaining in strength on a two-days-per-week program, a shift to three workouts a week is unlikely to make a positive difference, *and the explanation for your lack of progress rests elsewhere.* The boost in training frequency is targeted at producing greater size gains along with *sustained* strength increases.

c. The routines must be short. You should be done inside an hour—longer than that and you are either doing too much work or you are hanging around too long between sets.

21.19   While you may not be able to progress steadily over the long term on three workouts per week, you may be able to for 2–3 months periodically, and revert to two weight-training days per week at other times. But if you consistently gain better in size and strength on three workouts per week than on two, and you want the extra size, stick with the three workouts.

21.20   Some trainees have greater recovery ability than others, be it from genetics or the extent of your satisfaction of the components of recovery (or both). I do not know you, your lifestyle, motivation, and the control you have over your lifestyle. Lifestyle control, however, is usually more motivation-based than actual events-based—if you want a better physique badly enough, you will arrange your life accordingly so that you eat and sleep better.

21.21   The "Twice-a-week divided program . . . *modified*" is especially worth a try if you have been gaining strength well on a two-days-per-week program, but have not been gaining as much muscle as you would think should be associated with such strength gains. The increase in training frequency may make a significant difference.

## A long-term experiment

21.22    For an experiment to be worthwhile, you need to be consistent
         with satisfying the components of recovery. If on one program
         you are more consistent with getting a caloric and nutrient
         surplus, I would expect better progress on that program even
         if the actual training program is not as potentially valuable as
         another in the trial. So, with recovery in excellent order, try each
         of these schedules for *at least* six weeks apiece, and see if you
         notice any changes in strength gain and accompanying size gain.

21.23    You need to fine-tune the exercise selection and training days, for
         example, to suit you; and you may prefer to put the four
         schedules in a different order.

### Test schedule #1

21.24    *Twice-a-week divided program . . . modified (as described earlier)*

### Test schedule #2

21.25    *Twice-a-week divided program*
         **Monday**
         a.  Squat or squat equivalent
         b.  Stiff-legged deadlift from just below the knees
         c.  Calf raise
         d.  Ab work

         **Thursday**
         a.  Dip
         b.  Chin or pulldown
         c.  Overhead press
         d.  L-fly

### Test schedule #3

21.26    *Twice-a-week full-body program, same major exercises each time*
         **Monday**
         a.  Squat or squat equivalent
         b.  Stiff-legged deadlift from just below the knees
         c.  Dip
         d.  Chin or pulldown
         e.  Overhead press
         f.  L-fly

         **Thursday**
         a.  Squat or squat equivalent
         b.  Dip

   c.  Chin or pulldown
   d.  Overhead press
   e.  Calf raise
   f.  Ab work

*The exceptions to the twice-a-week frequency general rule are the stiff-legged deadlift and accessory exercises, which are only worked once a week each, to keep the routines short.*

## Test schedule #4
21.27   *Twice-a-week full-body program, different exercises each time*
### Monday
   a.  Squat or squat equivalent
   b.  Stiff-legged deadlift from just below the knees
   c.  Dip
   d.  Chin or pulldown
   e.  Overhead press
   f.  L-fly

### Thursday
   a.  Leg press
   b.  Back extension
   c.  Bench press
   d.  One-arm dumbbell row
   e.  Dumbbell press
   f.  Calf raise
   g.  Ab work

*A variation of the deadlift is performed only once a week here. Accessory work is only worked once a week for each involved area.*

21.28   The variety of schedules may yield consistent gains from program to program, be it from mental variety that keeps you "fresh" and motivated, or from the change in the actual training stimulation that keeps your gains coming. On the other hand, you may find that one or two of the schedules are noticeably more productive than the others.

## Strength *without* size, strength *with* size
21.29   HARDGAINER magazine, as well as my books and articles, have emphasized progressive strength gains as the principle means by which muscular bodyweight can be acquired. Although the precise mechanisms for how muscle is built are not fully understood, there is a correlation between added strength and

increased muscle mass. However, the correlation is often not linear, and it is possible to become considerably stronger *without* developing much bigger muscles.

21.30   An outstanding example of "strength without size" is Judd Biasiotto. Biasiotto, in 1986, squatted 575 pounds in competition at just 131 pounds bodyweight! He has also bench pressed 319 and deadlifted 529. For such a small man, these are staggering lifts, and show that there can be much more to strength demonstrations than size.

21.31   How strength and size are related varies among individuals, and is heavily linked to training methods *and* genetic factors. Better motor skills, advantageous tendon attachments and other superior structures/leverages for specific movements, greater willpower, etc., all combine to demonstrate strength without substantial muscular size.

21.32   Stronger muscles can mean bigger muscles (but not always), just like bigger muscles can mean stronger muscles (but not always). Maximum strength does not equate to maximum size, and neither does maximum size equate to maximum strength.

21.33   On specific exercises I have made substantial gains in strength while maintaining consistent form, *but with no increase in muscular size.* Many others have experienced the same sort of thing. In some exercises I have been able to out-lift much larger muscled trainees. While genetics play a role, training methods provide part of the explanation. While the training approach I used on those specific exercises (i.e., low reps or rest-pause high reps, hard single work sets, frequency of once-a-week maximum per exercise) was perfect for strength gains, it was ineffective for maximizing size gains—at least for me.

21.34   I have used volume training methods with no gains whatsoever in size or strength. And many of you have also tried volume training, without success. So flipping to volume training is not the solution for producing size gains for typical trainees.

21.35   The explanation for the non-linear non one-to-one relationship between strength and size, at least for many trainees, may lie in the composition of the muscles. Muscle cells are not made up of just the contractile elements (myofibrils) that produce strength. There are three major components of muscle cells—

the myofibrils, sarcoplasm (plasm within the cell) and mitochondria (the energy converters). The latter two yield muscle cell volume but are not contractile elements. Strength-focus training acts substantially on only the strength-yielding contractile components of the muscle cells.

21.36    Trainees who seem to respond in size pretty much linearly with strength may have a larger proportion of myofibrils in their muscle cells than other trainees.

21.37    To build size at an optimal rate—for all trainees—it may be necessary to address the components of muscle cells other than just the pure strength-yielding ones. But there is a big danger here—*try to do too much at the same time and you are likely to overtrain and thus kill progress in both size and strength.*

21.38    Many people seem to find that substantial strength gain is less difficult to achieve than substantial lean muscle gain. It may be that consistent practice of certain exercises in a specific strength-focus manner produces greater skill and neurological efficiency that yields greater strength *without* any enlargement of any volume-related element of muscle cells.

21.39    For function-first strength-focus trainees, muscle gain is of secondary importance. For some trainees, e.g., competitive lifters, strength gain is required *without* any size gain. But for many of you, lean muscle gain is the priority. Different trainees have different goals and values.

21.40    If you are more interested in size than strength—more concerned with appearance than function—you may need to train more frequently and perhaps in a different style too, to get closer to your particular genetic "ceiling." This does *not*, however, mean a lurch to mainstream routines. A bit more frequency, a bit more volume and a different set/rep format can *still* keep you in the confines of abbreviated training, albeit not as abbreviated as it can be for pure strength training.

## Enriching your training

21.41    Over the decades, bodybuilding has produced examples of men who have built very large muscles but without the strength that you would normally expect would accompany such large muscles. The training methods that account for this are typically called "pumping." The most striking examples of the success of this type of training are either genetic phenomena or drug assisted, or both. I am *not* advocating pure pumping.

21.42 If you are gaining strength well, but not getting much if any bigger, and your recovery machinery really is in good order, *you need to make some changes if you want to build size.*

21.43 My recommendation is that you first experiment with training frequency, and try things as given in the first part of this chapter. Then, if you still feel you are not getting the size gains you think your strength progress should produce, try further changes.

21.44 When strength building, adding just 10 pounds to your squat is not likely to make any measurable or visible difference to your quads. It is *substantial* strength gain that is more likely to produce significant size gain. If, however, you add 100 pounds to your squat with no noticeable size gain on your quads (or proportional increases in other exercises without any growth), that is when you need to make changes in your training *if* you want better size gains.

21.45 In general, and of course there are exceptions, here are perhaps the main variations between training with the emphasis on strength, and training with the emphasis on size:

**Strength focus**
a. low reps
b. long rests between sets
c. pauses between reps (on some movements by some trainees)
d. infrequent training
e. few work sets (low volume of work)

**Size focus**
a. higher reps
b. briefer rests between sets
c. very short or no pauses between reps
d. greater frequency of training
e. not so few sets (higher volume of work)

21.46 Some training approaches mix the two focuses. For example, classic 20-rep rest-pause squats combine high reps and long pauses between reps, and have produced many examples of substantial strength *and* size gains; and some strength afficionados perform many low-rep sets.

21.47    Compare how you train against the summary given above. For
         example, if you rest 5 minutes between sets of squats, always
         take a good few seconds pause between reps, do just a single
         work set of each exercise, and squat once every ten days, your
         training may have produced substantial strength but not
         necessarily substantial size.

21.48    A moderate increase in training frequency—as outlined in the
         first part of this chapter—and perhaps later on some
         adjustments in set and rep format, and rep performance (while
         keeping within the confines of abbreviated training), may make
         a *substantial* difference in terms of size gains. Whether strength
         gains will continue as before, or be moderated, is another
         matter, and will be determined by individual considerations
         (including genetic) and the particular training adjustments
         made. But, remember, tinker too much and you will kill gains
         in both size *and* strength. Make changes in a systematic trial-
         and-error basis. Keep what helps, drop what hinders.

## Practical examples
### Set-rep change #1
21.49    A possibility for increasing hypertrophy, *but while keeping
         strength gains moving as before*, is to add a couple of back-down
         sets to each exercise.

21.50    For an example of an equal-strength-and-size-focus approach
         (for want of a better description), I will use an illustration of 380
         for 2 sets of 5 reps in the barbell squat, with 5 minutes rest
         between all work sets, and several seconds break between reps.
         Reduce to just one work set, keep all the other variables
         constant, but add two back-down sets. Just 90 seconds after the
         380 x 5 in the squat, perform maximum reps with 250 pounds,
         and 90 seconds later do maximum reps with 250 once again.
         For the second of the back-down sets, your reps will be down
         relative to the first one.

> **If you are not already getting stronger on your current
> program, or know from experience *precisely* what
> builds strength for you, do not even think of trying
> the suggestions given in this chapter. If you cannot
> gain strength well, albeit slowly and steadily, then
> your training is hugely out of order and what you need
> to do to fix matters is not covered in this chapter.**

21.51   This approach has the advantage of maintaining the bedrock of strength-focus work, so that you keep plugging along getting stronger and stronger still (which is enjoyable and satisfying in its own right, of great functional value, and which still contributes to overall size), while mixing it with volume-focus supplementary work which you can vary over time—e.g., you can change rep count and rest periods.

21.52   *If the strength work remains similar to how it was on the strength-focus program, perhaps the training frequency should not change.* It would be the addition of the size-focus back-down sets that may offer the opportunity for size to accompany strength gain.

21.53   While a strength-focus program *performed with greater frequency* (as described in the early part of this chapter) may yield greater size gains, your *usual* training frequency but with the *addition* of the back-down sets (as just described in this "Set-rep change #1" section) may achieve a similar result. The latter may be the more practical, as it does not reduce the number of rest days between hits on the same exercise.

## Set-rep change #2

21.54   As a second set-rep change possibility, but one that is unlikely to build the strength of the first, say you have been progressing very nicely in strength, and have reached 380 for 2 sets of 5 in the barbell squat, with 5 minutes rest between work sets, and several seconds break between reps. The set/rep scheme and rep style are more favored to strength than size, and may not have produced the growth that was anticipated. To convert it into an approach that may have more of a size focus, the squat could, as an illustration, move to 275 pounds for 3 sets of 12, all sets done with no more than one second pause between reps, and only 90 seconds rest between sets. Only the final set would be *very* hard. Then you would apply the usual dictum of progressive poundages in good form, but while maintaining this very different albeit still abbreviated approach to training.

21.55   Being conditioned to lower reps, pauses between reps, and long inter-set rests, there may need to be a greater cutting back of poundage to begin with than in this illustration. With time, the weights will come back, and may be accompanied by size gains.

21.56   When you make a shift from a strength focus to a size focus (or from a strength focus to an equal strength and size focus), you may notice a dramatic effect on how your muscles feel as you train. If you have not been experiencing much soreness in your muscles from strength-focus training, if you switch to a size focus or equal size and strength focus, you may be in for substantial soreness in the days following your revised workouts.

## Important supplementary notes

21.57    What is excessive abbreviation of training for some trainees may be just the ticket for others. Different trainees need different interpretations of the same basic principles, and may need different variations at different stages of their training. But just because a bit more training volume and frequency can be good (if you have cut back excessively previously), that does not mean that a lot more will be better. *Training is more an art than a science*, and sensible experimentation is needed if you are to find what works best for you. You must, however, keep your training abbreviated, as typical trainees do not have the ability to deal with the type of routines that the gifted and drug-enhanced folk use and prosper on.

21.58    Do not misinterpret my advice and go jacking up your training to such an extent that you kill progress in all areas. *If you have been using conventional training methods, the last thing you need is to increase your training frequency or volume. You need to abbreviate.*

21.59    Full satisfaction of recovery is vital for optimum strength gains on a very abbreviated program, but it becomes *even more critical* on a less abbreviated size-focus or size-and-strength-focus program. If you have trouble satisfying recovery on a strength-focus program, do not switch to a different focus until you can get recovery in 100% good order (as outlined earlier in this chapter), or otherwise you are going to be disappointed.

21.60    I am not saying that light-weight pumping exercise on a daily basis will build a great physique. You still need to use some impressive poundages and have more rest days than training days. But *how* you use those weights—frequency of training, and set-rep format and style—can greatly affect *how much size those weights deliver.* If you are satisfied with the results you are getting from your training, do not change anything. But if you are not satisfied with your size gains (though you have gained lots of strength), you may need to switch from a total focus on manipulating training variables to achieve more weight on the bar, to a focus on achieving weight on the bar *and* size on your body. *A moderate increase in training frequency, and/or a change in set-rep format and style, may be all you need to turn weight on the bar into weight on your body.*

## The genetic factor

21.61    If you have trained for many years, and are very strong (by all standards except the really gifted folk), it is possible you are very close to your maximum *muscular* size. But you can never know for sure, so I would say that unless you have age or health limitations, and still want bigger muscles, you should still target them. That said, you will eventually reach a point—whatever that is—where you are very close to your natural limit for muscular size. However, even when you do reach it, you may still be able to build a good deal more strength (without much more size), so long as you are not limited by age or health. There is much more to training than building bigger muscles, especially once you are already well developed.

## How come the modified views?

21.62    I have been concerned that some trainees have taken the mentality of reduced frequency of training too far (though, in general, most trainees train too much). If you have found that you have been gaining strength steadily, but without much if any accompanying size, it may be that you have been training too infrequently. So experiment with increasing frequency, at least in some exercises (if you want more size).

21.63    Higher frequency ("higher" being *relative* to hitting each exercise only once every 7, 10 or even 14 days—which may still build strength) may promote better size gains; but train too often and you will build neither strength nor size. Here is where individual experimentation is needed. Please do not misinterpret my views. I am saying, for example, that training a given exercise three times every *two* weeks *may* increase size gains relative to training that exercise just once per week. I am *not* saying, for example, that hitting each exercise hard three times a week will give even better results—such a training frequency is overkill for even many genetic phenomena.

21.64    How come I have modified my point of view on this matter? I have always acknowledged individual variation, and the need (within reason) for individual experimentation on training frequency of each exercise. In this chapter I am giving increased emphasis on this point, and some definite suggestions for experimentation in order to find what works best for you. Reader feedback and personal experience, for sure, have contributed; and some folk claim there is some backup "science" too.

21.65    Some trainees have taken the "less is more" maxim too far. I want to encourage that *minority* of people to investigate the possibility that they may have done just that. "Less is more" is appropriate *only up to a certain point*, but what that point is varies among individuals. What may *not* be enough for some trainees, may be just right for some others to grow like weeds.

21.66    Experiment in a *careful* and *progressive* way. *But, once again, all the components of recovery must first be in 100% perfect order.* Doubling training frequency and adding back-down sets will be overkill for almost everyone. But perhaps just increasing frequency *or* volume *a little,* may be helpful, *but only if you have "overabbreviated" your training.*

21.67    Even within the framework of abbreviated training with a maximum of three weights workouts per week, there is considerable room for variation in order to find the particular approach that produces the results you want.

21.68    *Do not, however, think that poundage progression is no longer important,* and all that matters is training frequency, and set-rep format. Poundage progression is *very* important. *You still need progressive resistance, but the precise format of training you apply the "progressive poundages in good form" to (frequency, volume, rep count, etc.) can greatly influence how much size a given strength increase produces.*

## The food factor

21.69    Finally, some trainees have not been gaining any muscle (though they have gained some strength), at least in part because they have not been eating enough. Eating more (perhaps a lot more in some cases), not training excessively infrequently (or excessively frequently), avoiding *pure* strength-focus training methods such as very low reps, *yet still building strength*, are necessary for these people to gain substantial muscle mass *along with* gaining substantial strength. Strength gain does not always equal size gain, depending on how the strength was built, and the attention given to factors including nutrition. ▣

*I have said this before, but it warrants repetition:*

*"As Charles A. Smith told me shortly before his death, 'You never know how important good health is until you no longer have it.' Think about this. Dwell on it. Make it one with you while you still have your health, not when it is too late. Avoid all harmful habits, activities and environments. Look after yourself!"*

# 22. Beyond the Exterior

22.1    There is much more to looking good and feeling great than
        having big and strong muscles. If you are not healthy on the
        inside, then sooner or later you will be unable to maintain size
        and strength on the outside. *Your health is of supreme importance.*

22.2    Always being locked into the bigger and stronger mode, *even
        after you have already built impressive size and strength*, is
        something to avoid. I have known many trainees who have
        grasped the value of aerobic work, a health-producing diet,
        and reducing bodyfat, but yet forever put off making
        changes in their lifestyles because they first wanted to get
        even bigger and stronger.

22.3    Once you are over age thirty-five, the heavy diet and the
        training program free of aerobic work that packed on size and
        strength in your youth *will* make you bigger and stronger, *but
        at a cost*. Poor cardiorespiratory fitness takes its toll as you get
        into middle age and older, *perhaps even a fatal toll*. Excess
        bodyfat is harder to take off the older you get.

22.4    After you have hit age thirty-five, balance your total program
        and give *serious* attention to your diet and cardiorespiratory
        training. If you are already in your middle years, but a training
        novice, you need to build bigger and stronger muscles by using
        a balanced program right from the start.

22.5    As valuable as aerobic work can be, and as worthwhile as it is
        to be fit, being fit does not necessarily mean you are healthy.
        It is possible to be unfit and healthy, or fit and unhealthy.
        Factors including not smoking, not having high blood pressure,
        following a healthful diet, avoiding excessive stress, being
        happy with your work and life, and being lean are, in total,
        much more influential in affecting your health than is the
        single factor of aerobic work.

## Health tests

22.6      Regular blood and urine tests will let you see how you are doing internally. If you are under age thirty-five, have a blood and urine test every three years. If you are over thirty-five, have a test done annually. Consult a cardiologist or your physician for the procedure to follow that is most appropriate for you, and for help with interpreting the test results.

22.7      A very valuable and fascinating project is to monitor improvements in your test results following changes in your diet and exercise program. Chronicling changes for the better is great reward for the increased discipline given to your diet and exercise program.

22.8      Suppose you have been on a heavy diet for years, are over 15% bodyfat, and never do cardiorespiratory exercise. This is a common scenario among experienced bodybuilders and lifters. Get your blood and urine tested. Then overhaul your diet and exercise program. Substitute skim milk for whole milk; substitute virgin olive oil for all liquid oils, margarine and butter; consume more raw food; boost your fiber intake; add anti-oxidant food supplements, including vitamins C and E; cut out sugar and junk food; eat generously of foods rich in essential fatty acids (e.g., sardines, mackerel and sunflower seeds); reduce your bodyfat below 15%; and add moderate aerobic work to your exercise program three times a week. Should you be a smoker, then you must stop. Do this faithfully for six months and then get your blood and urine tested again. You should see a big improvement in your cholesterol, triglycerides, HDL, LDL and uric acid levels, among other markers. There will be an accompanying big improvement in your internal health. Then maintain this new profile of health markers by sticking with the overhauled diet and lifestyle.

## The danger of self-diagnosis

22.9      Do not self-diagnose a physical sickness or deficiency. Seek professional diagnosis, and more than one opinion if you are not satisfied with the first. Consider the following illustration.

22.10      Someone suggested that a factor behind my "hardgainingness" could be an underactive thyroid gland. The symptoms of an underactive thyroid gland include a substandard synthesis of protein, which perhaps could contribute to "hardgainingness." First I needed to see if I really had an underactive thyroid.

22.11   I did not seek a medical opinion. Instead I used a test I could do on myself. It involved taking my morning armpit temperature for several successive days. It turned out that my temperature is over a degree below the norm, which apparently *may* be a symptom of an underactive thyroid.

22.12   Concluding that I had an underactive thyroid I started some non-drug therapy (primarily herbal) to help correct the problem. After a few weeks I checked my temperature again, and found no change. So I increased the dosage of therapy.

22.13   Almost immediately my mood changed, and I became incredibly intolerant, aggressive and hostile. It was very scary to experience such a dramatic change of mood. But it was not until two days later that I realized there could be a connection with the increased level of therapy. I immediately stopped the therapy, and the next day my mood dramatically changed for the better.

22.14   Then I read a book on thyroid disorders. While I may have had one of the signs of an underactive thyroid, I had none of those listed in the book for that condition. Then I read the section dealing with an *over*active thyroid. I discovered that during the two days when I felt on the verge of losing control, I had a classic physical sign of an *over*active thyroid.

22.15   A little knowledge can be a dangerous thing. What you may think is a symptom or sign of a disorder may just be a condition unique to you that does not actually represent a disorder. Seek a medical confirmation of any condition you think you have before you take any action to alter that condition. Otherwise you risk doing more harm than good.

## Beyond the physical

22.16   Physical care of your body is not enough for health and well-being. Your emotional and mental state is a pivotal contributing factor. No matter how well you exercise and eat, if you are living with resentment, anger or other destructive emotions, you will be tearing yourself apart from within. Happiness is a vital part of physical health.

22.17   Face up to the events of life that cause you distress. Take action to heal old wounds, rather than let them fester. Let go of the past in order to be able to live contentedly in the present. And accept that sometimes it is better to be happy than to be right. Insisting on being right all the time will cause conflict and great distress. We are all flawed, and just as we have to accept our own imperfection, we must accept the imperfection of others. We live in the real world, not an ideal one.

22.18    Understand the background reasons for events. Accept that you played a part in the strife that is hurting you. Apply tolerance and compassion to others and *yourself*. Do not be overly hard on yourself. If you do not do all of this you will be constantly tortured by the past. This produces mental and physical distress, which leads to unhappiness and illness regardless of how fit and strong you may be.

22.19    Take action to improve your interpersonal relationships, and your working conditions. Truly appreciate what is going well in your life—i.e., count your blessings—rather than constantly focus on what is amiss with your life. And rather than get upset about what may be going awry with your life, take action to improve your circumstances. Of course this is easier said than done. But counter that with another cliché—where there is a will, there is a way.

22.20    As a start of the healing process, apply this Reiki maxim. As simple as it appears, put this maxim into practice and you can profoundly change how you live. Just focus on getting one day right at a time.

> *Just for today*
> *I'll not worry,*
> *I'll not be angry,*
> *I'll do my work honestly,*
> *I'll give thanks for my many blessings,*
> *And I'll be kind to my neighbor and all living things.* **BB**

---

**No matter how well you exercise and eat, if you are living with resentment, anger or other destructive emotions you will be tearing yourself apart from within. Happiness is a vital part of good health.**

# Perspective

*Though not written by a muscle and might buff, here are some wise words to help you keep the rigors of life in perspective.*

I woke up early today, excited over all I get to do before the clock strikes midnight. My job is to choose what kind of day I'm going to have.

Today I can complain because the weather is rainy, or I can be thankful that the grass is getting watered for free.

Today I can grumble about my health, or I can rejoice that I'm alive.

Today I can lament over all that my parents didn't give me when I was growing up, or I can feel grateful that they allowed me to be born.

Today I can cry because roses have thorns, or I can celebrate that thorns have roses.

Today I can mourn my lack of friends, or I can excitedly embark upon a quest to discover new relationships.

Today I can whine because I have to go to work, or I can shout for joy because I have a job to do.

Today I can complain because I have to go to school, or I can open my mind and fill it with rich new tidbits of knowledge.

Today I can murmur dejectedly because I have to do housework, or I can feel honored because I have shelter for my mind, body and soul.

Today stretches ahead of me, waiting to be shaped. And here I am, the sculptor who gets to do the shaping.

What today will be like is up to me. I get to choose what kind of day I'll have!

Have a great day . . . *unless you have other plans.*

– Unknown

*Having control, as each of us does, over the form, development and strength of our bodies is a marvelous power. Are you making the most of it?*

*Live for the moment and do not harp on about what you should have been doing in former years. No matter how many mistakes you have made, no matter how much training time you have wasted, and no matter how much you wish you could turn the clock back, what is done is done.*

*Today is the start of the rest of your life. You will never be as young as you are now. And there will never be a better time than today to start getting your life in perfect order. So start today to get in charge of your life!*

# 23. How to Get a Grip on Your Life, and Put All that You Have Learned from this Book into Action, *Now!*

23.1    Think of all the good ideas you have come up with, thought out well, believed in, planned, resolved to carry out...but did not. Think how much more you could have done with your life if only you had acted on your own good ideas or those of others. It may be good articles you could write, a worthwhile campaign you could get going, expertise to develop in a specific field, a business you could set up, new relationships to initiate, doing something important to improve your health, a valuable book you could write and self-publish, or the implementation of a radical but super-effective training strategy.

23.2    All of us, to varying degrees, realize but a small fraction of what we could have had we invested the courage, gumption and persistence needed to make a good idea happen in practice; and had we spent less time being interested in the successes of others but more time focusing on making our own successes.

23.3    Do not set yourself up for an old age tormented with, "I could have done much more with my life, if only I'd been more of a doer, instead of a watcher, thinker and procrastinator." While probably everyone has regrets in their old age, take measures *now* to ensure that you will have very few of them.

23.4    You can achieve *far more* than you think you can, in all walks of your life. Almost everyone underestimates what they can do. Some people are masters in arguing against the carrying out of their own good ideas, and listen too readily to people who have spent a lifetime suppressing their own potential.

23.5    Once you have a well-thought-out idea, give your all to making it bear fruit. Have no time for any criticism and nay saying others may pour on you. Realize that making your idea bear fruit necessitates overcoming obstacles, and being persistent and oh-so determined. *The satisfaction from achievement is not only in the end result, but in the journey.*

23.6    Those people who realize out-of-the-ordinary achievements are regular mortals like the rest of us. But they grabbed their good ideas and invested whatever was needed to make the ideas bear fruit. We can all do this. Achievement has *much more* to do with belief and sheer determination than talent and academic qualifications. There is a lot more than a grain of truth in the adage, "Success is 1% inspiration and 99% perspiration."

23.7    You can make at least some of your dreams come true. Even huge accomplishments are achieved by notching up lots of little accomplishments. But you have got to start, NOW! Life is in short supply and the years quickly slip by.

23.8    Start with your own training program. Having read this book you will have clicked, theoretically, with the value and effectiveness of hard work and progressive poundages on abbreviated routines of basic exercises. But will you give your all for a few years to such abbreviated training programs?

23.9    Imagine that food supplements had never been invented, and that there were no bodybuilding drugs and no equipment innovations beyond the basics of what a home gym needs. Then, with the unswerving application of what this book teaches, this "primitive" situation would deliver umpteen times more progress for the masses than what is actually being delivered today, despite the plethora of supposed and even actual advances.

23.10   Do not waste chunks of your life before finally learning this truth. So few people learn it, and nearly all who do must first waste years, if not decades of their lives. What usually happens is people assume resistance training cannot work for them, and thus give it up.

23.11   Really get into your training and see how much you can do to make it more productive, enjoyable and rewarding. Get each day right, again, and again, and again. Then you will get the weeks right, and the months. And then you will really start to get somewhere. Become the master of your time, and your life!

## Priorities and dedication

23.12    Having control, as each of us does, over the form, development and strength of our bodies is a marvelous power. Think about it for a few moments. But are you really making the most of it?

23.13    You need to give your training a very high priority in your life. *Make* the time for your workouts. Switch off the TV and get to sleep in good time. *Be* stubborn about ensuring you recuperate adequately. *Make* time to prepare good meals often enough to meet your nutritional needs. *Give* your body the chance to restore itself. *Find* time to do your stretching. *Exercise* the discipline to stay clear of things that will undermine your progress. *Develop* the fortitude to ignore the negative matters and people that get in the way of your training and your life in general.

23.14    Many if not most people believe they can tolerate rule breaking as far as health and training precepts are concerned. In your teens and twenties it may appear that you can get away with the corner cutting. But just wait a few years—then what you apparently could get away with will seriously mar your progress in muscle and might, and start to play havoc with your health.

23.15    While a few people can manage on less sleep than the typical person, they are few and far between. And most of those who think they need relatively little sleep are kidding themselves. They need their eight *or more* hours of sleep each night when in hard training, in order to make their fastest progress. *Do not short change yourself on sleep.*

23.16    Your training should be your number one leisure time activity if you are to realize your full potential. Or it has to be your *sole* leisure time activity if you get very little time to yourself. It is that demanding.

23.17    Of course the practical constraints of real life—e.g., sickness and heavy demands of work and family—have a tempering effect on even the most determined commitment to a training regimen. The more those demands obstruct your application, the poorer will be your progress in muscle and might.

23.18    No matter how rough your life gets, so long as you are truly disciplined you can nearly always find time for a very abbreviated training program, and fix things so that you get your feeds on time (some of them from pre-prepared liquid food stored in a flask), and get your full quota of sleep most nights.

## Individual experimentation

23.19    The studying of training and nutrition is great, and needed, but the purpose of it all is to help you build a stronger and better developed physique, not just educate you for the sake of it. *Apply the learning with every ounce of drive and desire you have got.*

23.20    Be sure you stick with a program long enough to pass fair judgement on it. You have to investigate something seriously, understand what you are doing, apply it to your own situation, fine-tune it, and then dedicate yourself to a few months of it before passing judgement, perhaps with further fine-tuning as you go along.

23.21    This book provides you with different interpretations of basic and abbreviated training because just one rendition does not suit everyone. Find an interpretation that works well for you— but a number of interpretations will probably work for you. This discovery involves experimentation. Once you have found an interpretation that works well for you, get on with applying it—again and again and again.

23.22    Do not worry if you are not training precisely like how someone else successfully trains. Do not agonize over your training not being "perfect." Do not intellectualize matters excessively. And never drop a productive program merely because you are tempted to try something else. Only change something that does not work.

23.23    Remember what I wrote in the segment *Failure of "One Size Fits All"* in Chapter 2:

Avoid seeking the "perfect" training routine. Once on that slippery slope you will join the mass of trainees who are buried in all the peripheral, downright irrelevant or even destructive aspects of training. Instead, knuckle down, *long-term,* to paying the necessary dues on basic, straight-forward, sound and abbreviated training programs as described in this book.

## Be on your guard!

23.24    When gains are not happening in the gym, and life seems to be all toil and no reward, watch out. That is when you will be most vulnerable to falling foul of bogus quick fixes to your problems. *Be on your guard!*

23.25    There are many tactics used by those who make money off the dreams of hard gainers. One of them is selling mega-hype training courses supposedly written by former contest winners who claim to have been hard gainers. Always keep in mind that a winner of a top-level bodybuilding or powerlifting championship was *never* a hard gainer. *Be on your guard!*

23.26    Some of these muscle peddlers claim they are hard gainers, and brag about how they overcame their "hardgainingness" using the training methods (and perhaps supplements) you can buy from them, sometimes at outrageous prices. But what these men do not tell you is that they overcame their genetic shortcomings with long-term drug abuse. Remember that the first casualty of steroid use is the truth. *Be on your guard!*

23.27    Most trainees waste years learning what does *not* work before finally applying what *does* work, though most give up long before reaching that point. This can lead to a reduction in ultimate size and strength potential, depending on the number of years wasted, and the age of the individual. This is made far worse if lasting injuries have been accumulated, which is often the case because so much dreadful advice on exercise technique is embedded in conventional training. *Be on your guard!*

23.28    Some people cannot gain in the gym because the *current* circumstances of their lives preclude gains—and this applies *even if* a perfect-for-hard-gainers training program is being used. When under *great* personal and emotional stress it is nigh-on impossible to make progress in muscle and might. But if you forget this, or are unaware of it, you will fall prey to deceptive arguments for sham solutions to your bodybuilding and strength training problems. *Be on your guard!*

23.29    As typical people, if we do not have all non-gym matters in at least *fairly* good order, but preferably very good order, then we can forget about gains. There is no room for compromise here. You must get the whole training-related package in good order.

23.30    If you are training seriously but have little or no appetite, then your life's total load is excessive, and/or you are grossly overtrained or under-rested. Not eating enough will only make matters worse. But if your body is physically incapable of responding to growth stimulation, then if you force feed you will just pack on fat.

23.31    It is not food, supplements or a new training routine you need when under this sort of stress. You need to reduce greatly the total stress in your life or, if that is out of your control for the present, maintain yourself as best you can and be patient as you wait until circumstances change for the better. Only then will matters related to gains-orientated training count.

23.32    The basics-first and abbreviated training format works, *if* it is implemented properly and in its entirety—with the *whole* package of considerations in sound order.

23.33    Three to five years of proper training can produce gains that most trainees may think impossible for a drug-free hard gainer. *Proper* training can make a hard gainer into an easy gainer, relatively speaking.

23.34    When counter arguments to basic, brief, intensive and practical training methods seem too good to be true, they almost certainly are. *Be on your guard!*

## The joy of training

23.35    Abbreviated, focused and basics-first training is a joy to perform because it brings workout-by-workout satisfaction from realizing small bits of progress. Effective training makes you feel good. You revel in it, and thus apply even more zeal. Then you get better gains. The confidence developed may carry over to other areas of your life. And the great value of focus and organization in the gym shows you the way to go outside of the gym.

23.36    When you have trained well, showered and eaten, you walk on water and experience the training high.

23.37    I have said it before, and I will keep on saying it: Hardly anyone makes the most of their chance to train. Too few trainees experience the training high.

## Never bemoan a blessing

23.38    When training intensity is high you may get the jitters prior to a workout. You may become fearful about your training. When this happens it is time for a change of perspective.

23.39    Get excited over the opportunity to push yourself hard in the gym. Revel in the blessing of good health that permits you to push yourself hard in the the gym. A day will come when you (and I) will not be able to go through the rigors of a hard workout, a day when you (and I) will not be able to savor the excitement and enjoyment that accompanies a workout.

23.40    This whole training "thing" is a good fortune only available to those who have the health, time and opportunity to do it.

23.41    Never bemoan the discipline that must accompany serious training. Never bemoan the discipline that must be applied to your diet and other components of recovery. To have the opportunity to apply all of this discipline is a great blessing.

23.42    You will not be able to train forever. Eventually you will not be able to apply dedication and determination to anything, let alone your training, diet and recovery. So make the absolute most of the present!

23.43    When you get the jitters prior to a rigorous workout, change the jitters into excitement—excitement over an opportunity to do something that is a privilege, and a reflection of your good health and well-being.

23.44    Never mind that you are not the champion you may have initially wanted to be. What matters is that you do your best to improve on where you are now. To improve a notch at your next workout, and at the following workout, and to keep doing that again and again, is the best you can do.

23.45    When you stumble along the way, take it in your stride but resolve to do better next time. Training is too great a privilege to get upset over a component that did not go exactly as planned.

23.46    Live your life one day at a time, doing your absolute best to get each day right, and while relishing all the single units of a lifetime of training. That is the route to achieving your own physical excellence and enjoying the journey there.

## Control your destiny

23.47    Live for the moment, and do not harp on about what you
         should have been doing in former years. No matter how many
         mistakes you have made, no matter how much training time
         you have wasted, and no matter how much you wish you
         could turn the clock back, what is done is done.

23.48    Today is the start of the rest of your life. You will never be as
         young as you are now. Learn from your mistakes and those of
         others, get in charge of your own destiny, and make the most
         of the now—make each day count. Get organized, get
         motivated, get working, and then get gaining.

23.49    The more time you have wasted on unproductive training
         routines and strategies in the past, the more urgent it is that
         you start getting your act together now.

23.50    You do not have to read much of this book before you realize
         what you have not been doing, but what you need to be doing
         if you are to start making great gains.

23.51    You have far more control over your own life and destiny than
         you probably give yourself credit for. Grab this control, and get
         doing what you know you need to be doing. There is so much
         more you can do with your life to make it more rewarding and
         enjoyable, if only you would challenge yourself to do more
         with it, and stop procrastinating well-planned action.

23.52    For example, if you do not like where you are training, and for
         sure it is holding you back, find a better gym. If there is not a
         decent gym in your neighborhood, then put your own together.
         Do not just wish you could do it; *do it*. Either by yourself, or by
         pooling resources with some training partners, you can put
         together a terrific home gym without having to lay out a lot of
         money or needing much space. See Chapter 6 for help.

23.53    Rather than finding reasons why something cannot be done,
         though you know it needs to be done, get on with doing it.
         See problems as challenges. And apply such an attitude change
         throughout your life—not just to training-related matters—and
         then delight in seeing your life change for the better.

23.54    Making the most of your life is not about earth-shaking
         achievements. It is about doing your best to be your best. This

is not measured merely in terms of what you actually achieve, but by the obstacles you overcame whilst striving to succeed.

23.55    Look after yourself. Cut out the things that are doing you harm. Do not wait till you learn the lesson the hard way: Without your health and well-being you cannot get anywhere in the gym. Be kinder to yourself. Ask a lot of yourself, but not the impossible. Push yourself hard, but do not push yourself over the limit. And when obstacles and problems hit you—as they will—never forget that your life is not determined by what happens to you, but by how you *respond* to what besets you.

23.56    Never let circumstances get the better of you—*you* get the better of them. Get in charge and control your destiny.

## The overall picture

23.57    While you are getting on with satisfying achievement, be sure not to be so busy that you forget to enjoy life as you go along. Slow down a little, step back and see life as an objective observer. Take the time to observe things around you, smile more, talk less, listen more. Too many people fail to make the most of their children, the treasure of a healthy body, and the actual fruits of their labors. They also fail to appreciate the everyday good things that are taken for granted.

23.58    When life draws to a close, when you no longer see much future for yourself, and when you dwell on your past, then you will wish you had made more of the moments as you were actually living them. Do not wait till then. Do it now!

23.59    Be obsessed, focused and consumed by your training *when you are in the gym*, and rest, eat and sleep well while out of the gym. Then get on with the rest of your life. Do not expect even stellar training achievements to bring order and happiness to your life. Great satisfaction in one limited area, yes, but nothing more. Suppose, for example, that you could squat 200 pounds more than you actually can now, and that you have 30 pounds more muscle. As terrific as that would be, would it make any difference to the events and relationships that have the greatest impact on your happiness?

23.60    As marvelous as training is, never forget that it is only a small part of the big picture. Those who are obsessed with training even when they are not in the gym expose themselves to the destructive side of training—neglect of personal relationships, family life, health, education and career.

23.61    You can get the most from training *without* it consuming your life. That is what this book is about. There is even an unexpected bonus from adopting the right perspective—you are much more likely to see through hype and deception, and use the rational programs that are the most productive.

## How to keep on track

23.62    Having arrived at the end of this book you now know exactly what to do to achieve your training goals. But an abundance of productive training information counts for nothing unless you act on it. Make it real by your own disciplined, conscientious, committed and so-very-serious application.

23.63    Having come this far you have established a relationship with sensible training methods that can last a lifetime. You have discovered a book to refer to again and again. And you have made a connection with me that I want to cement. This will ensure you never go off the rails of effective training.

23.64    While this book is thorough, there is still plenty to learn, especially about exercise technique and other people's interpretations of abbreviated and basics-first training. See the later pages of this book for details of how I can assist you further. If you are serious about making the most of your potential for muscle and might, keeping in touch is in your interest. It will spare you wasting your time and money on inferior or even useless training strategies.

23.65    I wish you much training success, and look forward to hearing of your successes. But before you finish studying this book, please read the following postscript.

You will not be able to train forever. Eventually you will not be able to apply dedication and determination to anything, let alone your training, diet and recovery. *So make the absolute most of the present!*

# Postscript:
# *Did You Deliver?*

23.66    Please read this postscript after finishing the book. Then reread
         it after having had at least three months to put into diligent
         practice what you have learned from this book. Regular
         reviewing of this postscript will help you to keep tabs on how
         well you are doing in applying what you have learned.

23.67    I am not trying to irritate you by checking up on you. I am
         being supportive because I want you to make the most of your
         training. This book has shown you how to build a superbly
         muscled, strong, fit, lean and healthy physique. But you have
         to *apply* the instruction for it to yield the benefits you want.

23.68    Have you nailed yourself to specific goals and deadlines as I
         have urged? Are you organized to succeed? Have you
         heightened your resolve? Are you making each day another
         small step towards realizing your targets? Have you become an
         achievement-orientated, goal-driven, success-attaining person?

23.69    One of the many advantages of having good hands-on training
         supervision is that there is someone there to get after you when
         you do not deliver the goods; and there is someone there to
         keep reminding you that you have got to keep delivering the
         goods, time after time after time. I am getting after you so as to
         ram home the importance of making each day count, so that
         you never get caught up in drifting and procrastinating.
         Achievement in life, be it training related or otherwise, is about
         getting a sequence of days, weeks and months in good order.

23.70    Did you get the last few months of your training life in good
         order? Did you stick with an abbreviated program of basic
         exercises? Did you avoid the distraction of other routines? Did
         you train consistently without skipping workouts? Did you
         train hard? Did you focus on progressive poundages? Did you
         discipline yourself to use good form in every single set? Did
         you use small poundage increments? Did you resist the urge to
         do something impetuous in the gym that would likely injure
         you? *Did you deliver the training goods?*

23.71    Did you organize your life so that you got enough sleep every
         night? Did you watch less TV so as to get more sleep? Did you,

as much as possible, avoid activities that would mar your progress in muscle and might? *Did you deliver the goods as far as rest and sleep were concerned?*

23.72    Did you eat well every day over the last few months? Did you eat five or six times each day? Did you satisfy your caloric needs each day? Did you substitute good food for junk? Did you avoid cutting corners with your diet? Did you monitor your waist and/or bodyfat level to ensure you are not eating yourself fat? Did you concentrate on food and not supplements? *Did you deliver the nutritional goods?*

23.73    Did you regularly perform a moderate and sensible stretching program? Did you apply trigger point therapy? Did you include moderate aerobic work in your weekly exercise program? Did you perform inversion therapy? Were you in a good emotional condition? *Did you deliver the components of total physical care?*

23.74    Over the last few months, did you exploit to the full the tremendous power you have to improve your physique, fitness and health? Were you 100% committed to doing the best that you possibly could? And did you stay clear of distractions?

23.75    Nail yourself to specific goals, and make things happen. Make every single day count, and make each week a perfect example of training, rest and nutritional satisfaction—and another important step forward to the realization of your goals. You *can* do this, week in and week out, so long as you set your mind to it. No matter how encyclopedic your knowledge of training and training-related matters may be, *it is only the application of that knowledge that will produce changes in your physique.*

23.76    It boils down to the commitment, dedication and self-discipline needed to satisfy the training, rest and nutritional components. Get committed, and then watch out for great gains. Half-hearted application produces little or no progress. Full-blooded, consistent commitment is the best way forward. Make the commitment, and make every day count—no more wasted days and opportunities.

23.77    Always remember that how you live your life is under *your* control. Take control! Then you will be all set to achieve your full potential for muscle and might. 🆑

*ACTION, NOT WORDS!*

*Put this book into disciplined, diligent and persistent practice. Study the book, grasp why conventional training is useless for most people, learn how to train properly, and then apply what you have discovered. Life is too short to waste a moment more. Let go of the unproductive ways! Time is pressing.*

## Your input, please

All books have room for improvement. Please provide feedback to help improve this book in a future edition. Let me know of any typos and errors you may find, and feel free to make any suggestions on how to improve the book.

Stuart McRobert
CS Publishing Ltd.
P.O. Box 20390
CY-2151 Nicosia
Cyprus

e-mail: cspubltd@spidernet.com.cy

# About the Author

Born in 1958, in Stockton-on-Tees, England, I have had an almost lifelong appreciation of muscle and might. I started resistance training at age 14, when I got a set of chest expanders as a Christmas present. Thus started an infatuation with resistance training. In 1973, at age 15, I started weight training, in a small "dungeon" gym at a local community center. That wonderful den became the focal point of my life until I left home to go to college in Liverpool, in 1978. Muscles were more important than everything else in my life. School work, social activities and sport all played second fiddle to the quest to build big muscles. If anything did not help in the quest, it was ditched.

Despite the 100% commitment, my initial gains were only very modest. After getting more "serious" about my training—i.e., increasing its volume, frequency and intensity—progress came to a total halt. Then started my fulsome appreciation of "hard gaining." Despite years of unrelenting total commitment to my training and the full bodybuilding lifestyle, the great physique that was promised did not develop. I was learning through great frustration that there was a lot more accounting for bodybuilding success than effort and dedication. As an archetypical hard gainer I was driven to *utter despair* over such paltry results relative to the effort and dedication I invested.

I gradually learned about the critical role of genetic factors, the need to use training routines appropriate to the individual, and the necessity of not imitating the training methods used by people who have tremendous genetic advantages.

Learning important truths about bodybuilding and strength training motivated me to share them with others. I wrote my first magazine article while at college in Liverpool, and had it published by Peary Rader in IRON MAN (in the June-July 1981 issue). In addition to writing further articles for IRON MAN, I started writing for a number of US- and UK-published bodybuilding magazines.

I graduated in 1982, but was unable to find a teaching post in England. I sought employment overseas, and in January 1983 I was appointed as a teacher at an international school in Nicosia, Cyprus. I stayed until summer 1984. Then I left due to an opportunity to visit the Hawaiian island of Molokai. I lived there for almost a year, and then returned to Cyprus in summer 1985. Shortly afterwards I married Maro, a Cypriot I had known since my first stay on the Mediterranean island, and decided to settle in Cyprus.

In 1989 I founded CS Publishing and started my own magazine, naturally called THE HARDGAINER (later changed to HARDGAINER.) At the time I lived in a two-bedroom apartment with my wife and two very young daughters. My office was also my daughters' bedroom. I was working as a full-time teacher while I established the business, and in addition was working for an advertising company in trade for services provided to CS Publishing. I was also helping in the rearing of the children. The first couple of years of running the business were incredibly rigorous.

During 1990–91 I wrote BRAWN, and in 1992 I started writing BEYOND BRAWN. In 1993 I was able to give up teaching and thus work solely for CS Publishing. In 1995–96 I put BEYOND BRAWN aside in order to write THE INSIDER'S TELL-ALL HANDBOOK ON WEIGHT-TRAINING TECHNIQUE. I then resumed work on BEYOND BRAWN. During 1997 I took a short "break" to write and design THE MUSCLE & MIGHT TRAINING TRACKER, and then returned to BEYOND BRAWN for the final leg.

I have the qualifications that are needed for providing training instruction for hard gainers and/or trainees with very demanding jobs and family lives. I am an archetypal hard gainer who has never used bodybuilding drugs. I have been an inveterate muscle and strength buff for most of my life. I have suffered the frustration and injuries that result from zealously following conventional training methods and abusive exercise techniques. I have been heavily involved in the raising of two children, and have worked 70–80 hours each week year round. And as described in Chapter 17 I have lifted some substantial iron to show that I am no armchair athlete or theoretician.

– Stuart McRobert

# Resources

## Little discs

1. PDA, 104 Bangor Street, Mauldin, SC 29662, USA (864-963-5640) www.fractionalplates.com
2. Watson Gym Equipment, Unit 8, Washington Road, West Wiltshire Trading Estate, Wiltshire BA13 4JP, England, (01373 859617, 0976752585) www.gymequipment.uk.com

## Magnetic little discs

PlateMates®, Benoit Built Inc., 12 Factory Cove Road, Boothbay Harbor, ME 04538, USA (207-633-5912) www.theplatemate.com

## Exercise equipment

1. Life Fitness/Hammer Strength, 2245 Gilbert Avenue Suite 305, Cincinnati, OH 45206, USA (513-221-2600) www.hammerstrength.com
2. IronMind® Enterprises Inc., P.O. Box 1228, Nevada City, CA 95959, USA (530-265-6725), www.ironmind.com
3. Watson Gym Equipment (see above)
4. PDA (see above)
5. Southern Xercise, Inc., P.O. Box 412, Cleveland, TN 37364, USA (423-476-8999, 800-348-4907) www.southernxercise.com
6. York Barbell Company, Inc., Box 1707, York, PA 17405, USA (717-767-6481) www.yorkbarbell.com

## Tru-Squat

Southern Xercise, Inc. (see above)

## Shrug bar (Trap Bar alternative)

In the US, contact PDA (see above)
In the UK, contact Watson Gym Equipment (see above)
*See page 16 for shrug/Trap Bar comparison.*

## Back Revolution

Meyer Distributing Co., 8580 Milliken Avenue, P.O. Box 3509, Rancho Cucamonga, CA 91729, USA (800-472-4221), www.meyerdist.com

## Books

Here are the books specifically referred to in BEYOND BRAWN:

1. Clark, N., NANCY CLARK'S SPORTS NUTRITION GUIDEBOOK (2nd edition), 1997, Human Kinetics, ISBN 0-87322-730-1

2. Erasmus, Udo, FATS THAT HEAL FATS THAT KILL (2nd edition), 1993, Alive Books, ISBN 0-920470-38-6

3. Prudden, B., MYOTHERAPY: BONNIE PRUDDEN'S COMPLETE GUIDE TO PAIN-FREE LIVING, First Ballantine Books Edition, 1985, ISBN 0-345-32688-1

4. Davies, C., THE TRIGGER POINT THERAPY WORKBOOK, New Harbinger Publications, 2001, ISBN 1572242507

5. Schneider, M. J., PRINCIPLES OF MANUAL TRIGGER POINT THERAPY, published by Michael J. Schneider, DC, 1994

## Johnny Gibson Gym Equipment

11 South Sixth Avenue, Tucson, AZ 85701, USA (520-622-1275)
web site: www.johnnygibson.com
e-mail: johnnygibson@earthlink.net
*Johnny Gibson's, established in 1952, manufactures a line-up of commercial strength, power and therapy equipment. It also sells used equipment from various suppliers, including Nautilus. Contact Johnny Gibson Gym Equipment for its catalog and a list of used gear in stock, or visit its web site.*

# This book's three companion texts . . .

This book, BEYOND BRAWN, is part one—and the core—of the series of four interrelated texts that make up **The Muscle & Might Master Method**. While each book can stand alone as an excellent instructional tool in its own right, *together* they provide the most complete and *responsible* package of instruction for achieving physique and strength goals. The four interrelated books are . . .

1. **BEYOND BRAWN**
2. **THE INSIDER'S TELL-ALL HANDBOOK ON WEIGHT-TRAINING TECHNIQUE**
3. **THE MUSCLE & MIGHT TRAINING TRACKER**
4. **FURTHER BRAWN**

## No Drugs, No Hype, No Bull & No Irresponsible or Impractical Training Routines. Instead, *AN HONEST APPROACH TO YOUR TRAINING*

Stuart McRobert's Muscle & Might Master Method is a series of interrelated instructional materials. You can use each component part separately—but to get the most out of your training, use them all together as an integrated whole. Though Stuart didn't "invent" the various parts of The Master Method, he put them together into a cohesive, interrelated, detailed and easy-to-learn whole. The Master Method is a responsible and individualistic approach, not a "one size fits all" one. For busy people of average genetic endowment, who are serious about their training but have a life outside of the gym, there really isn't any other choice. And there's no risk—our publications are BACKED BY AN UNCONDITIONAL MONEY-BACK GUARANTEE.

## How to use perfect exercise technique

You're ahead of the game as soon as you start using The Master Method, as described in *BEYOND BRAWN*. And you want to keep that competitive edge by performing each exercise *exactly* right. How to use perfect exercise form is covered in extensive and illustrated detail by *THE INSIDER'S TELL-ALL HANDBOOK ON WEIGHT-TRAINING TECHNIQUE*. Exercise form is such a serious subject that a whole book is needed to do it justice.

As incredible as it may seem, gyms are usually the worst places to learn about perfect exercise form. The myths, fallacies and dangerous techniques that are perpetuated in most gyms are astonishing. And most training publications and "personal trainers" are no better. The foolish "no pain, no gain" maxim has wreaked havoc in the training world. It's no wonder that so many people get hurt and frustrated with weight training, and give it up.

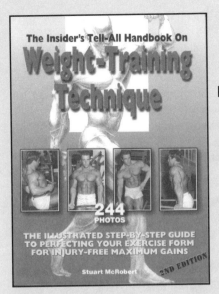

## Revised 2nd edition

## 224 big pages
## 244 photos

*"As a chiropractor with over 20 years of weight-training experience, I can honestly say that no other book comes even close to McRobert's for teaching safe and responsible exercise technique."*
– Dr. Gregory Steiner
Director of *Active Chiropractic*, Glasgow, UK

The perfect complement to *BEYOND BRAWN, THE INSIDER'S TELL-ALL HANDBOOK ON WEIGHT-TRAINING TECHNIQUE* contains 244 photographs and over 200 fully indexed big pages showing the right *and* wrong ways to perform all the most productive exercises—34 different exercises, and 50 of them, in fact, if you include the variations. In addition there is extensive commentary and advice from Stuart. This book also includes a thorough and intelligent flexibility program, how to use a video camera to perfect your exercise technique, how to compose form checklists, and more.

*TECHNIQUE* isn't just for beginners. No matter whether you're an advanced, intermediate or novice bodybuilder or strength trainee, this book will greatly increase your grasp of safe weight-training form. Become an expert on exercise technique. Then your *safe* training longevity is almost guaranteed. And unless you can train safely over the long term you'll never realize your goals.

If you're a visually oriented person who learns best when you can actually see what you're studying, *TECHNIQUE* is an absolute must read. And even if you learn better through other methods, having the pictures in front of you as you work out will be very beneficial.

No other book on exercise technique covers the subject matter so carefully, responsibly and with such attention to safety and training longevity.

*"I've been lifting weights for most of my life now. I'm no novice. So I was blown away when I realized, after reading your book, how much I DIDN'T know about proper exercise form."*
– *John Leschinski, Connell, Washington*

Each section offers clear, concise tips for setting up the equipment properly, assuming the safe and effective positions, performing the exercises step by step, and monitoring performance, along with photographs illustrating exactly what to do, and what *not* to do.

You can't afford to take a chance with using improper exercise form. The older you get, the more you'll realize the importance of using excellent exercise form. Don't wait until you have seriously hurt yourself before learning this lesson. Apply what *THE INSIDER'S TELL-ALL HANDBOOK ON WEIGHT-TRAINING TECHNIQUE* teaches, and you can train safely and productively for a lifetime.

## How to track your training progress

BEYOND BRAWN is best used with another of its companion volumes—*THE MUSCLE & MIGHT TRAINING TRACKER.*

*THE MUSCLE & MIGHT TRAINING TRACKER* is a 136-page workbook which contains everything you need in order to track your progress, day by day, month by month, and year by year. The systematic organization and focus upon achieving goals that an intelligently designed training journal enforces, will help you to improve your physique steadily and consistently. As simple as it is to use a training log, do not underestimate the critical role this can play in helping you to maximize your training productivity

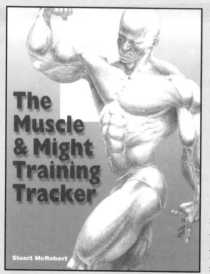

One training log will track your bodybuilding and strength-training progress for at least 24 months—that's a cost of just $1.00 per month. And this log is built for the job it's designed for. *This is no ordinary training diary.*

The log pages cover not only the specifics of your weight-training routines—exercises, sets, reps, poundages, and a comment area to note your performance and any issues you need to address—but also nutrition, sleep and body composition.

**1. Book lets you track your progress for at least two years**

**2. Big pages provide plenty of room for entering data**

**3. Robust paper provides strength to withstand heavy use**

**4. Spiral binding enables book to open flat for easy use**

**5. Design enables you to track your training AND recovery**

## USE THIS TRAINING LOG TO GET IN CHARGE OF YOUR PROGRESS

Most trainees are aware that they should record their workouts in a permanent way, but few actually do it. Even those trainees who keep some sort of training log usually fail to exploit its full potential benefits. This is one of the major reasons why most trainees get minimal results from their training. *This training log will make your data keeping easy.*

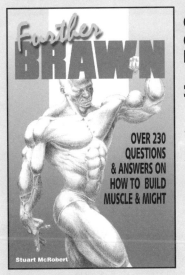

OVER 230 QUESTIONS & ANSWERS ON HOW TO BUILD MUSCLE & MIGHT

Stuart McRobert

## Over 230 questions & answers on how to build muscle & might

## 320 pages

Through our other books we tried to give readers all the information they need to achieve lifelong bodybuilding success. But over time we found there were questions that had slipped through unanswered. That's when we decided we had an obligation to address those questions, fill in the gaps, provide further information and wisdom, and in turn reinforce trainees' understanding of what it takes to hit the success target.

If you want to make the most of your training, even if you're a veteran trainee, the following will give you a flavor of what's in store. Here's just a very small sample of the 230+ questions answered in *FURTHER BRAWN*:

❑ I've read about a number of different ways to train in an abbreviated way, and I'm confused. How do I make sense of all the variation?

❑ After heavy 20-rep squatting, my heart rate is very high. Does this have the same effect on my cardio system that hard aerobic work would?

❑ How much protein can I assimilate at a given meal?

❑ What are "hard" aerobics? How can I incorporate them in my program?

❑ I'm losing my grip on the deadlift even though the rest of my body wants to carry on. Any ideas on how to solve this?

❑ I was wondering what you think of a CKD-type regime.

❑ How can I increase my hamstrings involvement in the stiff-legged deadlift?

❑ Is muscular soreness a good indicator that I've had a good workout?

❑ How much of an effect would a martial arts class two or three times a week have on the ability of a hard gainer to make strength and size gains?

❑ What are the differences between chiropractic, osteopathy and physiotherapy?

❑ Aren't you as guilty as some other people in being dogmatically rigid in your training views?

❑ I've heard reports of some people having heart attacks when engaged in intensive exercise, with a few of them actually dying. Is this for real?

❑ What's your opinion of a young trainee (beginner) following John McCallum's "Keys to Progress" series all the way through?

❑ Who influenced you most in the Iron Game, and how?

*Above are a mere 14 of the 230+ questions in FURTHER BRAWN. This sample is just the start. Apply what the book teaches, and you'll definitely take further strides towards your physique and strength goals, EVEN IF YOU'VE READ OUR OTHER BOOKS.*

---

# RISK-FREE ORDER FORM

**THE INSIDER'S TELL-ALL HANDBOOK ON WEIGHT-TRAINING TECHNIQUE**
❑   $24.95 US, or £15.95 UK

**THE MUSCLE & MIGHT TRAINING TRACKER**
❑   $19.95 US, or £11.95 UK

**FURTHER BRAWN**
❑   $24.95 US, or £15.95 UK

*For a single book, please add $5.00 or £3.00 for p&h.*
*Order any two books and there is no charge for p&h.*

Name _____

Address _____

_____ State & zip/code _____ Country _____

CS Publishing Ltd., P.O. Box 20390, CY-2151 Nicosia, Cyprus
*Please allow 3–5 weeks for delivery upon receipt of order in Cyprus*

*In the US, please pay by check or money order. Checks need to clear. No US or Canadian Postal Money Orders. In the UK, please pay by cheque or postal order.*

---

# Money-Back Guarantee

If you're not fully satisfied that our publications give you the know-how you need to take you towards your bodybuilding and strength-training goals, return within 60 days what you bought and you'll receive a full no-questions-asked refund.

---

# Online ordering at www.hardgainer.com

# Index

Numbers in parentheses refer to page, chapter and paragraph number, e.g., 79(4.23) refers to page 79, chapter 4, paragraph 23. "*See*" is a cross reference from a term that is *not* used in the index to the term, usually a synonym, where the information will be found, e.g., "Feeding. *See* Diet." "*See also*" is a reminder that related information is available under a different heading, e.g., "Eating. *See also* Diet."

# H

# T

# Notes

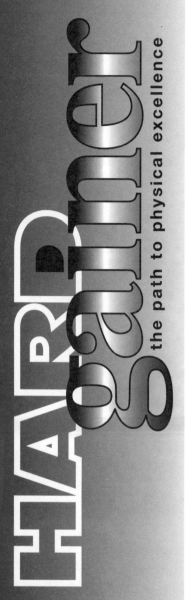

# HARD
# gainer

the path to physical excellence

**bastion of
no-nonsense
drug-free
training**

# FREE magazine!

Published by Stuart McRobert since 1989, HARDGAINER is probably the most instruction-dense, drug-free, bull-free, and hype-free training magazine on the market today, providing more practical and result-producing advice for drug-free bodybuilders and strength trainees than is available in any other magazine. It's crammed with practical advice and nuggets of wisdom to lead you to training success.

Here's some of what to expect from HARDGAINER. You'll get the undiluted truth—no exaggerated claims filled with puffery. What we say may not always sit easily with you. But you can count on one thing—it will be frank and down-to-earth. As the title implies, we speak to hard-gaining typical individuals—people like you. But average potential doesn't have to mean average achievements. In fact, an impressive physique and a terrific level of strength are well within your reach. The key is in the right approach. That's what HARDGAINER is about.

An 18-month/6-issue subscription costs US $35.00 (or UK £22.00).

You don't have to take our word for HARDGAINER being probably the most instruction-dense, practical, drug-free, bull-free and hype-free training magazine on the market. Write in and we'll send you a FREE sample copy of the magazine, with no strings attached.

HARDGAINER is a subscription-only magazine. You won't find it at newsstands. *So write in today, and grab yourself a free growing experience!*

---

Please send me a free sample copy of HARDGAINER.

Name _____

Address _____

_____

Code/zip and country _____

CS Publishing Ltd., P.O. Box 20390, CY-2151 Nicosia, Cyprus

# First Generation Classic

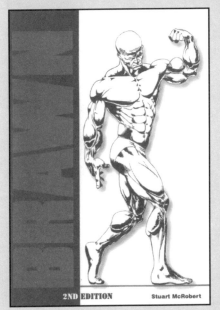

BRAWN
2ND EDITION          Stuart McRobert

**A**ll knowledge is built on that which preceded it. Before BEYOND BRAWN there was BRAWN, the 230-page precursor of the advanced version of wisdom, experience and insight. *BRAWN is now in its second edition.*

BRAWN focuses on genetic realities, appropriate role models, and most of the ins and outs of successful drug-free training. It is especially strong in the philosophical underpinning behind rational training. It also details *how* the genetically blessed are gifted, and shows why conventional training is so unproductive for typical people.

First you should read BEYOND BRAWN, and apply what it teaches. Later, you may want to read BRAWN.

Stuart McRobert's classic text is available in softcover for US $19.95 (or £11.95 in the UK), plus $5.00/£3.00 p&h, from CS Publishing Ltd., P.O. Box 20390, CY-2151 Nicosia, Cyprus.

"BRAWN bowled me over. It's an exceptional nuts and bolts compilation of productive training practices; so exceptional that it's avant-garde."
*Jan Dellinger*
*York Barbell Company*

"BRAWN has no hype, no bull and no commercial messages. It's the real thing and genuinely needed in this field."
*Dr. Ken E. Leistner*
*Co-founder of Iron Island Gym, New York*

"Instead of being yet another me-too bodybuilding book, McRobert's BRAWN is unique: Its tone is serious, its manner evangelical, but most important, its focus is on things that actually work for the average trainee. This is a very useful book, which can help a lot of people make tremendous bodybuilding progress."
*Randall J. Strossen, Ph.D.*
*Publisher of MILO*

"When it comes to training books I'm the world's harshest critic. So when I tell you that BRAWN is the first book I recommend to my clients, you will realize just how highly I rate this excellent book. It definitely sets the foundation and the standard for sensible and productive strength training."
*Bob Whelan, MS, MS, CSCS*
*President, Whelan Strength Training*

"One of the finest training books I've ever read."
*Richard Winett, Ph.D.*
*Publisher of MASTER TRAINER*

## In a nutshell

The essence of this book's instruction is summarized in Chapter 3. The points in that chapter may seem dictatorial. But if all of that chapter was written in stone, and laid down as *the law* in all gyms the world over, the instruction would work for so many people for so much of the time that it would probably be the most important contribution to Iron Game history.

*"Never would I have been allowed to waste time fiddling with my training according to fads. By denying me this freedom my mentor would have kept my attention where it needed to be, enabling me to make almost continuous gains. 'And what's training all about?' he would ask me each week, but never actually let me answer. 'Progressive poundages in good form, m'lad—getting bigger and stronger muscles.'"*

## How to order copies of this book

Individual softcover copies of this book are available at $24.95 plus $5.00 p&h. The hardcover edition costs $34.95 plus $5.00 p&h. Pay by check or money order. Checks need to clear. (In the UK the prices are £15.95 and £21.95 respectively, plus £3.00 p&h. Pay by cheque or postal order.) The discount schedule for multiple copies is available upon request. Please allow 4–6 weeks for delivery of books.

CS Publishing Ltd., P.O. Box 20390, CY-2151 Nicosia, Cyprus

CS Publishing Ltd., P.O. Box 1002, Connell, WA 99326, USA (tel. 509-234-0362)

web site: www.hardgainer.com

If you have not already done so, please write in for your free sample copy of HARDGAINER magazine.

CS Publishing Ltd., P.O. Box 20390, CY-2151 Nicosia, Cyprus